STEDMAN'S

OB-GYN
WORDS

SECOND EDITION

Edited by
Helen E. Littrell, CMT

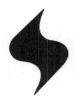

Stedman's

OB-GYN
WORDS

SECOND EDITION

Including:
Neonatology
Pediatrics
Genetics

Williams & Wilkins

BALTIMORE • PHILADELPHIA • HONG KONG
LONDON • MUNICH • SYDNEY • TOKYO

A WAVERLY COMPANY

Series Editor: Elizabeth B. Randolph
Associate Managing Editor: Maureen Barlow Pugh
Editor: Helen E. Littrell, CMT
Illustration Planner: Ray Lowman
Production Coordinator: Barbara J. Felton
Cover Design: Reuter & Associates

Copyright © 1995
Williams & Wilkins
351 W. Camden St
Baltimore, Maryland 21201-2436, USA

Printed in the United States of America

First Edition 1992

Library of Congress Cataloging-in-Publication Data

Stedman's OB-GYN words: including neonatology, pediatrics, genetics/ edited by Helen E. Littrell.—2nd ed.
   p. cm.—(Stedman's word book series)
   Developed from the database of Stedman's medical dictionary and supplemented by terminology found in
the current medical literature.
   Includes bibliographical references.
   ISBN 0-683-07967-0
1. Gynecology—Dictionaries. 2. Obstetrics—Dictionaries. I. Littrell, Helen E. II. Stedman, Thomas Lathrop,
1853-1938. Medical dictionary. III. Title: OB-GYN words IV. Series: Stedman's word book.
   [DNLM: 1. Obstetrics—dictionaries. 2. Gynecology—dictionaries.
WQ 13 S8124 1995
RG45.S74 1995
618'.03—dc20
DNLM/DLC
for Library of Congress
                                            95-4488
                                               CIP

               95 96 97 98 99
1 2 3 4 5 6 7 8 9 10

Contents

PREFACE TO THE SECOND EDITION vii

ACKNOWLEDGMENTS ix

EXPLANATORY NOTES xi

A-Z WORD LIST 1

APPENDICES A1

   1. Anatomical Illustrations A1

   2. Fetal Presentations A9

   3. OB/GYN Drug Names by Therapeutic Class A10

   4. Common instruments by OB/GYN Procedure A24

   5. Sample Reports of Common OB/GYN Procedures A31

Preface to the Second Edition

The terminology of obstetrics and gynecology frequently overlaps with that of several closely related specialties—neonatology, genetics, embryology, assisted reproduction, and yes, PEDIATRICS! Reliable, up-to-date word reference sources for these specialties, especially pediatrics, have been few and far between. For years, medical transcriptionists have had to rely for the most part on their "little black books" or their memory, neither of which were entirely satisfactory. Too many times we have had to guess at the spelling and hope for the best.

When Williams & Wilkins became aware of the great need for a truly comprehensive Ob-Gyn word book that would contain terminology of all of Ob-Gyn's integral specialties, they made plans to implement some major changes in the second edition of *Stedman's Ob-Gyn Words*. As the editorial staff contemplated exactly what this would entail, it became apparent that if they included *every* term related to obstetrics, gynecology, neonatology, genetics, embryology, assisted reproduction, and pediatrics, the book would be too big to handle easily.

Since the physical size of the book was an important consideration, the editors at Williams & Wilkins knew it was necessary to pare down to the core terms in these specialties. Working with medical transcriptionists and court reporters, they established guidelines about which terms to include and which ones to omit.

After a great deal of collaboration, painstaking research, and fine-tuning of the manuscript, we feel satisfied that here indeed is what we have been hoping to achieve—a comprehensive, user-friendly word book that completely covers its subject matter with the latest terminology available. I feel confident that *Stedman's Ob-Gyn Words, Second Edition* is a book that will meet the needs of not only medical transcriptionists, but a diverse group of other medical professionals as well.

It has been a rare privilege to be associated with Williams & Wilkins as an editor on this project. This is a company that listens to the input it receives from its readers, and responds by producing a superb word book series targeted to our needs.

Helen Littrell, CMT

Acknowledgments

An important part of our editorial process is the involvement of medical transcriptionists — as advisors, reviewers, and/or editors.

We extend a special thank you to Helen Littrell CMT who did an excellent job of editing and proofing the manuscript. Thanks also are due Catherine Baxter CMT who proofread the first edition of the book, helped compile the appendices, and spent hours verifying the new words we added to this second edition.

Thanks also to our *Stedman's Ob-Gyn Words* MT Editorial Advisory Board, consisting of Janice Deal RN, BSN, Deborah A. Frank MS, Dale Guedry Jr. CSR, Hazel Tank CMT, and Debbie Warshawski. These medical transcriptionists and court reporters served as editors and advisors, and spent hours perusing texts, journals, and manufacturer's information to compile the latest terms in obstetrics, gynecology, neonatology, pediatrics, and genetics.

Other important contributors to this revised edition include: Bonnie Bakal CMT, Theresa Lamberson CMT, Suzanne Minnick CMT, Kathy Rockel CMT, Laurie Spangler CMT, Ann Williams RRA, and Vicki Willms, all of whom gathered new words and/or provided invaluable suggestions. Once again, Barb Ferretti did a terrific job updating the database.

As with all our Stedman's word references, we have benefited from the suggestions and expertise of our many contacts in the medical transcriptionist community. Thanks to all our advisory board participants, reviewers and editors, AAMT meeting attendees, and others who have written in with requests and comments — keep talking, and we'll keep listening.

Explanatory Notes

Users of the first edition of *Stedman's OB-Gyn Words* will notice the greatly expanded coverage of this second edition. In addition to editing, updating, and expanding the obstetrics and gynecologic content from the first edition, we also have added pediatrics, neonatology. and genetics terminology. *Stedman's Ob-Gyn Words, Second Edition,* offers an authoritative assurance of quality and exactness to the wordsmiths of the health care professions — medical transcriptionists, medical editors and copy editors, health information management personnel, court reporters, and the many other users and producers of medical documentation.

Stedman's Ob-Gyn Words, Second Edition, can be used to validate both the spelling and the accuracy of terminology in obstetrics, gynecology, neonatology, pediatrics, and genetics. Coverage of OB/GYN includes gynecologic oncology, maternal-fetal medicine, endocrinology, and infertility. Thousands of diseases and syndromes, traditional and new operative procedures and techniques (including colposcopy, laparoscopy, hysterosalpingography), diagnostic ultrasound terms, medications, lab test names, and instrument names as well as abbreviations and acronyms are included in this book. For quick reference, appendices with anatomical illustrations, fetal presentations, drug names by therapeutic class, common instruments, and sample reports of common Ob-Gyn procedures are listed at the back of the book.

Because our goal has been to provide a comprehensive yet streamlined reference tool, we have omitted terminology that is not specific to these specialties. This holds true particularly for pediatrics terms, which could encompass a vast number of words related to gastroenterology, oncology, internal medicine, ophthalmology, etc. In deciding which pediatrics terms to include in this book, we have attempted to limit ourselves to those terms *exclusive* to pediatrics. In addition, some terms (such as anatomy and physiology terms) that are often dictated in these specialties are not included in this text as they can be found in a general medical dictionary.

This compilation of over 41,200 entries, fully cross-indexed for quick access, was built from a base vocabulary of over 25,700 medical words, phrases, abbreviations, and acronyms. The extensive A-Z list was developed from the database of *Stedman's Medical Dictionary* and supplemented by terminology found in current medical literature (please see list of References on page xiv).

Medical transcription is an art as well as a science. Both are needed to correctly interpret a physician's dictation, whose language is a product of education, training, and experience. This variety in medical language means that there are several acceptable ways to express certain terms, including jargon. This second edition of *Stedman's Ob-Gyn Words* provides variant spellings and phrasings for many terms. This, in addition to complete cross-indexing, makes *Stedman's Ob-Gyn Words, Second Edition,* a valuable resource for determining the validity of terms as they are encountered.

Alphabetical Organization

Alphabetization of entries is letter by letter as spelled, ignoring punctuation, spaces, prefixed numbers, Greek letters, or other characters. For example:

acid-fast staining methods
acid formaldehyde hematin
α-acid glycoprotein
acid hematin

In subentries, the abbreviated singular form or the spelled-out plural form of the noun main entry word is ignored in alphabetization.

Format and Style

All main entries are in **boldface** to speed up location of a sought-after entry, to enhance distinction between main entries and subentries, and to relieve the textual density of the pages.

Irregular plurals and variant spellings are shown on the same line as the singular or preferred form of the word. For example:

hypha, pl. **hyphae**

curette, curet

Possessives

Possessive forms have been dropped in this reference for the sake of consistency and to conform to the guidelines outlined by the American Association for Medical Transcription (AAMT) and other groups. It should be noted, however, that retaining the possessive is a question of style, not of accuracy, and thus is a matter of choice. To form the possessive of a word, simply add the apostrophe or apostrophe "s" to the end of the word.

Cross-indexing

The word list is in an index-like main entry-subentry format that contains two combined alphabetical listings:

(1) A *noun* main entry-subentry organization typical of the A-Z section of medical dictionaries like **Stedman's:**

cyst
adnexal c.
Bartholin c.
chocolate c.
dermoid c.
fetal ovarian c.

extractor
Bird vacuum e.
Kobayashi e.
Mityvac vacuum e.
Murless head e.
plastic cup vacuum e.

(2) An *adjective* main entry-subentry organization, which lists words and phrases as you hear them. The main entries are the adjectives or modifiers in a multi-word term. The subentries are the nouns around which the terms are constructed and to which the adjectives or modifiers pertain:

Douglas
D. cul-de-sac
D. mechanism
D. pouch
D. spontaneous evolution

multiple
m. birth
m. cervix
m. cyst
m. gestation

This format provides the user with more than one way to locate and identify a multi-word term. For example:

amenorrhea
    postpartum a.

postpartum
    p. amenorrhea

forceps
    Adson f.
    axis traction f.
    cephalic f.

Adson
    A. forceps
    A. ganglion scissors
    A. pick-ups

It also allows the user to see together all terms that contain a particular descriptor as well as all types, kinds, or variations of a noun entity. For example:

hormone
    h. abnormality
    adrenocortical h.
    h. assay
    bioactive h.
    calcitropic h.

ovulation
    o. age
    contralateral o.
    incessant o.
    o. induction
    paracyclic o.

Wherever possible, abbreviations are separately defined and cross-referenced. For example:

AID
    artificial insemination donor

artificial
    a. insemination donor (AID)

donor
    artificial insemination d. (AID)

References

In addition to the manufacturers' literature we gather at various medical meetings, scientific reports from hospitals, and our MT Editorial Advisory Board members' lists (from their daily work transcription), we used the following sources for new words for *Stedman's Ob-Gyn Words, Second Edition:*

Avery ME. Pediatric medicine, 2ed. Baltimore: Williams & Wilkins, 1994.

Cunningham. Williams obstetrics, 19ed. Norwalk: Appleton & Lange, 1994.

Devita V. Cancer: principles & practice of oncology, 4 ed. Philadelphia: J.B. Lippincott Company, 1993.

Lance LL. Quick Look Drug Book. Baltimore: Williams & Wilkins, 1995.

Nichols DH. Clinical problems, injuries & complications of gynecologic surgery, 2ed. Baltimore: Williams & Wilkins, 1988.

Nora JJ. Medical genetics: principles and practice, 4ed. Baltimore: Williams & Wilkins, 1994.

Sloane SB. The medical word book, 3ed. Philadelphia: WB Saunders Company, 1991.

Stedman's medical dictionary. 26th ed. Baltimore: Williams & Wilkins, 1995.

Stedman's ob-gyn words. Baltimore: Williams & Wilkins, 1992.

Tank HT. Neonatology word book, Modesto, CA: American Association for Medical Transcription, 1991.

Wall LL. Practical urogynecology. Baltimore: Williams & Wilkins, 1993.

Journals

Assisted Reproduction Reviews, Baltimore: Williams & Wilkins, 1994.

Contemporary OB/GYN, Montvale, NJ: Medical Economics, 1992–1995.

Infertility and Reproductive Medicine Clinics of North America. Philadelphia: W.B. Saunders Company, 1994.

Journal of Developmental and Behavioral Pediatrics, Baltimore: Williams & Wilkins, 1994.

Journal of Reproductive Medicine. St. Louis: J Reprod Med, 1992–1994.

Obstetrics & Gynecology. New York: Elsevier, 1992–1994.

Obstetrical & Gynecological Survey. Baltimore: Williams & Wilkins, 1994.

Pediatric Emergency Care. Baltimore: Williams & Wilkins, 1994.

Your Medical Word Resource Publisher

We strive to provide you with the most up-to-date and accurate word references available. Your use of this word book will prompt new editions, which will be published as often as justified by updates and revisions. We welcome your suggestions for improvements, changes, corrections, and additions—whatever will make this *Stedman's* product more useful to you. Please use the postpaid card at the back of this book and send your recommendations to the Reference Division at Williams & Wilkins.

A
    abortus
    alveolar
a
    arterial
A-a
    alveolar-arterial
      A-a gradient
a/A
    arterial to alveolar
(A-a)D$_{O2}$
    difference in partial pressures of
      oxygen in mixed alveolar gas
      and mixed arterial blood
AAGL
    American Association of
      Gynecologic Laparoscopists
Aarskog-Scott syndrome
Aarskog syndrome
Aase syndrome
AB
    abortion
    abortus
A & B
    apnea and bradycardia
      A & B spell
Abbe-McIndoe
    A.-M. procedure
    A.-M. vaginal reconstruction
Abbe-McIndoe-Williams procedure
Abbe vaginal construction
Abbe-Wharton-McIndoe procedure
Abbokinase
Abbott
    A. Laboratories
    A. LifeCare PCA Plus II
      infusion system
abbreviated atrioventricular
  conduction
Abderhalden-Fanconi syndrome
abdomen
    pendulous a.
abdominal
    a. adhesion
    a. approach
    a. auscultation
    a. ballottement
    a. binder
    a. cavity
    a. circumference (AC)

    a. delivery
    a. distention
    a. enlargement
    a. epilepsy
    a. examination
    a. fetal electrocardiography
    a. hernia
    a. hysterectomy
    a. hysteropexy
    a. hysterotomy
    a. irradiation
    a. muscle deficiency
    a. myomectomy
    a. percussion
    a. peritoneum
    a. pregnancy
    a. rescue
    a. sacropexy
    a. salpingo-oophorectomy
    a. salpingotomy
    a. stria
    a. strip radiotherapy
    a. tuberculosis
abdominocyesis
abdominohysterectomy
abdominohysterotomy
abdominopelvic
    a. irradiation
    a. scan
abdominovaginal hysterectomy
abembryonic
Aberdeen knot
aberrancy
    pubertal a.
aberrant
aberration
    chromosomal a.
    heterosomal a.
    newtonian a.
    penta-X chromosomal a.
    tetra-X chromosomal a.
    triple-X chromosomal a.
abetalipoproteinemia
ABG
    arterial blood gas
ablactation
ablation
    endometrial a.
    laser a.

ablation *(continued)*
    laser uterosacral nerve a. (LUNA)
    Nd:YAG laser a.
    ovarian a.
    rectoscopic endometrial a.
    rollerball endometrial a.
ablatio placentae
ablator
    endometrial a.
abnormal
    a. cortisol secretion
    a. decelerations
    a. embryo
    a. feedback signals
    a. fetal development
    a. labor
    a. menstruation
    a. response
    a. uterine bleeding
abnormality
    cervical a.
    chromosomal a.
    chromosomal structural a.
    congenital a.
    cord a.
    deflexion a.
    fetal a.
    fetal postural a.
    fetal thoracic a.
    fibrinogen a.
    genetic a.
    genitourinary a.
    gestational a.
    hormonal a.
    müllerian a.
    multiple endocrine a.'s (MEA)
    neurologic a.
    nonpalpable a.
    ovarian a.
    reproductive tract a.
    sex chromosomal a.
    skeletal a.
    soft tissue a.
    urinary tract a.
    uterine a.
    vaginal epithelial a.
    X-chromosome a.
ABO (blood groups A, AB, B, and O)
    ABO antigen
    ABO blood group system

ABO erythroblastosis
ABO hemolytic disease of the newborn
ABO incompatibility
abort
aborted ectopic pregnancy
aborter
    habitual a.
abortient
abortifacient
abortigenic
abortion (AB)
    Aburel a.
    accidental a.
    ampullar a.
    aneuploid a.
    complete a.
    criminal a.
    Csapo a.
    elective a.
    euploid a.
    habitual a.
    imminent a.
    incipient a.
    incomplete a.
    induced a.
    inevitable a.
    infected a.
    justifiable a.
    menstrual extraction a.
    missed a.
    recurrent a.
    recurrent euploidic a.
    recurrent spontaneous a. (RSA)
    repeated a.
    saline a.
    selective a.
    septic a.
    spontaneous a. (SAB)
    surgically-induced a.
    therapeutic a. (TAB)
    threatened a.
    tubal a.
abortionist
abortive
abortus (A, AB)
ABR
    auditory brainstem response
abruption
    placental a.
abruptio placentae

ABS
arterial blood sample
abscess
amebic a.
Bartholin a.
Bezold a.
Douglas a.
Dubois a.
epidural a.
milk a.
ovarian a.
parametric a.
parametritic a.
pelvic a.
perinephric a.
premammary a.
pyogenic a.
retroesophageal a.
retropharyngeal a.
retrotonsillar a.
stitch a.
subphrenic a.
tuboovarian a.
absence
a. seizure
uterine a.
vaginal a.
Absolok clip applicator
absolute
a. cardiac dullness

a. sterility
a. temperature
absorbable
a. gelatin sponge
a. staple
a. suture
absorptiometer
Hologic 1000 QDR dual-
energy a.
Lunar DPX dual-energy a.
absorptiometry
dual-energy photon a.
dual-energy x-ray a.
(DEXA)
dual-photon a.
single-energy photon a.
single-photon a.
x-ray a.
absorption
calcium a.
a. fever
fluorescent treponemal
antibody a. (FTA-ABS)
abstinence
a. score
Abt-Letterer-Siwe syndrome
Aburel abortion
abuse
alcohol a.
child a.

NOTES

abuse *(continued)*
    maternal drug a.
    sexual a.
AC
    abdominal circumference
ACA
    anticentromere antibody
acanthocytosis
acantholysis bullosa
acanthosis nigricans
ACAPI
    anterior cerebral artery
      pulsatility index
acardiac
    a. fetus
    a. twin
acardius
    fetus a.
acatalasemia
acatalasia
accelerated starvation
accelerator
    betatron electron a.
    linear a.
Accelon Combi cervical biosampler
access
    fetoplacental a.
    uterine a.
accessory
    a. breast
    a. chromosome
    a. müllerian funnel
    a. nipple
    a. ovary
    a. placenta
    a. spleen
    a. tragus
    a. yolk
accident
    cerebrovascular a. (CVA)
    obstetrical a.
accidental
    a. abortion
    a. fetal injury
    a. hemorrhage
    a. pregnancy
accompanying mood state
accouchement
    a. forcé
accoucheur
Accoustix conductivity gel
accretio cordis

accretion
    bone a.
Accu-Chek
    A.-C. Easy glucose monitor
    A.-C. II Freedom blood
      glucose monitor
    A.-C. II glucometer
    A.-C. test
AccuPoint hCG Pregnancy Test Disk
accuracy
    assay a.
    diagnostic a.
Accurbron
Accurette
    A. endometrial suction
      curette
    A. microcurettage
Accuscope colposcope
Accuscope II
Accustat pulse oximeter
Accutane
ACD
    area of cardiac dullness
      ACD level
ACE
    angiotensin-converting enzyme
acebutolol
acenocoumarol
acentric
    a. chromosome
acephalia
acephalobrachia
acephalocardia
acephalochiria
acephalogaster
acephalopodia
acephalorrhachia
acephalostomia
acephalothoracia
acephalus
Aceta
acetaminophen
acetate
    calcium a.
    cyproterone a.
    demedroxyprogesterone a.
      (DMPA)
    desmopressin a. (DDAVP)
    flecainide a.
    gonadorelin a.
    goserelin a.
    leuprolide a.

medroxyprogesterone a.
(MPA)
megestrol a.
nafarelin a.
norethindrone a.
quingestanol a.
sermorelin a.
acetazolamide
acetic acid
acetohexamide
acetone
acetonide
  fluocinolone a.
  triamcinolone a.
acetonuria
acetophenazine
acetophenetidin
acetophenide
  dihydroxyprogesterone a.
acetowhite
  a. epithelium
  a. reaction
acetoxyprogesterone derivative
acetylcholine
  a. chloride
acetylcholinesterase (ACHE, AchE)
acetyldigitoxin
acetylsalicylic acid
achalasia
Achard syndrome
Achard-Thiers syndrome
ACHE, AchE
  acetylcholinesterase
acheilia
acheiria, achiria
acheiropodia
acheiropody, achiropody
achiria (var. of acheiria)
acholic
  a. stool
achondrogenesis
  a. syndrome
achondroplasia
  a. syndrome
achondroplastic dwarfism
achordia
achromasia

achromia
achromiens
  incontinentia pigmenti a.
Achromobacter lwoffi
Achromycin
  A. V
achrondoplastic dwarf
acid
  acetic a.
  acetylsalicylic a.
  amino a.
  D-amino a.
  L-amino a.
  aminocaproic a.
  ε-aminocaproic a. (*var. of*
    epsilon-aminocaproic a.)
    (EACA)
  arachidonic a.
  arginine-glycine-aspartic a.
    (arg-gly-asp)
  arginosuccinic a.
  arylalkanoic a.
  arylcarboxylic a.
  arylpropionic a.
  ascorbic a.
  a. aspiration syndrome
  bichloracetic a.
  bile a.
  boric a.
  branched-chain amino a.
  carbonic a.
  clavulanic a.
  deoxyadenylic a. (dAMP)
  deoxycytidylic a. (dCMP)
  deoxyguanylic a. (dGMP)
  deoxyribonucleic a. (DNA)
  deoxythymidylic a. (dTMP)
  dichloroacetic a.
  diethylenetriamine
    pentaacetic a. (DPTA)
  diisopropyl-iminodiacetic a.
    (DISIDA)
  dimercaptosuccinic a.
  a. elution test
  epsilon-aminocaproic a.,
    ε-aminocaproic a. (EACA)
  ethacrynic a.

NOTES

5

acid *(continued)*
    ethylenediaminetetraacetic a.
    flufenamic a.
    folic a.
    folinic a.
    formiminoglutamic a.
      (FIGLU)
    free fatty a.
    fusanic a.
    hydriodic a.
    hydroxybenzeneazobenzoic a.
      (HABA)
    5-hydroxyindoleacetic a. (5-
      HIAA)
    21-hydroxyindoleacetic a.
      (21-HIAA)
    iocetamic a.
    iopanoic a.
    linoleic a.
    lipid-associated sialic a.
    lysergic a.
    mandelic a.
    mefenamic a.
    messenger ribonucleic a.
      (mRNA)
    nalidixic a.
    nicotinic a.
    noncarbonic a.
    nonvolatile a.
    pantothenic a.
    para-aminomethylbenzoic a.
      (PAMBA)
    para-aminosalicylic a. (PAS,
      PASA)
    phenylpyruvic a.
    a. phosphatase
    retinoic a.
    ribonucleic a. (RNA)
    salicylsalicylic a.
    sialic a.
    Slow Fe with folic a.
    sodium citrate with citric a.
    tolfenamic a.
    tranexamic a.
    transfer ribonucleic a.
      (tRNA)
    trichloroacetic a.
    2,4,5-
      trichlorophenoxyacetic a.
    uric a.
    valproic a.
    volatile a.

acid-base
    a.-b. balance
    a.-b. equilibrium
    a.-b. measurement
    a.-b. status
    a.-b. value
acidemia
    fetal a.
    glutaric a.
    isovaleric a.
    lactic a.
    metabolic a.
    methylmalonic a.
    mixed umbilical arterial a.
    pyroglutamic a.
    trihydroxycoprostanic a.
acidic fibroblast growth factor
    (FGFa)
acidification
    renal a.
acidosis
    diabetic a.
    fetal a.
    hyperchloremic renal a.
    hyperchromic a.
    lactic a.
    metabolic a.
    perinatal a.
    renal tubular a. (RTA)
    respiratory a.
acids/bioflavonoids
    ascorbic a.
acid-Schiff
    periodic a.-S.
aciduria
    β-aminoisobutyric a.
    hereditary orotic a.
    methylmalonic a.
    xanthurenic a.
Aci-Jel vaginal jelly
Acinetobacter lwoffi
ACIP
    Advisory Committee on
      Immunization Practices
aCL
    anticardiolipin antibody
aclasis
    diaphyseal a.
acne
    a. conglobata
    halogen a.
    a. neonatorum
    a. vulgaris

ACOG
American College of
Obstetricians and
Gynecologists
acorn cannula
Acosta classification
acoustic
a. blink reflex
a. enhancement
a. impedance
a. meningioma
a. neuroma
a. reflex
a. shadow
a. stimulation study
a. stimulation test (AST)
a. trauma
acoustical interference
ACPS
acrocephalopolysyndactyly
acquired
a. agammaglobulinemia
a. hemolytic anemia
a. hypogammaglobulinemia
a. immune deficiency
syndrome (AIDS)
a. immunodeficiency
syndrome (AIDS)
a. immunodeficiency
syndrome-related virus
(ARV)
Acrad HS catheter
acrania
acroblast
acrobrachycephaly
acrocentric chromosome
acrocephalopolysyndactyly (ACPS)
acrocephalosyndactyly (type I-V)
(ACS)
acrocephaly
acrochordon
acrocyanosis
acrodermatitis
a. enteropathica
papular a. of childhood
(PAC)
acrodynia

acrodysostosis syndrome
acrofacial dysostosis
acromastitis
acromegaly
acromesomelia
acromion presentation
acromphalus
acropustulosis
a. of infancy
acrosin
acrosomal cap
acrosome
a. reaction
acrosome-intact sperm
acrosphenosyndactyly
acrosyndactyly
acrotism
ACS
acrocephalosyndactyly (type I-V)
ACT
activated clotting time
Actamin
act-FU-Cy
actinomycin D, 5-fluorouracil,
cyclophosphamide
ACTH
adrenocorticotropic hormone
ACTH deficiency
ACTH insufficiency
ACTH stimulation
ACTH stimulation test
Acthar
ActHIB H. influenzae type B
vaccine
Actidil
actin
actin-myosin interaction
Actinomyces
A. israelii
actinomycin D
a. D., 5-fluorouracil,
cyclophosphamide (act-FU-
Cy)
actinomycosis
action
fetal heart a.
gene a.

NOTES

action *(continued)*
    law of mass a.
    luteolytic a.
    mediating a.
    self-priming a.
    uterine a.
activated
    a. clotting time (ACT)
    a. estrogen receptor
    a. partial thromboplastin
      time (APTT)
activation
    egg a.
activator
    lymphocyte a.
    plasminogen a. (PA)
    Platelin Plus A.
    urokinase-type
      plasminogen a. (u-PA)
active
    a. bowel sounds
    Free & A.
    a. labor
    a. phase
    a. phase arrest
    a. phase of labor
    a. range of motion
      (AROM)
    a. third-stage management
activin
activity
    antigen a.
    colony-stimulating a. (CSA)
    elevated enzyme a.
    endometrial cycling a.
    enzyme a.
    fetal a.
    fetal cardiac a.
    fetal somatic a.
    lupus anticoagulant a.
    lymphotoxin antitumor a.
    Manning score of fetal a.
    mitogenic a.
    opioid a.
    ovarian a.
    peripheral androgen a.
    phospholipase a.
    proline aminopeptidase a.
    sexual a.
    tonicocolonic seizure a.
    uterine a.
    withdrawal-like a.
actocardiotocograph fetal monitor

Actrapid insulin with Ultratard
actuarial survival
Acular
acuminata
    condylomata a.
    verruca a.
acupuncture
Acuson
    A. computed sonography
    A. 128 Doppler ultrasound
acuta
    Juliusberg pustulosis
      vacciniformis a.
    pityriasis lichenoides et
      varioliformis a.
acute
    a. anaphylaxis
    a. cystitis
    a. fatty liver
    a. fatty liver disease
    a. fatty liver of pregnancy
    a. intermittent porphyria
    a. interstitial pneumonia
    a. laryngotracheal bronchitis
    a. lymphocytic leukemia
    a. neonatal herpes
    a. nonlymphocytic leukemia
    a. otitis media (AOM)
    a. renal failure
    a. rheumatic fever (ARF)
    a. tubular necrosis (ATN)
    a. urethral syndrome
acute disseminated histiocytosis X
acute-phase serum study
Acuvel
acyclic pelvic pain
acyclovir
acyesis
acystia
AD
    autosomal dominant
ADA
    American Diabetes Association
      ADA diet
adacrya
adactyly
Adair-Dighton syndrome
Adair-Veress needle
Adalat
Adam complex
Adams
    A. advancement

A. advancement of round
    ligaments
A. test for scoliosis
Adams-Stokes syndrome
Adapin
adaptation
    maternal ocular a.
ADC
    AIDS dementia complex
ADC Medicut shears
ADD
    attention deficit disorder
addiction
    alcohol a.
    cocaine a.
    drug a.
    opioid a.
Addison disease
addisonian
    a. crisis
    a. pernicious anemia
    a. syndrome
additivity
    intralocal a.
adelocephaly
adelomorphous
adenine
    a. arabinoside
adenitis
    cervical a.
    mesenteric a.
    sclerosing a.
    vestibular a.
adenoacanthoma
    endometrial a.
    lymph node
      endometriotic a.
adenocarcinoma
    cervical clear cell a.
    ciliated cell endometrial a.
    clear cell a.
    endometrial a.
    endometrial clear cell a.
    endometrial secretory a.
    mesonephric a.
    metastatic a.
    ovarian clear cell a.

papillary a.
secretory a.
serous a.
vaginal a.
vaginal clear cell a.
vulvar adenoid cystic a.
adenofibroma
adenofibromyoma
adenofibrosis
adenohypophysis
adenohypophysitis
    lymphocytic a.
adenoid
    a. cystic carcinoma
    a. facies
adenoidectomy
adenoiditis
adenoleiomyofibroma
adenoma
    apocrine a.
    chromophobic a.
    ductal a.
    growth hormone-secreting a.
    islet cell a.
    lactating a.
    a. malignum
    a. of nipple
    ovarian tubular a.
    parathyroid a.
    pituitary a.
    prolactin-secreting a.
    a. sebaceum
    suspected pituitary a.
    testosterone-secreting
      adrenal a.
    virilizing a.
adenomatoid
    a. oviduct tumor
    a. tumor
adenomatosis
    erosive a. of nipple
    familial multiple
      endocrine a.
    fibrosing a.
adenomatous
    a. endometrial hyperplasia

NOTES

adenomatous *(continued)*
    a. hyperplasia
    a. polyp
adenomegaly
adenomere
adenomyoma
adenomyomatosis
adenomyosis
    stromal a.
    a. uteri
adenopathy
    axillary a.
    cervical a.
    postinflammatory a.
adenosalpingitis
adenosarcoma
    müllerian a.
adenosine
    a. monophosphate (AMP)
    a. phosphate
    a. triphosphate (ATP)
adenosis
    blunt duct a.
    fibrosing a.
    microglandular a.
    sclerosing a.
    vaginal a.
adenosquamous carcinoma
adenoviral pneumonia
adenovirus
adenylate cyclase
adenyl cyclase
adermia
adermogenesis
ADH
    antidiuretic hormone
adhalin gene
ADHD
    attention deficit hyperactivity
    disorder
adherens
    zonula a.
adherent placenta
adhesiolysis
adhesion
    abdominal a.
    amniotic a.'s
    banjo-string a.
    a. barrier
    cell-extracellular matrix a.
    fiddle-string a.
    intrauterine a.
    a. lysis

    peritubal a.
    piano-wire a.
    platelet a.
    sperm-egg a.
adhesive
    Biobrane a.
    a. disease
    a. endometriosis
    a. vaginitis
    a. vulvitis
Adie syndrome
Adipex-P
adipocere
adiponecrosis subcutanea
    neonatorum
adipose tissue
adiposogenital
    a. syndrome
adipsia
adjusted gestational age
adjustment
    psychosocial a.
adjuvant
    a. chemoradiation therapy
    a. chemotherapy
    Freund a.
    a. radiotherapy
    a. therapy
ad lib feeding
administration
    oral a.
    parenteral a.
    pulsatile GnRH a.
    sequential a.
    transdermal a.
    transnasal a.
    vaginal a.
adnata
    alopecia a.
adnexa (*pl. of* adnexum)
    transposed a.
adnexal
    a. cyst
    a. infection
    a. mass
    a. metastasis
    a. torsion
    a. tumor
adnexectomy
adnexitis
adnexopexy
adnexum, pl. adnexa
adolescence

adolescent
  a. breast
  a. gynecology
  A. and Pediatric Pain Tool (APPT)
  a. pregnancy
  a. sterility
adolescentis
  Bifidobacterium a.
adoption
adoptive immunotherapy
adrenal
  a. androgen
  a. androgen secretion
  a. cell rest tumor
  a. cortex
  a. crisis
  a. gland
  a. gland morphology
  a. hyperandrogenism
  a. hyperandrogenism marker
  a. hyperplasia
  a. insufficiency
  Marchand a.'s
  a. morphologic consideration
  a. neoplasm
  a. steroid
  a. tumor
  a. virilism
  a. virilizing syndrome
adrenalectomy
Adrenalin
adrenaline injection
adrenarche
  precocious a.
  premature a.
β-adrenergic
  β-a. agent
  β-a. agonist
  β-a. receptors
adrenergic
  a. blocker
  a. drug
  a. receptors
  a. stimulator
α-adrenergic receptors

adrenocortical
  a. function
  a. hormone
  a. insufficiency
  a. steroid
  a. steroidogenesis
adrenocorticotropic,
adrenocorticotrophic
  a. hormone (ACTH)
adrenocorticotropin
  chorionic a.
adrenogenital
  a. syndrome (AGS)
adrenoleukodystrophy
adrenomegaly
Adriamycin
  A. PFS
  A. RDF
Adrucil
ADS
  anonymous donor sperm
Adson
  A. forceps
  A. ganglion scissors
  A. pickups
Adsorbocarpine
adult-onset
  a.-o. congenital adrenal hyperplasia
  a.-o. diabetes mellitus (AODM)
adult respiratory distress syndrome (ARDS)
Advance
  A. formula
advanced
  a. carcinoma
  a. maternal age
advancement
  Adams a.
Advantage ultrasound
adverse
  a. effect
  a. outcome
Advisory Committee on Immunization Practices (ACIP)
adynamia episodica hereditaria

NOTES

adynamic ileus
AEC
   ankyloblepharon-ectodermal
     dysplasia-clefting
   AEC syndrome
AEGIS sonography management
  system
AENNS
   Albert Einstein Neonatal
     Developmental Scale
AEP
   auditory evoked potentials
aequales
   gemini a.
Aequitron 9200 apnea monitor
AER
   aldosterone excretion rate
aeration of lung
aerobe
aerobic metabolism
Aerochamber
aerocolpos
Aerolate
   A. III
   A. Jr.
   A. SR S
Aerolone
aerophore
Aeroseb-Dex
aerosol
   Breezee Mist A.
   cromolyn sodium
     inhalation a.
   a. therapy
aerosolized medication
aeruginosa
   Pseudomonas a.
aestivale
   hydroa a.
AF
   amniotic fluid
   Lotrimin AF
AFAFP
   amniotic fluid alpha-fetoprotein
afetal
affective disorder
Affinity bed
Affirm
   A. VPIII test
   A. VP microbial
     identification system
AFI
   amniotic fluid index

afibrinogenemia
   congenital a.
Afko-Lube
AFP
   alpha-fetoprotein
   AFP X-tra
Afrinol
AFS
   American Fertility Society
afterbirth
afterload
   a. applicator
   a. colpostat
   a. tandem
afterpain
A/G
   albumin/globulin
   A/G ratio
AGA
   appropriate for gestational age
agalactia
agalactiae
   Streptococcus a.
agalactorrhea
agalactosis
agalactous
agammaglobulinemia
   acquired a.
   Bruton a.
   X-linked a.
aganglionic megacolon
aganglionosis
age
   adjusted gestational a.
   advanced maternal a.
   appropriate for
     gestational a. (AGA)
   bone a.
   childbearing a.
   coital a.
   developmental a. (DA)
   estimated gestational a.
     (EGA)
   fertilization a.
   fetal a.
   gestational a. (GA)
   Greulich and Pyle bone a.
   growth-adjusted
     sonographic a. (GASA)
   large for gestational a.
     (LGA)
   maternal a.
   menstrual a.

ovulatory a.
paternal a.
postconceptional a.
postovulatory a.
small for gestational a.
(SGA)
agenesia corticalis
agenesis
callosal a.
diaphragmatic a.
gonadal a.
müllerian a.
nuclear a.
ovarian a.
pulmonary a.
renal a.
sacral a.
vaginal a.
agenitalism
agent
β-adrenergic a.
alkylating a.
anticancer a.
antifibrinolytic a.
antifolic a.
antineoplastic a.
antiplatelet a.
antiprostaglandin a.
beta-adrenergic a.
beta$_2$-adrenergic a.
A. Blue
chemotherapeutic a.
cycle-nonspecific a.
cycle-specific a.
cytotoxic a.
delta a.
fibrinolytic a.
hyperosmotic a.
infertility a.
myelosuppressive a.
nonalkylating a.
A. Orange
Osteomark a.
pressor a.
progestational a.
sclerosing a.

teratogenic a.
tocolytic a.
agglutination
a. inhibation test
labial a.
latex a.
agglutinin
lens culinaris a.
pisum sativum a. (PSA)
ricinus communis a.
Aggregate Neurobehavioral Student Health & Education Review System (ANSER)
aggregation
platelet a.
aging gamete
agitated depression
aglossia-adactylia syndrome
aglossia congenita
aglossostomia
agnathia
agonadal
agonadism
agonal respirations
agonist
beta-adrenergic a.
β-receptor a.
calcium a.
cholinergic a.
dopamine a.
dopamine receptor a.
dopaminergic a.
GnRH a.
gonadotropin-releasing
hormone a.
agranulocytosis
Kostmann infantile a.
AGS
adrenogenital syndrome
Ahlfeld sign
Ahumada-Del Castillo syndrome
AI
artificial insemination
Aicardi syndrome
AID
artificial insemination by donor

NOTES

13

AIDS
acquired immune deficiency
syndrome
acquired immunodeficiency
syndrome
AIDS dementia complex
(ADC)
transfusion-related AIDS
(TRAIDS)
AIDS-related complex (ARC)
AIH
artificial insemination by
husband
AIHA
autoimmune hemolytic anemia
AIM
area of interest magnification
AIN
anal intraepithelial neoplasia
air
a. bronchogram
a. leak syndrome
airway
a. conductance
a. resistance
a. suction
AI 5200 S Open Color Doppler
imaging system
AJCC
American Joint Committee for
Cancer Staging
AK-Chlor
akinesia algera
Akineton
AKTob
alacrima
Alagille syndrome
Alajouanine syndrome
alanine aminotransferase
alar flaring
alarm
Sioux a.
alba
pityriasis a.
pneumonia a.
Albers-Schönberg syndrome
Albert Einstein Neonatal
Developmental Scale (AENNS)
Albert-Smith pessary
albescens
retinopathy punctata a.
Albini nodule

albinism
cutaneous a.
Forsius-Eriksson type
ocular a.
tyrosinase-negative
oculocutaneous a.
tyrosinase-positive
oculocutaneous a.
albinismus circumscriptus
albinoidism
oculocutaneous a.
albopapuloid variant
Albright
A. disease
A. syndrome
albuginea
tunica a.
albumin
plasma a.
serum a.
albumin/globulin (A/G)
a.g. ratio (A/G ratio)
albuminuria
albuterol
ALCAPA
anomalous left coronary artery
from pulmonary artery
ALCAPA syndrome
Alcock canal
alcohol
a. abuse
a. addiction
blood a.
ethanol, ethyl a. (EtOH)
a. ingestion
nicotinyl a.
a. related (AR)
alcoholism
maternal a.
Alconefrin
Aldactone
Alder anomaly
Alder-Reilly anomaly
Aldomet
Aldoril
aldosterone
a. excretion rate (AER)
aldosteronism
juvenile a.
Aldrich syndrome
Aldridge
A. rectus fascia sling
A. sling procedure

Aldridge-Studdefort urethral suspension
aleukia
    congenital a.
Aleve
Alexander
    A. disease
    A. operation
Alexander-Adams
    A.-A. hysteropexy
    A.-A. uterine suspension
alfa
    dornase a.
alfa-n3
    interferon a.-n.
alfentanil
Alferon N
algera
    akinesia a.
algomenorrhea
Algo newborn hearing screener
alimentation
    intravenous a.
    parenteral a.
Alimentum
    A. feeding
A-line
    arterial line
Alka-Butazolidin
alkalemia
alkaline phosphatase
alkaloid
    levorotatory a.
    plant a.
    Veratrum a.
    Vinca a.
alkalosis
    metabolic a.
    respiratory a.
Alka-Mints
alkaptonuria
Alka-Seltzer
Alkeran
alkylating
    a. agent
    a. chemotherapy

allantoic
    a. cyst
    a. duct
    a. sac
    a. stalk
allantoidoangiopagous twins
allantoidoangiopagus
allantois
allele
    multiple a.'s
    premutation a.
    silent a.
allelic
    a. exclusion
    a. gene
Allemann syndrome
Allen
    A. fetal stethoscope
    A. laparoscopic stirrups
Allen and Capute neonatal neurodevelopmental examination
Allen-Doisy test
Allen-Masters syndrome
Allerest
allergen
allergic dermatitis
allergy
    sperm a.
alligator
    a. forceps
    a. skin
Allis
    A. clamp
    A. forceps
Allis-Abramson
    A.-A. breast biopsy
    A.-A. breast biopsy forceps
alloantibody
alloantigen
allodiploid
allogeneic
    a. antigen
    a. disease
    a. fetal graft
allogenicity

NOTES

allograft
    a. survival
alloimmune
    a. factor
    a. mechanism
    a. neonatal
      thrombocytopenic purpura
    a. thrombocytopenia
alloimmunity
alloimmunization
allopolyploidy
all-or-none phenomenon
allosome
    paired a.
allotropism
allotype
allowance
    recommended dietary a.
Allport retractor
Aloka
    A. OB/GYN ultrasound
    A. 650 scanner
    A. SSD-720 real-time
      scanner
    A. ultrasound system
alopecia
    a. adnata
    a. areata
    a. congenitalis
    a. hereditaria
Alpers disease
alpha
    a. antitrypsin level
    a. error
    a. helix
    a. interferon
    a. particle
    Prostin F2 a.
    a. thalassemia
    transforming growth
      factor a. (TGFα)
alpha-1
    a.-antitrypsin
    a. PI
    a. protease inhibitor (alpha-
     1 PI)
    a. thymosin product
17-alpha-acetoxyprogesterone
  derivative
alpha-adrenergic
    a.-a. blocker
    a.-a. stimulator

alpha-chain disorder
Alphaderm
17-alpha-ethinyl testosterone
alpha-fetoprotein, α-fetoprotein
  (AFP)
    amniotic fluid a.-f. (AFAFP)
    a.-f. elevation
    maternal serum a.-f.
     (MSAFP)
alpha-melanotrophin
Alphamine
alphaprodine
alpha-recombinant interferon
Alport syndrome
alprazolam
Alstrom sign
ALTE
    apparent life-threatening event
alteration
    uterine activity a.
alternative hypothesis
altretamine
aludrine
Alupent
Alurate
aluteal
alveolar (A)
    arterial to a. (a/A)
    a. partial pressure (PA)
    a. soft part sarcoma
alveolar-arterial (A-a)
    a.-a. oxygen diffusing
     capacity
    a.-a. pressure difference
     (p(A-a)O$_2$)
alveolus, pl. alveoli
    pulmonary a.
alymphocytosis
alymphoplasia
amantadine
amastia
amaurosis
    a. congenita
    a. fugax
    Leber congenital a. (LCA)
amaurotic familial idiocy
amazia
amazon thorax
ambenonium
Ambien
ambient
    a. oxygen concentration

ambiguity
  genital a.
  sexual a.
ambiguous genitalia
amboceptor
Ambu
  A. bag
  A. infant resuscitator
  A. respirator
ambulation
ambulatory
  a. care
  a. uterine contraction test
Amcill
amebiasis
amebic
  a. abscess
  a. dysentery
  a. vaginitis
amelia
Amen
amenia
amenorrhea
  athletic a.
  dietary a.
  emotional a.
  eugonadotropic a.
  exercise-induced a.
  hypergonadotropic a.
  hyperprolactinemic a.
  hypogonadotropic a.
  hypophysial a.
  hypothalamic a.
  jogger's a.
  lactation a.
  ovarian a.
  pathologic a.
  physiologic a.
  postmenopausal a.
  postpartum a.
  postpill a.
  primary a.
  secondary a.
  traumatic a.
amenorrhea-galactorrhea syndrome
amenorrheal, amenorrheic
Americaine

American
  A. Association of
    Gynecologic Laparoscopists
    (AAGL)
  A. College of Obstetricians
    and Gynecologists (ACOG)
  A. Diabetes Association
    (ADA)
  A. Fertility Society (AFS)
  A. Joint Committee for
    Cancer Staging (AJCC)
  A. Society of
    Anesthesiologists
    classification
amethopterin
ametria
AMF
  autocrine motility factor
Amfetamine
AMH
  anti-müllerian hormone
Amicar
Amiel-Tison
  A.-T. score
  A.-T. test
amikacin
  a. sulfate
Amikin
amiloride
amino
  a. acid
  a. acid metabolism
aminoacidemia
aminoacidopathy
aminoaciduria
aminoaciduriasis
aminocaproic acid
ε-aminocaproic acid (EACA)
Amino-Cerv pH 5.5 cervical Creme
aminoglutethimide
aminoglycoside
β-aminoisobutyric aciduria
Amino-Opti-E
aminopeptidase
  leucine a.
aminophylline

NOTES

17

aminoprine
aminopterin
aminopyrine
Aminosyn-PF supplement
amino-terminal peptide
aminotransferase
    alanine a.
    aspartate a.
amiodarone
Amipaque
Amitid
Amitone
Amitril
amitriptyline
Amko vaginal speculum
ammonemia (*var. of* ammoniemia)
Ammon fissure
ammoniac
    sal a.
ammoniemia, ammonemia
ammonium
    a. bromide
    a. chloride
amnestic response
amnii
    hydrops a.
amniocentesis
    early a. (EA)
    genetic a.
amniochorion
amniocyte
amniogenic cells
amniography
    a. in hydatidiform mole
Amniohook
amnioinfusion
amnioma
amnion
    a. nodosum
    a. ring
    a. rupture
amnionic
    a. caruncle
amnionitis
    silent a.
amniorrhea
amniorrhexis
amnioscope
amnioscopy
Amniostat fetal lung maturity
   screening
Amniostat-FLM test

amniotic
    a. adhesions
    a. band amputation
    a. band anomalad
    a. banding syndrome
    a. bands
    a. cavity
    a. fluid (AF)
    a. fluid alpha-fetoprotein
    (AFAFP)
    a. fluid cell culture
    a. fluid embolism
    a. fluid embolus
    a. fluid embolus syndrome
    a. fluid fluorescence
    polarization
    a. fluid index (AFI)
    a. fluid level
    a. fluid pocket
    a. fluid quantitation
    a. fluid syndrome
    a. fluid volume
    a. infection syndrome
    a. infection syndrome of
    Blane
    a. sac
    a. sheet
amniotome
    Baylor a.
amniotomy
amobarbital
A-mode ultrasound
amoebic colitis
amorphous fetus
amorphus
    fetus a.
amotio placentae
amoxapine
amoxicillin
Amoxil
AMP
    adenosine monophosphate
    assisted medical procreation
AmpErase electrocautery
amphetamine
amphigonous inheritance
amphotericin B
ampicillin
    a. sodium/sulbactam sodium
    a. trihydrate
Amplicor
    A. Chlamydia Assay
    A. HIV-1 test kit

A. PCR diagnostics
A. PCR kit
amplification
DNA a.
gene a.
Y-specific DNA a.
amplitude
oscillation a.
ampulla of oviduct
ampullar
a. abortion
a. pregnancy
amputation
amniotic band a.
birth a.
cervical a.
congenital a.
intrauterine a.
Jabouley a.
spontaneous a.
Amreich vaginal extirpation
Amrinone
amrinone lactate
Amsacrine (mAMSA)
Amsterdam
A. dwarfism
A. infant ventilator
amyelencephalia
amyelencephalous
amyelia
amyeloidosis
amyelous
amygdalin
amylase
serum a.
amylase-creatinine clearance ratio
amyl nitrite
amylobarbitone
amyloidosis
amylophagia
amyoplasia
a. congenita
amyotonia congenita
Amytal
Anabolin
anacatadidymus
anadidymus

anaerobe
anaerobic
a. vaginosis
anaerobius
Peptococcus a.
Anafranil
anagen
anakatadidymus
anal
a. atresia
a. canal
a. incontinence
a. intraepithelial neoplasia
(AIN)
a. reflex
a. sphincter
a. sphincter disruption
a. squamous intraepithelial
lesion (ASIL)
a. wink
analgesia
caudal a.
conduction a.
continuous epidural a.
epidural a.
narcotic a.
patient-controlled a.
peridural a.
perineal a.
regional a.
spinal a.
analgesic
narcotic a.
analogue
gonadotropin-releasing
hormone a.
luteinizing hormone-releasing
hormone a.
oxytocin a.
tetracycline a.
analysis, pl. analyses
automated multiple a.
blood a.
cell block a.
chromosomal a.
clinicopathological a.
a. of covariance (ANCOVA)

NOTES

analysis *(continued)*
    cytogenic a.
    endonuclease a.
    karyotype a.
    linkage a.
    molecular genetic a.
    multivariant a.
    postoperative symptom a.
    restriction endonuclease a.
    saturation a.
    semen a.
    a. of variance (ANOVA)
analyzer
    AVL 9110 pH a.
    Coulter Channelyser cell a.
    HemoCue blood glucose a.
    HemoCue blood
      hemoglobin a.
    Osteomeasure computer-
      assisted image a.
    Serono SR1 FSH a.
    Sonoclot coagulation a.
    SRI automated
      immunoassay a.
anamnestic response
anaphase
    a. lag
anaphylactic shock
anaphylactoid purpura
anaphylaxis
    acute a.
    recurrent a.
anaplastic carcinoma
Anaprox
    A.-DS
anasarca
    fetoplacental a.
anaspadias
Anaspaz
anastomosis, pl. anastomoses
    Clado a.
    colorectal a.
    cornual a.
    isthmointerstitial a.
    microsurgical tubocornual a.
    onlay patch a.
    ureterotubal a.
    ureteroureteral a.
anatomy
    fetal a.
    fetal intracranial a.
    immune system a.
    intracranial a.

Anavar
Ancef
ancestor
    leading a.
Ancobon
Ancotil
ANCOVA
    analysis of covariance
ancylostomiasis
Andernach ossicle
Andersen disease
Anderson marker
Andogsky syndrome
Andrews infant laryngoscope
Andro
androblastoma
Andro-Cyp
androgen
    adrenal a.
    a. antagonist
    a. dynamics
    excess a.
    a. excess
    a. insensitivity syndrome
    a. interaction
    a. receptor
    a. resistance
    a. resistance syndrome
    a. secretion
androgen-dependent carcinoma
androgenesis
androgenic
androgenized woman
androgenous
androgen-producing tumor
androgynism
androgynous
androgyny
android
    a. obesity
    a. pelvis
Android-F
Andro-L.A.
Androlone
    A.-D
Andronate
Andropository-200
androstane
    5α-a.-3α,17β-diol glucuronide
      (3α-diol-G)
3α-androstanediol glucuronide
androstenediol
androstenedione

androsterone
a. glucuronide
Androvite
anechoic tissue
anectasis
anembryonic gestation
anemia
acquired hemolytic a.
addisonian pernicious a.
angiopathic hemolytic a.
aplastic a.
autoimmune acquired
hemolytic a.
autoimmune hemolytic a.
(AIHA)
Blackfan-Diamond a.
blood-loss a.
congenital a.
congenital hypoplastic a.
congenital nonregenerative a.
congenital nonspherocytic
hemolytic a.
Cooley a.
crescent cell a.
Czerny a.
Diamond-Blackfan congenital
hypoplastic a.
Diamond-Blackfan juvenile
pernicious a.
elliptocytic a.
erythroblastic a.
familial erythroblastic a.
Fanconi a.
globe cell a.
Heinz body a.
hemolytic a.
hereditary nonspherocytic a.
Herrick a.
a. hypochromica
siderochrestica hereditaria
hypoplastic a.
iron deficiency a. (IDA)
Jaksch a.
juvenile pernicious a.
Larzel a.
macrocytic a. of pregnancy
Mediterranean a.

megaloblastic a.
microcytic a.
a. neonatorum
ovalocytary a.
pernicious a. (PA)
physiologic a.
pregnancy-associated
hypoplastic a.
a. of prematurity
a. pseudoleukemica
infantum
pyridoxine-responsive a.
Runeberg a.
sickle cell a.
sideroblastic a.
Von Jaksch a.
anemic
a. effect
anemicus
nevus a.
anencephalic
anencephaly
anergy
Anestacon
anesthesia
caudal a.
conduction a.
epidural a.
extradural a.
general a.
inhalation a.
local a.
lumbar epidural a.
maternal a.
obstetric a.
paracervical a.
peridural a.
perineal a.
pudendal a.
regional a.
saddle block a.
spinal a.
anesthesiologist
anesthetic
eutectic mixture of
local a.'s (EMLA)
gas a.

NOTES

anesthetic *(continued)*
    a. gas exposure
    local a.
    volatile a.
    walking epidural a.
Anesthetist
    Certified Registered
      Nurse A. (CRNA)
anestrous
aneugamy
aneuploid
    a. abortion
aneuploidy
    recurrent a.
    XXXXY a.
aneurysm
    aortic a.
    arterial a.
    dissecting aortic a.
    intracranial a.
    ruptured cerebral a.
    saccular a.
ANF
    atrial natriuretic factor
Angelman syndrome
angiitis
angina
angiocardiogram
    Elema a.
angioedema
angiogenesis
angiogenic growth factor
angiography
    pulmonary a.
angiokeratoma
    a. circumscriptum
    Mibelli a.
    a. of Mibelli
    vulvar a.
angiolysis
angioma
    cerebral a.
    dural spinal a.
    intradural spinal a.
    spider a.
    spinal a.
angiomatoid tumor
angiomatosis
    encephalofacial a.
    encephalotrigeminal a.
angiomyoma of oviduct
angioneurotic edema

angio-osteohypertrophy
    a. syndrome
angiopathic hemolytic anemia
angiosarcoma
    uterine a.
angiotensin
    a. II
angiotensin-converting enzyme
  (ACE)
angiotensinogen
angle
    urethral a.
    urethrovesical a.
anhedonia
anhidrotic ectodermal dysplasia
anhydrohydroxyprogesterone
Anhydron
ani (*pl. of* anus)
anideus
    embryonic a.
anileridine
anion gap
aniridia
anisindione
anisocoria
anisodactyly
anisomastia
anisomelia
anisotropine
ankle clonus
ankyloblepharon-ectodermal
  dysplasia-clefting (AEC)
ankylocheilia
ankylocolpos
ankylodactyly
ankyloglossia
ankyloproctia
ankylosing spondylitis
anlage, pl. anlagen
annexectomy
annexitis
annexopexy
annular
    a. band
    a. placenta
    a. tubule
annulare
    granuloma a.
annulati
    pili a.
ano
    fissure in a.
anococcygeal raphe

anogenital wart
anomalad
    amniotic band a.
    holoprosencephaly a.
    Robin a.
anomalous
    a. left coronary artery from
      pulmonary artery
      (ALCAPA)
    a. left coronary artery from
      pulmonary artery syndrome
    a. pulmonary venous
      connection
    a. uterus
anomaly
    Alder a.
    Alder-Reilly a.
    branchial a.
    cardiac a.
    cervical a.
    Chédiak-Higashi a.
    Chiari a.
    chromosomal a.
    coloboma, heart anomaly,
      choanal atresia,
      retardation, and genital
      and ear a.'s (CHARGE)
    congenital a.
    Duane a.
    Ebstein a.
    fetal a.
    fetal vascular a.
    genetic a.
    intracranial dural
      vascular a.
    May-Hegglin a.
    Moebius a.
    müllerian a.
    multiple congenital a.'s
    orthopaedic a.
    Pelger-Huet a.
    Peters a.
    Poland a.
    sex chromosomal a.
    Shone a.
    Sprengel a.
    Uhl a.

    umbilical cord a.
    Undritz a.
    urogenital a.
    uterine a.
    VACTERL a.
    vaginal a.
    vascular a.
    vertebral, anal, cardiac,
      tracheal, esophageal, renal,
      limb a.
anonymous donor sperm (ADS)
anophthalmia
anorchia
anorchism
anorectal stenosis
anorectic
    a. reaction
Anorex
anorexia
    a. nervosa
anorgasmic
anosmia
anotia
ANOVA
    analysis of variance
anovarianism
anovular
    a. menstruation
anovulation
    persistent a.
anovulatory
    a. bleeding
    a. infertility
    a. patient
anoxia
    fetal a.
    a. neonatorum
anoxic-ischemic encephalopathy
Ansaid
Ansaldo AU560 ultrasound
ANSER
    Aggregate Neurobehavioral
      Student Health & Education
      Review System
Anspor
Answer
    A. Plus

NOTES

Antabuse
antacid
antagonism
antagonist
    androgen a.
    calcium a.
    folic acid a.
    follicle-stimulating
      hormone a.
    gonadotropin-releasing
      hormone a.
    narcotic a.
    opioid receptor a.
antagonist-induced gonadotropin
  deprivation
antecedent
    cerebral palsy a.
    plasma thromboplastin a.
      (PTA)
anteflex
anteflexed
    anteverted and a. (AV/AF)
anteflexion
antenatal
    a. anti-D immunoglobulin
    a. diagnosis
    a. patient
    a. phenobarbital treatment
    a. screening
    a. ultrasound
antepartum
    a. bleeding
    a. care
    a. hemorrhage
    a. monitor
anteposition
anterior
    a. asynclitism
    a. cerebral artery pulsatility
      index (ACAPI)
    a. chamber cleavage
      syndrome
    a. commissure
    a. lie
    occiput a. (OA)
    a. pelvic exenteration
    a. pituitary-like hormone
    a. and posterior (A&P)
    a. and posterior repair
    a. repair
    a. retrosternal hernia of
      Morgagni
    a. urethritis

anterolateral fontanel
anteroposterior (AP)
    a. diameter of the pelvic
      inlet
anteversion
anteverted
    a. and anteflexed (AV/AF)
anthelix, antihelix
anthrax
    cutaneous a.
    pulmonary a.
anthropoid pelvis
anthropometric measurement
antiarrhythmic
antibacterial therapy
antibiotic
    beta-lactam a.
    beta-lactamase-resistant
      antistaphylococcal a.,
      β- lactamase-resistant
      antistaphylococcal a.
    prophylactic a.
antibody
    anticardiolipin a. (aCL)
    anticentromere a. (ACA)
    antigliadin a.
    anti-HIV a.
    anti-idiotype a.
    anti-Kell a.
    anti-Lewis a.
    anti-M a.
    antimitochondrial a.
    antinuclear a.
    antipaternal
      antileukocytotoxic a.
    antiphospholipid a.'s (aPLs)
    antisperm a.
    blood group a.
    circulating platelet a.
    conjugated a.
    cytophilic a.
    fluorescent treponema a.
     (FTA)
    Frei a.
    hemagglutinating
     inhibition a. (HIA)
    humoral a.
    IgM a.
    Kveim a.
    lupus anticoagulant a.
    maternal a.
    monoclonal a.
    natural a.

ovarian a.
phospholipid a.
platelet-associated a.
polyclonal a.
a. reaction site
a. response
a. screening
serum a.
species-specific a.
sperm a.
tissue-specific a.
xenogeneic a.
anticancer agent
anticardiolipin
    a. antibody (aCL)
anticentromere antibody (ACA)
anticholinergic
    a. drug
anticholinesterase
anticoagulant
    lupus a.
    a. therapy
anticoagulation
anticodon
anticonvulsant
    a. drug
anti-D
    a.-D. gamma globulin
    a.-D. immune globulin
    a.-D. immunoglobulin
antidepressant
    a. therapy
    tricyclic a.
antidiuretic hormone (ADH)
antiembolism stocking
antiemetic therapy
antiestrogen
antiestrogenic effect
antiferritin antibody linked to iodine-131
antifibrinolytic agent
antifolic agent
antifungal drug therapy
antigalactagogue
antigalactic
antigen
    ABO a.

a. activity
allogeneic a.
Australia a.
a. binding site
CA-125 a.
cancer a. (CA)
carcinoembryonic a. (CEA)
carcinoembryonic a.-125 (CEA-125)
carcinoma a.
cell surface a.
a. determinant
direct fluorescent a. (DFA)
Forssman a.
Goa a.
hepatitis B a. (HBAg)
hepatitis B surface a. (HBsAg)
heterophil a.
histocompatibility a.
histocompatibility locus a.
human leukocyte a. (HLA)
human lymphocyte a.
H-Y a.
incompatible blood group a.
M a.
major histocompatibility a.
MHC a.
nuclear a.
oncofetal a.
ovarian carcinoma a.
p24 a.
pancreatic oncofetal a. (POA)
platelet a.
red cell a.
Rh a.
a. screen
surface a.
T6 a.
thymic lymphocyte a. (TL)
a. tolerance
transplantation a.
tumor a.
tumor-associated a. (TAA)
tumor-specific transplantation a. (TSTA)

NOTES

antigen-antibody complex
antigenic
    a. modulation
    a. paralysis
antigenicity
    tumor a.
antigen-sensitive cell
antigliadin antibody
antiglobulin test
antiglomerular basement membrane
   antibody disease
antigonadotropin
antihelix (*var. of* anthelix)
antihelminthic therapy
antihemophilic factor
antihistamine
anti-HIV antibody
antihypertensive
    a. drug
    a. therapy
anti-icteric
anti-idiotype antibody
anti-Kell antibody
anti-Lewis antibody
antiluteogenic
antimalarial drug
anti-M antibody
antimetabolite
antimicrobial
    beta-lactam a.
    a. therapy
Antiminth
antimitochondrial antibody
antimongolism
antimongoloid
anti-müllerian hormone (AMH)
antineoplastic
    a. agent
    a. drug
antinuclear antibody
antiparasitic drug therapy
antipaternal antileukocytotoxic
   antibody
antiphospholipid
    a. antibodies (aPLs)
    a. syndrome
antiplatelet agent
Antipress
antiprogesterone
antiprogestin
antiprostaglandin
    a. agent
antipsychotic drug

antipyretic
antireceptor
antiserum, pl. antisera
    SB-6 a.
antishock trousers
antisialagogue
antispasmodic
antisperm antibody
antistreptolysin titer
antithrombin
    a. II
    a. III
antithymocyte globulin
antithyroid
    a. drug
    a. drug therapy
antitreponemal test
Anti-Tuss
antiviral therapy
Antley-Bixler syndrome
antral
    a. follicle
    a. stenosis
antrum, pl. antra
anuria
anus, pl. ani
    ectopic a.
    imperforate a.
    levator ani
    patent a.
    pruritus ani
    a. of Rusconi
    vaginal ectopic a.
    vestibular a.
    vulvovaginal a.
AODM
    adult-onset diabetes mellitus
AOM
    acute otitis media
aorta, pl. aortae
    coarctation of a.
    descending a.
    fetal a.
    overriding a.
aortic
    a. aneurysm
    a. bruit
    a. insufficiency
    a. laceration
    a. node
    a. node metastasis
    a. regurgitation
    a. root diameter

a. stenosis
a. valve disease
a. valve insufficiency
aorticopulmonary (*var. of*
aortopulmonary)
aortitis
aortocardiotocograph
aortography
aortopulmonary, aorticopulmonary
a. septum
a. shunt
a. window
AP
anteroposterior
A&P
anterior and posterior
A&P repair
apareunia
ape hand
Apert
A. disease
A. syndrome
Apert-Crouzon
A.-C. disease
A.-C. syndrome
apex, pl. apices
a. of vagina
Apgar
A. rating
A. scale
A. score
A. timer
APGO
Association of Professors of
Gynecology and Obstetrics
aphasia
global a.
Wernicke a.
aphtha, pl. aphthae
Bednar aphthae
aphthous
a. stomatitis
a. ulcer
APIB
Assessment of Preterm Infants
Behavior

apices (*pl. of* apex)
A.P.L.
aplasia
a. axialis extracorticalis
congenita
a. cutis congenita
gonadal a.
Leydig cell a.
nuclear a.
retinal a.
thymic a.
thymic-parathyroid a.
aplastic
a. anemia
a. crisis
a. leukemia
a. pancytopenia
aPLs
antiphospholipid antibodies
apnea
a. alarm mattress
a. and bradycardia (A & B)
initial a.
late a.
a. monitor
a. neonatorum
a. of prematurity
reflexic a.
sleep a.
vasovagal reflex a.
apneustic
apocrine
a. adenoma
a. cyst
a. gland
a. miliaria
apodia
apolipoprotein
apoplectic
apoplexy
parturient a.
uteroplacental a.
apoprotein
a. A
apoptosis
apparatus, pl. apparatus

NOTES

apparatus *(continued)*
 Heyns abdominal
  decompression a.
apparent life-threatening event
 (ALTE)
appearance
 bull's eye sonographic a.
 cushingoid a.
 ground-glass a.
 meconium ileus a.
 peau d'orange a.
 snowstorm a.
 strawberry a.
appendectomy
appendiceal fecalith
appendicitis
 suppurative a.
appendix
Apple Medical bipolar forceps
application
 topical iodine a.
applicator
 Absolok clip a.
 afterload a.
 Bloedorn a.
 cesium a.
 Ernst radium a.
 Falope ring a.
 Filshie clip a.
 Filshie clip
  minilaparotomy a.
 Fletcher-Suit a.
 radioactive a.
 ring a.
 Ter-Pogossian cervical a.
apposition
 a. of skull suture
approach
 abdominal a.
 transrectal a.
appropriate for gestational age
 (AGA)
APPT
 Adolescent and Pediatric Pain
  Tool
Apresoline
aprobarbital
aproctia
apron
 Hottentot a.
 pudendal a.
aprosopia
aprotinin

APTT
 activated partial thromboplastin
  time
Aquachloral
 A. Supprettes
Aquaflex ultrasound gel pad
Aquagel lubricating gel
AquaMEPHYTON
Aquaphyllin
Aquasol A
Aquasol E
Aquasonic 100 ultrasound
 transmission gel
Aquatensen
aqueductal
 a. stenosis
Aquest
AR
 alcohol related
 autosomal recessive
arabinoside
 adenine a.
 cytosine a.
arabinosylcytosine
arachidic bronchitis
arachidonic
 a. acid
 a. acid level
 a. acid metabolites
arachnidism
arachnodactyly
 congenital contractural a.
  (CCA)
arachnoiditis
Aralen
Aramine
Aran-Duchenne disease
arborization
 pulmonary a.
arbor vitae
arbovirus
ARC
 AIDS-related complex
arcade
 mitral a.
arch
 branchial a.
 neural a.
 pubic a.
 Zimmerman a.
archencephalon
archenteron
archenteronoma

archiblast
archigastrula
architectural disturbance
architecture
    histologic a.
    pelvic a.
arcuate
    a. artery
    a. ligament of pubis
    a. nucleus
    a. uterus
arcus tendineus
ARDS
    adult respiratory distress
    syndrome
area
    body surface a. (BSA)
    a. of cardiac dullness
      (ACD)
    a. of interest magnification
      (AIM)
    skip a.
areata
    alopecia a.
areflexia
Arenavirus
areola, pl. areolae
    a. umbilicus
areolar
Arey rule
ARF
    acute rheumatic fever
Arfonad
arg-gly-asp
    arginine-glycine-aspartic acid
arginase deficiency
arginine
    a. glutamate
    a. hydrochloride
    a. vasopressin
    a. vasotocin
arginine-glycine-aspartic acid
  (arg- gly-asp)
arginine-insulin
argininemia
argininosuccinicacidemia
argininosuccinicaciduria

arginosuccinic acid
argon
    a. beam coagulator
    a. laser
Argonz-Del Castillo syndrome
Argyle arterial catheter
argyrophilic granule
arhinia (*var. of* arrhinia)
Arias-Stella
    A.-S. effect
    A.-S. phenomenon
    A.-S. reaction
Aristocort
Arlidin
ARM
    artificial rupture of membranes
arm
    a. board
    a. of chromosome
    chromosome a.
    nuchal a.
    a. position
    a. presentation
    a. recoil
Army-Navy retractor
Arnold-Chiari
    A.-C. deformity
    A.-C. malformation
    A.-C. syndrome
Arnoux sign
AROM
    active range of motion
    artificial rupture of membranes
aromatase
aromatization
array
    superficial linear a. (SLA)
arrest
    active phase a.
    cardiac a.
    circulatory a.
    a. disorder
    follicular development a.
    a. of labor
    preterm labor a.
    respiratory a.

NOTES

arrest *(continued)*
    sinus a.
    transverse a.
arrested development
Arrestin
arrhenoblastoma
arrhinencephalia
arrhinencephaly
arrhinia, arhinia
arrhythmia
    cardiac a.
    fetal a.
    sinus a.
arrival
    born on a. (BOA)
ART
    assisted reproductive technology
Artane
arterenol
arterial (a)
    a. to alveolar (a/A)
    a. aneurysm
    a. blood gas (ABG)
    a. blood pressure
    a. blood sample (ABS)
    a. calcification
    a. carbon dioxide pressure (tension) ($PaCO_2$)
    a. line (A-line, art line, art line)
    a. linear density
    a. occlusive disease
    a. oxygen pressure (tension) (PaO_2)
    a. partial pressure (Pa)
    a. thrombosis
    a. vascular bed
    a. vascular disease
    a. waveform
arteriogram
    pelvic a.
arteriography
arteriohepatic dysplasia
arteriosclerosis
    infantile a.
ArterioSonde
arteriosus
    ductus a. (DA)
    patent ductus a. (PDA)
    truncus a.
arteriovenous
    a. fistula
    a. malformation
    a. oxygen difference
    a. shunt
arteritis umbilicalis
artery
    anomalous left coronary artery from pulmonary a. (ALCAPA)
    arcuate a.
    azygos a.
    basal a.
    cervical a.
    circumflex a.
    coiled a.
    colic a.
    deep circumflex iliac a.
    endometrial spiral a.
    epigastric a.
    femoral a.
    femoral circumflex a.
    fetal cranial a.
    great a.'s
    hemorrhoidal a.
    hypogastric a.
    ileocolic a.
    iliac a.
    inferior mesenteric a.
    lumbar a.
    mesenteric a.
    middle sacral a.
    obturator a.
    ovarian a.
    Parrot a.
    pelvic a.
    posterior inferior communicating a. (PICA)
    pudendal a.
    radial a.
    spiral a.
    superficial external pudendal a. (SEPA)
    superior mesenteric a.
    transposition of great a.'s (TGA)
    umbilical a. (UA)
    uterine a.
    vaginal a.
    vertebral a.
arthritis, pl. arthritides
    juvenile rheumatoid a. (JRA)
    monarticular a.

polyarticular juvenile
rheumatoid a.
psoriatic a.
pyogenic a.
rheumatoid a. (RA)
septic a.
arthrochalasis multiplex congenita
arthrogryposis
a. multiplex
a. multiplex congenita
Arthropan
Arthus reaction
Articu-Lase laser mirror
artifact
deodorant a.
artificial
a. fever
a. insemination (AI)
a. insemination by donor
(AID)
a. insemination donor
a. insemination by husband
(AIH)
a. intravaginal insemination
a. pacemaker
a. rupture of membranes
(ARM, AROM)
a. temperature
a. vagina
art line
arterial line
ARV
acquired immunodeficiency
syndrome-related virus
Arvee model 2400 infant apnea
monitor
aryepiglottic fold
arylalkanoic acid
arylcarboxylic acid
arylpropionic acid
AS
Crysticillin AS
Duracillin AS
Pentids-P AS
Pfizerpen AS
asaccharolyticus
Peptococcus a.

ascariasis
ascensus
ascertainment
total a.
Aschheim-Zondek (AZ)
A.-Z. test
aschistodactylia
ascites
chylous a.
lues a.
tumor a.
ascorbic
a. acid
a. acids/bioflavonoids
Ascriptin
A. A/D
ASCUS
atypical squamous cells of
undetermined significance
ASCUS smear
ASD
atrial septal defect
Asendin
aseptic
a. fever
a. meningitis
a. temperature
Asepto syringe
asexual
a. dwarfism
Asherman syndrome
Ashkenazi Jew
ASIL
anal squamous intraepithelial
lesion
Asmalix
asoma
aspartate
a. aminotransferase
Aspen laparoscopy electrode
AspenVAC smoke evacuation
system
aspergillosis
bronchopulmonary a.
ocular a.
pulmonary a.
Aspergum

NOTES

aspermia
asphyxia
    autoerotic a.
    birth a.
    blue a.
    fetal a.
    a. livida
    a. neonatorum
    a. pallida
    perinatal a.
    sexual a.
asphyxiating
    a. thoracic dysplasia
    a. thoracic dysplasia
      syndrome
    a. thoracic dystrophy
    a. thoracodystrophy
      syndrome
asphyxiation
    intrapartum a.
aspirate
    nasopharyngeal a.
    surveillance tracheal a.
aspiration
    a. biopsy
    cyst a.
    fine-needle a. (FNA)
    a. of gastric contents
    gastric fluid a.
    meconium a.
    menstrual a.
    microsurgical epididymal
      sperm a. (MESA)
    needle a.
    a. pneumonia
    a. pneumonitis
    a. prophylaxis
    vacuum a.
aspirator
    Aspirette endocervical a.
    Cavitron USA NS100
      ultrasonic surgical a.
    ENDO-ASSIST sponge a.
    endocervical a.
    endometrial a.
    GynoSampler endometrial a.
    Sharplan USA ultrasonic
      surgical a.
    Vabra cervical a.
    vacuum a.
Aspirette endocervical aspirator
asplenia
    a. syndrome

assault
    sexual a.
assay
    a. accuracy
    Amplicor Chlamydia A.
    biologic a.
    CA-125 a.
    enzyme a.
    enzyme-linked
      immunosorbent a. (ELISA)
    estradiol a.
    hamster egg penetration a.
    hemizona a.
    hormone a.
    immunologic a.
    immunoradiometric a.
      (IRMA)
    IMx Estradial A.
    limulus amebocyte lysate a.
    Lyme enzyme-linked
      immunosorbent a.
    a. marker
    microhemagglutination a.
      (MHA)
    PCR a.
    PIVKA-II a.
    radioreceptor a.
    RAMP hCG a.
    receptor a.
    sandwich a.
    a. sensitivity
    serum a.
    a. specificity
    sperm penetration a.
    stem cell a.
    TDx-FLM A.
    TDxFLx A.
    thyroid-stimulating
      hormone a.
    tumor-cloning a.
    ViraType HPV DNA
      typing a.
assessment
    Dubowitz Neurological A.
    Erhardt Developmental
      Prehension A.
    gestational age a.
    high-risk pregnancy a.
    morphologic a.
    periodic patient a.
    psychometric a.
    Scanlon A.

TOVA ADD/ADHD a.
  ultrasound a.
Assessment of Preterm Infants Behavior (APIB)
assignment
  gender a.
  sex a.
assimilation pelvis
assisted
  a. breech delivery
  a. cephalic delivery
  a. conception
  a. medical procreation (AMP)
  a. reproduction
  a. reproductive technology (ART)
  a. zonal hatching (AZH)
association
  American Diabetes A. (ADA)
  a. constant
Association of Professors of Gynecology and Obstetrics (APGO)
assortative mating
AST
  acoustic stimulation test
astasia-abasia
Astech meter
asteroid bodies
asthenospermia
asthma
  bronchial a.
  maternal a.
  thymic a.
AsthmaHaler
AsthmaNefrin
asthmaticus
  status a.
astigmatism
Astler-Coller modification of Dukes classification
astomia
Astramorph PF
Astrand 30-beat stopwatch method
astrocytoma

AstroGlide personal lubricant
Astrup blood gas value
asymmetrical conjoined twins
asymmetric tonic neck reflex (ATNR)
asymmetrus
  janiceps a.
asymmetry
  a. of face
  facial a.
  nasolabial fold a.
asymptomatic
  a. bacteriuria
  a. infection
  a. infertility
  a. mild endometriosis
  a. myoma
  a. viral shedding
asynapsis
asynclitic
  a. position
  a. position of fetus
asynclitism
  anterior a.
  posterior a.
Atabrine
atactica
  heredopathia a.
Atarax
ataxia
  cerebellar a.
  Friedreich a.
  a. telangiectasia
ataxia-telangiectasia
  a.-t. syndrome
atelectasis
  congenital a.
  linear a.
  plate-like a.
  primary a.
  secondary a.
atelectatic
atelencephalia
atelia
ateliosis
ateliotic dwarfism
atelocardia

NOTES

atelocephaly-atelocheilia
atelocheiria
ateloglossia
atelognathia
atelomyelia
atelopodia
atelostomia
atenolol
a-thalassemia intermedia
atheosis
    congenital a.
atherosclerosis
atherosis
athetoid
athlete's foot
athletic amenorrhea
athyreotic cretinism
athyroid, athyroidism
athyrotic hypothyroidism
Ativan
ATL/ADR Ultramark 4/9 HDI
  ultrasound
atlantodidymus
ATN
    acute tubular necrosis
ATNR
    asymmetric tonic neck reflex
atomic
    a. absorption
      spectrophotometry
    a. milk
atonic
    a. seizure
atonic-astatic diplegia
atony
    uterine a.
atopic
    a. dermatitis
    a. erythroderma
atopy
atovaquone
ATP
    adenosine triphosphate
atraumatic forceps
atresia
    anal a.
    biliary a.
    choanal a.
    duodenal a.
    esophageal a.
    a. folliculi
    ileal a.
    jejunoileal a.

mitral a.
pulmonary artery a.
pyloric a.
tricuspid a.
vaginal a.
atretic
    a. cervix
    a. follicle
atretocormus
atretocystia
atretogastria
atria (*pl. of* atrium)
atrial
    a. bigeminy
    a. contraction
    a. fibrillation
    a. flutter
    a. natriuretic factor (ANF)
    a. natriuretic peptide
    a. septal defect (ASD)
    a. septostomy
    a. septostomy via balloon
    a. tachycardia
atrioventricular (AV)
    a. block
    a. conduction delay
    a. discordance
    a. node
    a. reciprocating tachycardia
    a. septal defect
    a. septum
    a. shunt
at-risk pregnancy
atrium, pl. atria
Atromid-S
atrophia bulborum hereditaria
atrophic
    a. change
    a. vaginitis
atrophicus
    lichen sclerosus et a. (LS)
atrophy
    Dejerine-Sottas a.
    dentatorubral-
      pallidoluysian a.
    endometrial a.
    Fazio-Londe a.
    infantile spinal muscular a.
    juvenile spinal muscular a.
    linear a.
    Parrot a. of newborn
    peroneal muscle a.
    postmenopausal a.

skin a.
traction a.
urogenital a.
vaginal a.
vulvar a.
Werdnig-Hoffmann
  muscular a.
atropine
attack
  transient ischemic a. (TIA)
attention
  a. deficit disorder (ADD)
  a. deficit hyperactivity
    disorder (ADHD)
attenuating tissue
Attenuvax
attitude
  fetal a.
  postpartum a.
attrition
  follicular a.
  sperm a.
Attwood staining method
atypia
  bowenoid a.
  koilocytic a.
  vulvar a.
atypical
  a. cell
  a. epithelium
  a. glandular cells of
    undetermined significance
  a. squamous cells of
    undetermined significance
    (ASCUS)
  a. vessel colposcopic pattern
[198]**Au**
  gold-198
Audio Doppler D920
audiogram
audiometer
  Pilot a.
audiometry
  behavioral a.
auditory
  a. brainstem response
    (ABR)

a. evoked potentials (AEP)
a. evoked response
Auerbach plexus
Aufricht nasal retractor
augmentation
  labor a.
  a. mammaplasty
  oxytocin a.
  Pitocin a.
  submucosal urethral a.
augmented breast
Augmentin
augnathus
aura
aural temperature
Aureomycin
aureus
  Staphylococcus a.
aurothioglucose
auscultation
  abdominal a.
  chest percussion and a.
  periodic a.
Australia antigen
autism
autistic
autoamputation
autoantibody
  thyroid a.
  typhoid a.
autoantigen
autochthonous tumor
autocrine
  a. communication
  a. motility factor (AMF)
autodilation
  Frank nonsurgical
    perineal a.
autoerotic asphyxia
autograft
autoimmune
  a. acquired hemolytic
    anemia
  a. disease
  a. factor
  a. hemolytic anemia (AIHA)
  a. mechanism

NOTES

autoimmune *(continued)*
    a. oophoritis
    a. thrombocytopenic purpura
autoimmunity
autoinoculation
autologous
    a. blood
    a. blood donation
    a. bone marrow reinfusion
    a. transfusion
autolysis
automated multiple analysis
automaticity
automatic walking
autonomic
    a. nervous system
    a. seizure
    a. walking reflex
autopolyploid
autoprothrombin I
autoradiography
Autoread
    A. centrifuge hematology
      system
autosite
autosomal
    a. chromosome disorder
    a. deletion
    a. dominant (AD)
    a. dominant disorder
    a. dominant inheritance
    a. dominant trait
    a. gene
    a. heredity
    a. monosomy
    a. recessive (AR)
    a. recessive disorder
    a. recessive inheritance
    a. recessive trait
    a. trisomy
autosome translocation
autotransfusion
Auvard speculum
AV
    atrioventricular
    AV malformation
    AV shunt
AV/AF
    anteverted and anteflexed
    AV/AF uterus
AVC suppository
Aventyl
average radiation dose

Avitene
avium-intracellulare
    Mycobacterium a.-i.
Aviva mammography system
AVL 9110 pH analyzer
Axenfeld syndrome
axes (*pl. of* axis)
axetil
    cefuroxime a.
axial resolution
axilla, pl. axillae
axillary
    a. adenopathy
    a. hematoma
    a. lymphadenopathy
    a. lymph node
    a. skin lesion
    a. tail
    a. tail of Spence
    a. temperature
    a. view
axis, pl. axes
    conjugate a.
    embryonic a.
    gonadal a.
    HPA a.
    hypothalamic-hypophyseal-
      ovarian-endometrial a.
    hypothalamic-pituitary a.
    hypothalamic-pituitary-
      gonadal a.
    pelvic a.
    a. of pelvis
    pituitary a.
    a. traction
axis-traction forceps
Axotal
Ayercillin
Aygestin
Ayr
    A. saline drops
    A. saline nasal mist
Ayre
    A. spatula
    A. spatula-Zelsmyr
    Cytobrush technique
AZ
    Aschheim-Zondek
Azactam
azasteroid
azatadine
azathioprine

AZH
    assisted zonal hatching
azidothymidine (AZT)
azithromycin
    a. dihydrate
azlocillin
Azmacort
azo
    a. dye
    A. Gantanol
    A. Gantrisin
Azo-Gamazole
azoospermia

Azorean disease
Azo-Standard
azotemia
    prerenal a.
Azovan Blue
AZT
    azidothymidine
Aztec
    A. ear
    A. idiocy
A.-Z. test
aztreonam
azygos artery

NOTES

β
- β chain
- β melaninogenicus

B
- B cell
- B chromosome
- B complex vitamins
- B lymphocyte

Babcock clamp
BABE OB ultrasound reporting system
babesiosis
Babinski
- B. reflex
- B. sign

Babinski-Fröhlich syndrome
Babkin reflex
Babson chart
Baby
- B. Doe regulations

baby
- blue b.
- blueberry muffin b.
- boarder b.
- bottle-fed b.
- breast-fed b.
- cocaine b.
- collodion b.
- crack b.
- giant b.
- jittery b.
- juice b.
- nipple-fed b.
- test-tube b.
- b. Tischler biopsy punch
- well-hydrated b.
- well-perfused b.

BABYbird
- B. II respirator
- B. II ventilator

Babyflex
- B. heated ventilation system
- B. ventilator

BAC
- blood alcohol concentration

bacampicillin
Bacarate
Baciguent
bacillary dysentery

Bacille
- B. bilié de Calmette-Guérin (BCG)
- B. bilié de Calmette-Guérin vaccine

bacillus, pl. bacilli
- b. Calmette-Guérin (BCG)
- b. Calmette-Guérin vaccine
- Döderlein b.
- Ducrey b.
- Gram-negative bacilli
- Gram-positive bacilli

bacitracin
backache
backcross
- b. mating

Backhaus clamp
back-up position
baclofen
Bacon-Babcock operation
bacteremia
- polymicrobial b.

bacteremic shock
bacteria (*pl. of* bacterium)
- Gram-negative b.
- Gram-positive b.

bacterial
- b. contamination
- b. count
- b. cystitis
- b. endocarditis
- b. enteritis
- b. growth
- b. infection
- b. pneumonia
- b. recovery
- b. toxin
- b. vaginosis (BV)

bacteriology
bacteriuria
- asymptomatic b.

Bacteroides
- B. capillosus
- B. corrodens
- B. distasonis
- B. fragilis
- B. ovatus
- B. thetaiotaomicron

bacteroidosis
Bactocill

Bactrim
Bact-T-Screen
Badenoch urethroplasty
Baden procedure
BAEP
    brainstem auditory evoked
      potentials
BAER
    brainstem auditory evoked
      responses
bag
    Ambu b.
    b.-and-mask ventilation
    Barnes b.
    Cardiff resuscitation b.
    Champetier de Ribes b.
    Hope resuscitation b.
    b. and mask
    Voorhees b.
    b. of waters (BOW)
bagged mask ventilation
bagging
Baggish hysteroscope
Bagshawe protocol
Bair Hugger patient warming
  system
baker leg
BAL
    blood alcohol level
balance
    acid-base b.
    electrolyte b.
    fetal acid-base b.
    sodium b.
    transcapillary fluid b.
balanced translocation
balanic hypospadias
balanitic hypospadias
balanitis
    b. circinata
    b. circumscripta
      plasmacellularis
    plasma cell b.
    b. of Zoon
Baldy operation
Baldy-Webster
    B.-W. procedure
    B.-W. uterine suspension
Balfour
    B. bladder blade
    B. retractor
ball
    Bichat fat b.

cauterizing b.
b. electrode
fungus b.
Ballantyne-Runge syndrome
Ballantyne-Smith syndrome
Ballard
    B. chart
    B. examination
    B. test
Ballentine clamp
Baller-Gerold syndrome
balloon
    atrial septostomy via b.
    b. catheter technique
    Rashkind b.
    b. septectomy
    b. septostomy
    Soft-Wand atraumatic tissue
      manipulator b.
    b. tuboplasty
    b. valvulotomy
ballottable
ballottement
    abdominal b.
    uterine b.
Balmex
Balminil
Baloser hysteroscope
Balthazar Scales of Adaptive
  Behavior
Baltic myoclonus
Bamberger fluid
Banana
    Kanana B.
banana sign
bananas, rice cereal, applesauce,
  and toast (BRAT)
band
    amniotic b.'s
    annular b.
    BB b.
    C b.
    chorioamniotic b.'s
    chromosome b.
    G b.
    hymenal b.
    b. keratopathy
    Ladd b.'s
    limbic b.'s
    MB b.
    MM b.
    oligoclonal b.'s
    Q b.

R b.
Silastic b.
Streeter b.'s
T b.
bandage
Kerlix gauze b.
Kling b.
b. scissors
Band-Aid operation
banding
centromeric b.
chromosomal b.
chromosome b.
Giemsa b.
b. pattern
pulmonary artery b.
quinacrine b.
reverse b.
Bandl
pathologic retraction ring of B.
B. ring
banjo-string adhesion
bank
sperm b.
banked breast milk
Banthine
Banti syndrome
bar
Denis Browne b.
Mercier b.
Barbita
barbiturate
b. poisoning
Bard
B. Biopty cut needle
B. Biopty gun
Bardet-Biedl syndrome
Bard-Parker blade
barium
b. enema
b. study
barium-impregnated plastic intrauterine device
Barkan infant lens
barking cough

Barlow
B. disease
B. hip dysplasia test
B. maneuver
B. syndrome
Barnes
B. bag
B. cerclage
B. curve
B. zone
baromacrometer
baroreceptor
baroreflex response
barotrauma
Barr body
barrel-shaped
b.-s. cervix
b.-s. lesion
barren
barrier
adhesion b.
b. contraception
b. contraceptive
B. gown
Interceed absorbable adhesion b.
B. laparoscopy drape
b. method
B. pack
placental b.
Sil-K OB b.
TC-7 adhesion b.
Barron pump
Bart
hemoglobin B.
B. hemoglobin
B. syndrome
Bartholin
B. abscess
B. cyst
B. cystectomy
B. duct
B. gland
B. gland carcinoma
bartholinitis
Bartholomew rule of fourths
Barton forceps

NOTES

Bartter syndrome
barymazia
basal
    b. artery
    b. body temperature (BBT)
    b. body temperature chart
    b. body thermometer
    b. cell carcinoma
    b. cell epithelioma
    b. cell nevus syndrome
    b. ganglion
    b. lamina
    b. plate
base
    b. deficit
    b. excess
    b. medication
    b. pair
baseline
    b. fetal heart rate
    b. tonus
    b. value
    b. variability of fetal heart
      rate
basement
    b. membrane
    b. membrane zone (BMZ)
bas-fond
basicaryoplastin
basichromatin
basilemma
Basis
    B. breast pump
    B. soap
basophilic leukemia
Bassen-Kornzweig
    B.-K. disease
    B.-K. syndrome
Basset radical vulvectomy
bastard
Bastiaanse-Chiricuta procedure
bat ear
bath
    belly b.
    B. respirator
    sitz b.
bathing trunk nevus
bathrocephaly
batrachian position
Batten-Mayou disease
battered
    b. child syndrome
    b. fetus syndrome

    b. wife syndrome
    b. woman
battering cycle
battery
    Vulpe Assessment B.
battledore placenta
Baudelocque
    B. diameter
    B. operation
    B. uterine circle
Baumberger forceps
Baum bumps
Bayer Timed-Release-Arthritic Pain
    Formula
bayesian hypothesis
Bayley-Pinneau table
Bayley Scale of Infant
    Development (BSID)
Baylor
    B. amniotic perforator
    B. amniotome
Bayne Pap Brush
bayonet leg
BB band
BBB syndrome
BBT
    basal body temperature
BCDDP
    Breast Cancer Detection
      Demonstration Project
BCG
    Bacille bilié de Calmette-Guérin
    bacillus Calmette-Guérin
      BCG vaccine
BCP
    birth control pill
beading
beads
    DEAE b.
beaked pelvis
BEAM
    brain electrical activity map
bean
    castor b.
Bear
    B. Cub infant ventilator
    B. Hugger warming blanket
    B. NUM-1 tidal volume
      monitor
    B. respirator
bearing down
bearing-down pain

beat
> escape b.'s
> b.'s per minute (bpm)

Beath pin
Beatson ovariotomy
beat-to-beat
> b.-t.-b. variability
> b.-t.-b. variability of fetal
> heart rate
> b.-t.-b. variation of fetal
> heart rate

Beau line
Because
> B. vaginal foam

Beccaria sign
Beck disease
Becker muscular dystrophy
Beckwith syndrome
Beckwith-Wiedemann syndrome
Béclard sign
beclomethasone
> b. diproprionate
> b. propionate

Beclovent
Beconase
bed
> Affinity b.
> arterial vascular b.
> bumper b.
> Ohio b.
> pulmonary vascular b.
> b. rest

Bednar aphthae
bedwetting
beef insulin
Beesix
Béguez César disease
Behavior
> Assessment of Preterm
> Infants B. (APIB)
> Balthazar Scales of
> Adaptive B.

behavioral
> b. audiometry
> b. genetics

Behçet syndrome

Bell
> B. palsy
> B. staging criteria

bell
> Gomco b.

belladonna
Bell-Buettner hysterectomy
Bellergal
belly
> b. bath
> b. bath therapy

Benadryl
Benahist
Bendectin
Bendopa
bendroflumethiazide
Benemid
benign
> b. breast disease
> b. cyst
> b. cystic ovarian teratoma
> b. familial chronic
> pemphigus
> b. familial neonatal
> convulsions (BFNC)
> b. familial neonatal seizure
> b. infantile familial
> convulsions (BIFC)
> b. lesion
> b. mass
> b. mesothelioma of genital
> tract
> b. nevus
> b. ovarian neoplasm
> b. papillomavirus infection
> b. tumor

Bennett
> B. PR-2 ventilator
> B. respirator
> B. small corpuscles

Benoject
Benson baby pylorus separator
Bentyl
benzathine
> b. benzylpenicillin
> b. penicillin G

NOTES

Benzedrine
benzocaine
benzodiazepine
benzoin
benzthiazide
benztropine mesylate
Benzylpenicillin
beractant
   b. surfactant
Berger
   B. paresthesia
   B. renal disease
beriberi
Berkeley
   B. suction machine
   B. Vacurette
Berkow formula for burns
Berkson-Gage calculation
Bernay uterine packer
Bernoulli trial
Besnier prurigo of pregnancy
Best disease
bestiality
beta
   b. chain
   b. error
   free b.
   b. interferon
   b. ray
   transforming growth
     factor b. (TGFβ)
beta-1 integrin
beta-2 integrin
beta-adrenergic, β-adrenergic agonist
   b.-a. agent
   b.-a. agonist
   b.-a. drug
beta$_2$-adrenergic agent
beta-blocker
beta carotene
Betachron E-R
Betadine
beta-endorphin, β-endorphin
beta-lactam
   b.-l. antibiotic
   b.-l. antimicrobial
beta-lactamase-resistant
  antistaphylococcal antibiotic
Betalin S
beta-lipotrophin
Betaloc
betamethasone
   b. valerate

Betapen-VK
beta-subunit
   human chorionic
     gonadotropin b.-s. (β-HCG)
betatron electron accelerator
Betaxin
bethanechol, bethanecol
   b. chloride
Bethesda
   B. classification system
   B. Pap smear classification
Betke-Kleihauer test
Betke stain
Betnelan
Beverly-Douglas lip-tongue
  adhesion technique
Bewon
Bexophene
bezoar
Bezold abscess
BFNC
   benign familial neonatal
   convulsions
bG
   Chemstrip b.
Biamine
bias
   detection b.
biatriatum
   cor triloculare b.
BICAP
   Bipolar Circumactive Probe
   BICAP cautery
   BICAP probe
bicarbonate
   sodium b.
bicarbonate-carbonic acid system
bicephalus
Bichat fat ball
bichloracetic acid
Bicillin
   B. L-A
Bicitra
BiCoag forceps
bicornuate, bicornate
   b. uterus
bicuspid aortic valve
bidet
bidirectional PDA
bidiscoidal placenta
Biederman sign
Bielschowsky-Jansky disease
Bielschowsky syndrome

Biemond syndrome
Bierer ovum forceps
BIFC
   benign infantile familial
   convulsions
bifid
   b. pelvis
   b. scrotum
   b. uterus
   b. uvula
bifida
   spina b.
Bifidobacterium
   B. adolescentis
   B. bifidum
   B. infantis
bifidum
   Bifidobacterium b.
   cranium b.
biforate uterus
bigeminal pregnancy
bigeminy
   atrial b.
Biglieri syndrome
biischial diameter
bilaminar blastoderm
BiLAP bipolar laparoscopic probe
bilateral
   b. acoustic
      neurofibromatosis
   b. ectopic pregnancy
   b. left-sidedness
   b. myocutaneous graft
   b. myringotomy tubes
      (BMT)
   b. ovarian neoplasm
   b. salpingo-oophorectomy
      (BSO)
   b. simultaneous tubal
      pregnancies
   b. uropathy
bile acid
bile-plug syndrome
bili
   b. lights
   b. mask

biliary
   b. atresia
   b. cirrhosis
   b. hypoplasia
Biliblanket phototherapy
bilirubin
   b. blanket
   b. encephalopathy
   b. infarct
bilirubinometry
bili-Timer
Bill
   B. maneuver
   B. traction handle forceps
Billings method
Billroth tumor forceps
biloba
   placenta b.
biloculare
   cor b.
Bilopaque
Biloptin
bimanual
   b. pelvic examination
   b. version
binary process
binder
   abdominal b.
   breast b.
   Dale abdominal b.
   obstetrical b.
   scultetus b.
binding
   breast b.
   fragment antigen b.
   protein b.
   b. protein
   b. site
binomial distribution
binovular twin
bioactive
   b. hormone
bioassay
BioBands bracelet
bioblast
Biobrane adhesive
Biobrane/HF dressing

NOTES

45

Biocept-5 pregnancy test
Biocept-G pregnancy test
biochemical study
biochemistry
biofeedback therapy
bioflavonoids
Biogel glove
Biojector
biologic
    b. assay
    b. response modifier (BRM)
biological sampling
Biomerica
biometric profile
biometry
    fetal b.
Biomydrin
biophysical
    b. profile (BPP)
    b. profile score
biopsy
    Allis-Abramson breast b.
    aspiration b.
    cervical cone b.
    chorionic villus b. (CVB)
    coin b.
    cone b.
    b. dating
    embryo b.
    endometrial b.
    excisional b.
    fine-needle aspiration b.
    hot b.
    Kevorkian punch b.
    Keyes punch b.
    kidney b.
    lymph node b.
    mirror image breast b.
    needle b.
    out-of-phase endometrial b.
    Pipelle b.
    b. probe
    punch b.
    renal b.
    stereotactic breast b.
    trophectoderm b.
    vulvar b.
Biopty cut needle
biosampler
    Accelon Combi cervical b.
BioStar strep A 1A test

biosynthesis
    prostaglandin b.
    steroid b.
biosynthetic defect
Bio-Tab
biotin
biotinidase
Biotirmone
biparental inheritance
biparietal diameter (BPD)
bipartita
    placenta b.
bipartite
    b. uterus
biperiden
biphenyl
    polychlorinated b.
biplane
    b. cineangiography
    b. intracavitary probe
    b. seriography
bipolar
    b. cautery
    B. Circumactive Probe
    (BICAP)
    b. electrocautery
    b. electrode
    b. laparoscopic forceps
    b. taxis
    b. version
bipotential
bipotentiality
bipronucleate
Birbeck granule
Bird
    B. Mark 8 respirator
    B. vacuum extractor
bird-beak jaw
bird-headed
    b.-h. dwarfism
    b.-h. dwarf of Seckel
    b.-h. dwarf syndrome
Birnberg bow
birth
    b. amputation
    b. asphyxia
    b. canal
    b. canal laceration
    b. care center
    b. certificate
    b. control
    b. control pill (BCP)
    date of b. (DOB)

b. defect
dry b.
b. fracture
gravida, para, multiple
  births, abortions, live b.'s
  (GPMAL)
home b.
b. injury
multiple b.'s
b. paralysis
premature b.
preterm b.
b. rate
b. trauma
twin b.
b. weight (BW)
year of b. (YOB)
birthing
  b. chair
  b. room
birthmark
bisacodyl
biscoumacetate
  ethyl b.
Bi-Set catheter
Bishop
  B. score
  B. score of cervical
    ripening
bishydroxycoumarin
Biswas Silastic vaginal pessary
bitartrate
  dihydrocodeine b.
bite
  stork b.
bitemporal diameter
bitterling test
bivalent chromosome
bivalve speculum
biviua
  Prevotella b.
Bixler hypertelorism
black
  b. jaundice
  b. line
  b. tongue
blackened speculum

Blackfan-Diamond
  B.-D. anemia
  B.-D. syndrome
bladder
  b. blade
  b. bubble
  b. catheter
  b. drill
  b. dysfunction
  b. flap
  b. function
  b. habits
  hypotonic b.
  b. laceration
  b. muscle stress test
  b. neck
  b. neck elevation test
  b. neck mobility
  b. neck obstruction
  b. neck stenosis
  b. neck suspension
  neurogenic b.
  b. outlet syndrome
  b. retractor
  b. retraining
  stammering b.
  b. tumor
  urinary b.
BladderScan BVI2500
blade
  Balfour bladder b.
  Bard-Parker b.
  bladder b.
  E-Mac laryngoscope b.
  ENDO-ASSIST retractable b.
  Gott-Balfour b.
  Gott-Harrington b.
  Gott-Seeram b.
  Miller b.
Blair-Brown procedure
Blalock-Hanlon
  B.-H. operation
  B.-H. procedure
Blalock-Taussig
  B.-T. operation
  B.-T. procedure
  B.-T. shunt

NOTES

blanching
    laser b.
Blane
    amniotic infection syndrome
      of B.
blanket
    Bear Hugger warming b.
    bilirubin b.
blastema
    metanephric b.
blastocele
blastocyst
    b. implantation
    b. splitting
blastocyte
blastoderm
    bilaminar b.
    embryonic b.
    trilaminar b.
blastodisk
blastogenesis
blastolysis
blastoma
    nodular renal b.
blastomere
    b. separation
blastomycosis
blastotomy
blastula
bleed
    herald b.
bleeding
    abnormal uterine b.
    anovulatory b.
    antepartum b.
    breakthrough b.
    b. diathesis
    dysfunctional uterine b.
      (DUB)
    estrogen breakthrough b.
    estrogen-progesterone
      withdrawal b.
    estrogen withdrawal b.
    intermenstrual b.
    pelvic b.
    postcoital b.
    postmenarchal b.
    postmenopausal b.
    preadolescent vaginal b.
    progesterone breakthrough b.
    progesterone withdrawal b.
    b. site
    b. site ligation

    third trimester b.
    b. time
    uterine b.
    vaginal b.
    withdrawal b.
Bleier clip
blennorrhagia
blennorrhagic
blennorrhea
blennorrheal
Blenoxane
bleomycin
    cisplatin, vinblastine, and b.
    b. sulfate
Bleph-10
blepharitis
blepharophimosis
blepharospasm
blighted ovum
blind loop syndrome
BLIS
    breast leakage inhibitor system
bloc
    en b.
Blocadren
Bloch-Sulzberger syndrome
block
    atrioventricular b.
    bundle branch b.
    Cerrobend b.'s
    complete atrioventricular b.
    complete heart b.
    congenital heart b.
    dorsal penile nerve b.
    extradural b.
    heart b.
    lead b.'s
    nerve b.
    paracervical b.
    pudendal b.
    saddle b.
    subarachnoid b.
    Wenckebach heart b.
blockade
    spinal b.
blockage
    neuromuscular b.
    proximal tubal b.
blocker
    adrenergic b.
    alpha-adrenergic b.
    calcium channel b.

cyproheptadine receptor b.
ganglionic b.
blocking factor
Bloedorn applicator
blood
    b. alcohol
    b. alcohol concentration
    (BAC)
    b. alcohol level (BAL)
    b. analysis
    autologous b.
    b. chimerism
    b. component
    b. component therapy
    cord b.
    b. count
    b. culture
    designated donor b.
    difference in partial
      pressures of oxygen in
      mixed alveolar gas and
      mixed arterial b.
      $((A-a)D_{O2})$
    donor-specific b.
    b. dyscrasia
    b. ethanol
    fetal b.
    b. flow $(\dot{Q})$
    b. gas determination
    b. gases
    b. glucose
    b. group
    b. group antibody
    b. group immunization
    b. grouping
    intervillous b.
    b. level
    b. loss
    maternal peripheral b.
    b. mole
    oxygenated fetal b.
    oxygen concentration in
      pulmonary capillary b.
      (C_cO_2)
    b. patch
    b. pigment stain
    b. pressure

    b. product
    b. sampling
    b. spot
    b. sugar
    b. sugar monitoring
    b. transfusion
    b. typing
    b. urea nitrogen (BUN)
    b. vessel formation
    b. volume
    whole b.
Bloodgood disease
blood-loss anemia
blood-type test
bloody show
Bloom syndrome
blot
    Eastern b.
    Southern b.
    Western b.
Blount disease
blow-by oxygen
blue
    Agent B.
    b. asphyxia
    Azovan B.
    b. baby
    b. cone monochromatism
    b. diaper syndrome
    b. dome cyst
    methylene b.
    b. navel
    b. nevus
    postpartum b.'s
    b. ring pessary
    b. rubber-bleb nevus
      syndrome
    b. sclera
    b. spot
    toluidine b.
    Urolene B.
blueberry
    b. muffin baby
    b. muffin nodule
    b. muffin spot
Blumberg sign
Blumer shelf

NOTES

blunt
    b. duct adenosis
    b. probe
    b. trauma
BMD
    bone mineral density
BMI
    body mass index
B-mode ultrasound
BMT
    bilateral myringotomy tubes
BMZ
    basement membrane zone
BNBAS
    Brazelton Neonatal Behavioral
    Assessment Scale
BOA
    born on arrival
board
    arm b.
    papoose b.
boarder baby
Boari flap
bobbing
    ocular b.
Bochdalek hernia
Bodian-Schwachman syndrome
body
    asteroid b.'s
    Barr b.
    Call-Exner b.
    dense b.
    Döhle b.
    Donovan b.
    b. fluid
    foreign b.
    Golgi b.'s
    b. habitus
    Heinz b.'s
    Howell-Jolly b.'s
    ketone b.'s
    Lostorfer b.'s
    b. mass index (BMI)
    b. mass index nomogram
    Nissl b.'s
    owl's eye inclusion b.'s
    perineal b.
    polar b.
    psammoma b.
    Schaumann b.'s
    Schiller-Duvall b.
    b. stalk
    b. surface area (BSA)

    b. surface area calculation
    b. temperature
    b. weight
    Winkler b.
boggy uterus
Bogros space
Bohn
    B. epithelial pearls
    B. equation
Bohr effect
Bolt sign
Bombay phenotype
Bonamine
bonding
    mother-infant b.
bone
    b. accretion
    b. age
    b. age standard of Greulich
      and Pyle
    b. attenuation coefficient
    brittle b.'s
    b. formation
    innominate b.
    ivory b.'s
    b. loss
    marble b.'s
    b. marrow
    b. marrow failure
    b. marrow puncture
    b. marrow toxicity
    b. marrow transplantation
    b. mass
    b. mineral content
    b. mineral density (BMD)
    b. resorption
    b. tumor
    b. turnover
    weightbearing b.
    wormian b.'s
Bonine
Bonnaire method
Bonnano catheter
Bonnevie-Ullrich syndrome
Bonney
    B. abdominal hysterectomy
    B. blue stress incontinence
      test
Bontril
bony metastasis
Bookwalter retractor
booster
    tetanus toxoid b.

BOR
brachial otorenal syndrome
brachio-otorenal syndrome
BOR syndrome
border
shaggy heart b.
borderline
b. diabetes
b. epithelial ovarian
carcinoma
b. epithelial ovarian
neoplasm
b. epithelial ovarian tumor
b. malignant epithelial
neoplasm
Bordetella
B. genus
B. *pertussis*
Borg Physical Activity Scale
boric acid
Börjeson-Forssman-Lehmann
syndrome
Börjeson syndrome
borne
Bornholm disease
born on arrival (BOA)
Borrelia burgdorferi
Borsieri sign
bosselated
bossing
frontal b.
botryoid
b. pseudosarcoma
b. sarcoma
bottle
b. feed
b. tooth decay
bottle-fed baby
botulism
Bouchut respiration
bougie
Holinger infant b.
Bouin solution
bound
b. estradiol
b. testosterone
Bourneville disease

Bourns
B. infant respirator
B. LS104-150 infant
ventilator
boutonierre incision
Bovie
B. cauterization
B. cautery
B. unit
bovina
facies b.
bovine
b. dermal collagen
b. face
b. facies
b. mucus penetration test
pegademase b.
b. surfactant
BOW
bag of waters
bow
Birnberg b.
bowel
b. function
b. habits
hyperechoic b.
b. obstruction
perforated b.
b. preparation
small b.
b. sounds
Bowen double-bladed scalpel
bowenoid
b. atypia
b. papulosis
bowing reflex
bowleg
Bowman layer
box
Hogness b.
negative-pressure b.
Bozeman
B. operation
B. position
B. uterine dressing forceps
Bozeman-Fritsch catheter

NOTES

BPD
   biparietal diameter
   bronchopulmonary dysplasia
bpm
   beats per minute
   breaths per minute
BPP
   biophysical profile
   BPP score
brace
   Cruiser hip abduction b.
   Rhino Triangle b.
bracelet
   BioBands b.
brachial
   b. birth palsy
   b. otorenal syndrome (BOR)
   b. plexus
   b. plexus injury
   b. plexus palsy
brachio-otorenal syndrome (BOR)
Brachmann-de Lange syndrome
Bracht maneuver
brachycephaly
brachydactyly
brachymelia
brachypelvic, brachypellic
brachysyndactyly
brachytherapy
   intracavitary b.
Bradley method of prepared
   childbirth
bradyarrhythmia
bradycardia
   apnea and b. (A & B)
   fetal b.
   sinus b.
bradycardiac
bradygenesis
bradykinin
bradylexia
bradymenorrhea
bradyspermatism
bradytocia
Bragg-Paul respirator
Bragg peak
brain
   b. damage
   b. death
   b. disorder
   b. electrical activity map
     (BEAM)
   fetal b.

   b. peptide
   b. sparing
brain-death syndrome
brainstem, brain stem
   b. auditory evoked
     potentials (BAEP)
   b. auditory evoked
     responses (BAER)
2-Br-alpha-ergocryptine mesylate
branched-chain amino acid
brancher deficiency
branchial
   b. anomaly
   b. arch
   b. arch syndrome
   b. cleft
   b. cleft remnant
   b. cyst
   b. ducts
   b. fistula
branchiomere
Brandt-Andrews maneuver
Brandt syndrome
brash
   weaning b.
BRAT
   bananas, rice cereal, applesauce,
     and toast
   BRAT diet
Braune canal
Braun episiotomy scissors
Braun-Schroeder single-tooth
   tenaculum
brawny edema
Braxton Hicks
   B. H. contraction
   B. H. sign
   B. H. version
Brazelton Neonatal Behavioral
   Assessment Scale (BNBAS)
breakage
   chromosome b.
breakdown
   endometrial b.
   germinal vesicle b. (GVBD)
   wound b.
breakthrough bleeding
breast
   accessory b.
   adolescent b.
   augmented b.
   b. binder
   b. binding

b. biopsy tissue
b. bud
caked b.
b. cancer
B. Cancer Detection Demonstration Project (BCDDP)
b. carcinoma
b. care
b. change
childhood b.
b. cyst
b. disease
b. embryology
engorged b.
b. engorgement
b. fed
b. feeding
fibrocystic b.
b. flush
irritable b.
keeled b.
lactating b.
b. leakage inhibitor system (BLIS)
b. malignancy
b. milk
b. milk jaundice
nonlactating b.
pigeon b.
b. prosthesis
b. pump
b. self-examination (BSE)
b. stimulation contraction test (BSCT)
breast-fed baby
breathing
    fetal b.
    intermittent positive pressure b. (IPPB)
    periodic b.
    synchronous b.
breaths per minute (bpm)
Brecht feeder
breech
    b. delivery
    b. extraction

b. head
b. presentation
Breeze
    B. respirator
    B. ventilator
Breezee Mist Aerosol
bregma
    b. of skull
bregmatodymia
bregmocardiac reflex
Breisky-Navratil retractor
Brenner tumor
Brentano syndrome
Breonesin
brephic
brephoplastic
brephotrophic
Brethaire
Brethine
bretylium tosylate
Bretylol
Breuer-Hering inflation reflex
Breus mole
Brevibloc
Brevicon
Brevital
Bricanyl
Bricker procedure
bridge
    membrane b.
Briggance Diagnostic Inventory of Early Development
brim
    pelvic b.
brine flotation method
bris
Brissaud
    B. dwarfism
    B. infantilism
brittle
    b. bones
    b. diabetes
BRM
    biologic response modifier
broad
    b. ligament

NOTES

broad *(continued)*
  b. ligament hernia
  b. ligament pregnancy
broad-based gait
broad-spectrum antibiotic therapy
Broca pouch
Brockenbrough technique
Broders index
bromide
  ammonium b.
  calcium b.
  distigmine b.
  ipratropium b.
  mepenzolate b.
  methantheline b.
  pancuronium b.
  Peacock b.
  potassium b.
  pyridostigmine b.
  sodium b.
  strontium b.
  triple b.
bromocriptine
  injectable b.
  b. mesylate
  b. resistance
  b. therapy
bromocriptine-resistant prolactinoma
bromodiphenhydramine
bromopheniramine maleate
Brompton cocktail
bromsulfophthalein (BSP)
bronchi (*pl. of* bronchus)
bronchial
  b. asthma
  b. bud
bronchiectasis
bronchiolectasia
bronchiolitis
bronchitis
  acute laryngotracheal b.
  arachidic b.
  chronic obstructive b.
  epidemic capillary b.
bronchobiliary
  b. fistula
bronchogenic
bronchogram
  air b.
bronchopneumonia
bronchopulmonary
  b. aspergillosis
  b. dysplasia (BPD)

  b. lavage
  b. malformation
bronchoscope
  Holinger infant b.
  Storz infant b.
bronchoscopy
bronchospasm
bronchus, pl. **bronchi**
  elastic recoil of the b.
Bronitin
  B. Mist
Bronkaid
  B. Mist
Bronkephrine
Bronkodyl
Bronkometer
Bronkosol
Bronson
  B. chewable prenatal
    vitamins
bronze
  b. baby syndrome
  b. diabetes
Brouha test
Broviac catheter
brow
  b. position
  b. presentation
brow-anterior position
brow-down
  b.-d. position
  b.-d. presentation
brown
  b. baby syndrome
  b. fat nonshivering
    thermogenesis
  B. uvula retractor
  B. vertical retraction
    syndrome
Brown-Adson tissue forceps
Brown-Symmers disease
Brown-Wickham technique
brow-posterior position
brow-up position
brucellosis
Brudzinski sign
Bruehl-Kjaer transvaginal
  ultrasound probe
Bruhat
  B. laser fimbrioplasty
  B. technique
Bruininks-Oseretsky Test of Motor
  Proficiency

bruit
    aortic b.
    carotid b.
    placental b.
Brunschwig operation
brush
    Bayne Pap B.
    cytology b.
    b. cytology
    endocervical sampling b.
    Stormby b.
Brushfield spot
Brushfield-Wyatt syndrome
Bruton
    B. agammaglobulinemia
    B. disease
Bryant traction
Bryce-Teacher ovum
BSA
    body surface area
B-scanner
    real-time B.-s.
    static B.-s.
BSCT
    breast stimulation contraction
    test
BSE
    breast self-examination
BSID
    Bayley Scale of Infant
    Development
BSO
    bilateral salpingo-oophorectomy
BSP
    bromsulfophthalein
bubble
    bladder b.
    b. boy disease
    gastric b.
    b. isolation unit
    b. isolette
    b. stability test
bubbly lung syndrome
bubo
    bullet b.
    chancroidal b.
    climatic b.

    primary b.
    tropical b.
    venereal b.
    virulent b.
bubonic
buccal fat pad
Bucladin-S Softabs
buclizine
bud
    breast b.
    bronchial b.
    end b.
    limb b.
    metanephric b.
    syncytial b.
    tail b.
    ureteric b.
Budd-Chiari syndrome
Buddha-like habitus
Buddha stance
budesonide
Budin rule
buffalo hump
Buffaprin
buffered aspirin
Bufferin
Buffinol
buffy coat component
Buhl disease
Buist method
bulb
    Rouget b.
    sinovaginal b.
    b. suctioning
    b. syringe
    vestibular b.
bulbar polioencephalitis
bulbitis
bulbocavernosus
    b. fat flap
    b. muscle
bulbocavernous reflex
bulbourethral
    b. gland
bulimia
    b. nervosa
bulky carcinoma

NOTES

bullet bubo
bullosa
    acantholysis b.
    epidermolysis b.
    varicella b.
bullous
    b. congenital ichthyosiform
      erythroderma
    b. dermatosis
    b. impetigo
    b. myringitis
    b. pemphigoid
bull's eye sonographic appearance
bumetanide
Bumex
Bumm curette
bump
    Baum b.'s
bumper bed
BUN
    blood urea nitrogen
bundle
    b. branch block
    b. of His
buphthalmia
bupivacaine
Burch
    B. colposuspension
    B. colpourethropexy
    B. modification
    B. procedure
burden
    genetic b.
    tumor b.
Burger triangle
Burkitt lymphoma
burn
    Berkow formula for b.'s
Burnet acquired immunity
burning vulva syndrome
Burow solution
burp
    wet b.
burping

bursa-dependent system
bursa of Fabricius
buserelin
busulfan, busulphan
butabarbital
Butalan
butalbital
Butalgen
Butanefrine
butaperazine
Butazolidin
Butazone
butoconazole
    b. nitrate
butorphanol
    b. tartrate
    b. tartrate nasal spray
butoxide pyrethrins and piperonyl
butriptyline hydrochloride
butterfly
    b. drain
    b. flap
    b. needle
    b. rash
button
    peritoneal b.
buttonhole incision
buttonholing
butyrophenone
BV
    bacterial vaginosis
BVI2500
    BladderScan B.
BW
    birth weight
Byers flap
Byler disease
bypass
    cardiopulmonary b.
    gastric b.
    jejunoileal b.
    b. surgery
Byrd-Drew method

C-500
　Optimox C.
c (*var. of* cal)
CA
　cancer antigen
　cardiac-apnea
　　CA 15-3 breast cancer
　　　marker
　　CA 72-4 cancer marker
　　CA 19-9 GI cancer marker
　　CA 195 GI cancer marker
　　CA 50 GI cancer marker
　　CA monitor
CA-125
　cancer antigen-125
　　CA-125 antigen
　　CA-125 assay
　　CA-125 endometrial cancer
　　　marker
Ca
　calcium
Cabot
　　C. cannula
　　C. trocar
cachectic infantilism
cachectin
cachexia
　cancer c.
cacogenesis
cacomelia
CAF
　cell adhesion factor
　cyclophosphamide, doxorubicin,
　　and 5-fluorouracil
café au lait spot
caffeine
　c. therapy
Caffey
　　C. disease
　　C. syndrome
Caffey-Kenny disease
Caffey-Silverman syndrome
Caffey-Smyth-Roske syndrome.
CAH
　congenital adrenal hyperplasia
cake
　omental c.
caked breast
cal, c
　calorie
Calan

calcaneovalgus
　talipes c.
calcaneovarus
　talipes c.
calcaneus
　talipes c.
Cal Carb-HD
Calci-Chew
Calciday-667
calcifediol
Calciferol
calcificans
　chondrodystrophia fetalis c.
calcification
　arterial c.
　coarse c.
　dystrophic c.
　granulomatous c.
　malignant c.
　popcorn-like c.
　skin c.
　sutural c.
　vascular c.
calcified fetus
Calcimar
Calci-Mix
calcinosis
　c. cutis, Raynaud
　　phenomenon, sclerodactyly,
　　telangiectasia (CRST)
　c. cutis, Raynaud
　　phenomenon, esophageal
　　motility disorders,
　　sclerodactyly, telangiectasia
　　(CREST)
calciotropic
Calciparine
calcitonin
　c.-salmon
calcitriol
calcitropic hormone
calcium (Ca)
　c. absorption
　c. acetate
　c. agonist
　c. antagonist
　c. bromide
　c. carbonate
　c. channel blocker
　c. citrate

calcium *(continued)*
    c. cyclamate
    docusate c.
    c. glubionate
    c. gluconate
    c. heparin
    c. ion
    ionized c. (iCa)
    c. pantothenate
    c. polycarbophil
    c. supplement
calculation
    Berkson-Gage c.
    body surface area c.
calculus, pl. calculi
    mammary c.
    renal calculi
    urate c.
    urinary c.
    uterine c.
Calderol
Caldwell-Moloy classification
calf compression unit
caliectasis
californium
    c.-252 (^{252}Cf)
calipers
    Harpenden c.
    Tenzel c.
cal/kg/day
    calories per kilogram per day
Calkins sign
Call-Exner body
callosal agenesis
Calmette-Guérin
    Bacille bilié de C.-G.
      (BCG)
    bacillus C.-G. (BCG)
calmodulin
calorie (cal, c)
    c.'s per kilogram per day
      (cal/kg/day)
    c.'s per ounce (cal/oz)
20-calorie formula
cal/oz
    calories per ounce
Cal-Plus
Caltrate 600
Caltrate, Jr.
Calvé-Legg-Perthes syndrome
Calymmatobacterium granulomatis
CAM
    cell adhesion molecule

child-adult mist
chorioallantoic membrane
cystic adenomatous
  malformation
  CAM tent
Cameco syringe pistol aspiration
  device
camera
    ETV8 CCD ColorMicro
      video c.
Camey ileocystoplasty
cAMP
    cyclic adenosine monophosphate
Camper fascia
camphor
camphorated oil
camptodactyly, campylodactyly
camptomelia
camptomelic
    c. dysplasia
    c. syndrome
campylodactyly *(var. of*
  camptodactyly)
camsylate
    trimethaphan c.
Camurati-Englemann syndrome
canal
    Alcock c.
    anal c.
    birth c.
    Braune c.
    cervical c.
    endocervical c.
    inguinal c.
    Kovalevsky c.
    Lambert c.'s, c.'s of Lambert
    neurenteric c.
    c. of Nuck, Nuck c.
    parturient c.
    Steiner c.'s
    uterovaginal c.
    vesicourethral c.
canalicular period
canaliculus
Canavan disease
cancer
    c. antigen (CA)
    c. antigen-125 test
    breast c.
    c. cachexia
    cervical c.
    cervical stump c.
    c. chemotherapy

clear cell vaginal c.
colorectal c.
C. Committee of College of
American Pathologists
endometrial c.
epithelial c.
gynecologic c.
intraepithelial endometrial c.
invasive c.
invasive cervical c.
lung c.
microinvasive cervical c.
c. nests
occult c.
ovarian c.
rectal c.
c. and steroid hormone
(CASH)
C. and Steroid Hormone
study
testicular c.
c. therapy
thyroid c.
vaginal c.
cancer antigen-125 (CA-125)
candicidin
Candida
C. albicans
C. glabrata
C. tropicalis
candidal
c. diaper dermatitis
c. vulvovaginitis
candidiasis
vaginal c.
vulvovaginal c.
candidosis
intertriginous c.
mucocutaneous c.
candle
cesium c.
urethral c.
candy-cane stirrups
Canesten
canker
cannabis
cannulate

cannulation
cantharides
cantharidin
canthomeatal line
Cantil
Cantor tube
Cantrell syndrome
CAP
cyclophosphamide, doxorubicin,
cisplatin
cap
acrosomal c.
cervical c.
cradle c.
Dutch c.
Oves Cervical C.
ProtectaCap c.
capacitation
sperm c.
capacity
alveolar-arterial oxygen
diffusing c.
corticosteroid-binding
globulin-binding c.
(CBG- BC)
cystometric c.
fetal blood oxygen-
carrying c.
functional residual c. (FRC)
iron-binding c. (IBC)
lung c.
c. of lung (CL)
maximum breathing c.
oxygen-diffusing c.
plasma iron-binding c.
pulmonary diffusing c.
total iron-binding c. (TIBC)
total lung c. (TLC)
urinary concentrating c.
vital c.
Capasee diagnostic ultrasound
system
CAPD
continuous ambulatory
peritoneal dialysis
capillary
c. blood gas (CBG)

NOTES

capillary *(continued)*
 c. blood sampling
 c. erection
 c. refill time
capillosus
 Bacteroides c.
capita *(pl. of* caput)
capitis
 pediculosis c.
 tinea c.
Capoten
capped uterus
caproate
 hydroxyprogesterone c.
 17-hydroxyprogesterone c.
 17α-hydroxyprogesterone c.
capsularis
capsule
 Crosby-Kugler pediatric c.
 Heyman c.'s
 Uro-Mag c.'s
 Virilon c.
captopril
capture
 ovum c.
caput, pl. **capita**
 c. medusae
 c. quadratum
 c. succedaneum
carbachol
carbamazepine
Carbamide
carbarsone
carbazole
carbenicillin
carbetocin
Carb-HD
 Cal C.-H.
carbimazole
carbinoxamine maleate
carbogen
carbohydrate
 c. homeostasis
 c. intolerance
 c. metabolism
 c. tolerance
Carbolith
carbon
 arterial c. dioxide pressure
  (tension) ($PaCO_2$)
 c. dioxide (CO_2)
 c. dioxide laser

 c. dioxide tension
 c. monoxide poisoning
carbonate
 calcium c.
carbonic acid
carboplatin
carboprost tromethamine
carboxamide
 dimethyl-triazeno-
  imidazole c. (DTIC)
carboxyl terminal peptide (CTP)
carbuncle
Carcassone perineal ligament
carcinoembryonic
 c. antigen (CEA)
 c. antigen-125 (CEA-125)
carcinogen
 chemical c.
carcinogenesis
carcinoid
 nonappendiceal c.
 c. syndrome
 c. tumor
carcinoma, pl. **carcinomas,**
 carcinomata
 adenoid cystic c.
 adenosquamous c.
 advanced c.
 anaplastic c.
 androgen-dependent c.
 c. antigen
 Bartholin gland c.
 basal cell c.
 borderline epithelial
  ovarian c.
 breast c.
 bulky c.
 cecal c.
 cervical c.
 c. of cervix
 clear cell endometrial c.
 colloid c.
 colon c.
 contralateral synchronous c.
 ductal c.
 embryonal c.
 endometrial c.
 endometrioid c.
 epithelial ovarian c.
 FAB staging of c.
 fallopian tube c.
 focal lobular c.
 glassy cell c.

gynecological c.
hepatocellular c.
infiltrating c.
infiltrating small-cell
  lobular c.
inflammatory c.
intracystic papillary c.
intraductal c.
intraductal papillary c.
invasive c.
juvenile c.
lobular c.
lung c.
medullary c.
mesometanephric c.
mesonephric c.
metaplastic c.
metastatic c.
microinvasive c.
mucinous c.
multicentric c.
oat cell c.
ovarian c.
ovarian small-cell c.
papillary c.
papillary endometrial c.
papillary serous cervical c.
preclinical c.
recurrent c.
renal cell c.
scirrhous c.
secretory c.
serous c.
signet ring cell c.
c. in situ (CIS)
small cell c.
squamous cell c.
tubular c.
uterine papillary serous c.
vaginal c.
verrucous c.
vulvar c.
vulvovaginal c.
well-circumscribed c.
Wolfe classification of
  breast c.

wolffian duct c.
yolk sac c.
carcinoma in situ (CIS)
carcinosarcoma
  uterine c.
card
  Guthrie c.
  Sono-Gram fetal ultrasound
    image c.
cardiac
  c. anomaly
  c. arrest
  c. arrhythmia
  c. catheterization
  c. dysrhythmia
  c. failure
  c. flow
  c. function
  c. glycoside
  c. massage
  c. output
  c. tamponade
cardiac-apnea (CA)
  c.-a. monitor
cardiac-limb syndrome
Cardiff resuscitation bag
Cardilate
cardinal
  c. ligament
  c. movements
  c. points
cardinal-uterosacral ligament
cardiogenic shock
cardiomyopathy
  peripartum c.
  postpartum c.
cardioplegia
  cold potassium c.
cardioprotective effect
cardiopulmonary
  c. bypass
  c. collapse
  c. resuscitation (CPR)
Cardioquin
cardiorespiratory function
cardiorespirogram (CR-gram)
cardiospasm

NOTES

cardiotachometer
cardiothymic shadow
cardiotocogram
    terminal c.
cardiotocograph
cardiotocography
    intrapartum c.
cardiovascular (CV)
    c. complication
    c. effect
    c. system
carditis
Care-24
    Similac Special C.
care
    ambulatory c.
    antepartum c.
    breast c.
    followup c.
    Kangaroo C.
    obstetrical c.
    postoperative c.
    postpartum c.
    preconception c.
    prenatal c.
    prepregnancy c.
caries
    dental c.
carina, pl. carinae
carinatum
    pectus c.
carmine
    indigo c.
Carmol
Carnation Follow-Up
carneous
    c. degeneration
    c. mole
carnitine
    c. deficiency
    c. transferase enzyme
      disorder
Caroli disease
carotid bruit
carotin
Carpenter syndrome
carphenazine maleate
carp mouth
carrier
    embryo c.
    ENDO-ASSIST endoscopic
      ligature c.
    fragile X c.

    heterozygous c.
    latent c.
    Miya hook ligature c.
    c. protein
    Raz double-prong ligature c.
    translocation c.
Cart
    Sensorimedics Horizon
      Metabolic C.
cartilage
    fetal c.
Cartwright blood group
caruncle
    amnionic c.
    myrtiform c.
    urethral c.
caruncula, pl. carunculae
    c. hymenalis, pl. carunculae
      hymenales
    c. myrtiformis,
      pl. carunculae myrtiformes
Carus
    C. circle
    C. curve
casanthranol
cascara sagrada
case
    index c.
casein hydrolysate
caseosa
    vernix c.
caseous
CASH
    cancer and steroid hormone
    classic abdominal Semm
      hysterectomy
    CASH study
Casodex
Casser fontanel
casserian
    c. fontanel
cast
    decidual c.
    hyaline c.
    uterine c.
Castaneda procedure
casting
    Cerrobend c.'s
castor bean
CAT
    computed axial tomography
catadidymus
Cataflam

catagen phase
catamenia
catamenial
catamenogenic
cataplexy
Catapres
cataract
    cerulean c.
    infantile c.
catarrhal
    c. jaundice
cat cry
cat-cry syndrome
catecholamine
    endogenous c.'s
catechol estrogen
cat-eye syndrome
catgut suture
cathartic
    saline c.
cathepsin
    c. D
catheter
    Acrad HS c.
    Argyle arterial c.
    Bi-Set c.
    bladder c.
    Bonnano c.
    Bozeman-Fritsch c.
    Broviac c.
    central venous c. (CVC)
    central venous pressure c.
    coudé c.
    Cystocath c.
    Davis bladder c.
    double-balloon c.
    Drew-Smythe c.
    Ehrlich c.
    femoral arterial c.
    Foley c.
    French Gesco c.
    Gesco c.
    hystersalpingography c.
    intrauterine pressure c.
      (IUPC)
    KDF-2.3 intrauterine c.
    Labotect c.

LeRoy ventricular c.
Malecot c.
Mentor c.
Millar microtransducer
    urethral c.
percutaneous central
    venous c. (PCVC)
percutaneous nephrostomy c.
peripherally-inserted
    central c. (PICC)
peritoneal c.
Pezzer c.
Quinton dual-lumen c.
radial arterial c.
Raimondi c.
c. specimen
Stamey c.
suction c.
suprapubic c.
Swan-Ganz c.
Tenckhoff c.
c. toes
transurethral c.
umbilical artery c. (UAC)
umbilical vein c. (UVC)
Vabra c.
venous c.
whistle-tip c.
c.-within-a-catheter
Word-Bartholin gland c.
Word bladder c.
catheterization
    cardiac c.
    femoral artery c.
    pulmonary artery c.
    transvaginal tubal c.
    umbilical artery c.
    umbilical vein c.
    urinary c.
cat-scratch
    c.-s. disease
    c.-s. fever
Cattell Infant Intelligence Scale
caudal
    c. analgesia
    c. anesthesia
    c. duplication

NOTES

caudal *(continued)*
    c. dysplasia syndrome
    c. regression syndrome
      (CRS)
caul
causal
    c. embryology
    c. independence
cauterization
    Bovie c.
cauterizing ball
cautery
    BICAP c.
    bipolar c.
    Bovie c.
    c. conization
    Endoclip c.
    laparoscopic c.
    monopolar c.
    ovarian c.
    Oxycel c.
cava (*pl. of* cavum)
    inferior vena c.
    superior vena c.
    vena c.
cavernous
    c. hemangioma
    c. lymphangioma
    c. plexus
    c. sinus thrombosis
CAVH
    continuous arteriovenous
    hemofiltration
Cavitron USA NS100 ultrasonic
surgical aspirator
cavity
    abdominal c.
    amniotic c.
    exocelomic c.
    oral c.
    pelvic c.
    peritoneal c.
    thoracic c.
    uterine c.
cavovalgus
    talipes c.
cavum, pl. cava
cavus
    pes c.
    talipes c.
C band
CBCL
    Child Behavior Checklist

CBG
    capillary blood gas
    cord blood gas
    corticosteroid-binding globulin
CBG-BC
    corticosteroid-binding globulin-
    binding capacity
cc
    cubic centimeters
CCA
    congenital contractural
    arachnodactyly
CCAM
    congenital cystic adenomatoid
    malformation
CCD Spirette
CCHD
    cyanotic congenital heart disease
cc/hr
    cubic centimeters per hour
cc/kg/d
    cubic centimeters per kilogram
    per day
CcO_2
    oxygen concentration in
    pulmonary capillary blood
CCSG
    Children's Cancer Study Group
CCUP
    colpocystourethropexy
CDAP
    continuous distending airway
    pressure
CDC
    Centers for Disease Control
CD_8 cell
CD_4 cell
CDE blood group system
CDH
    congenital dislocated hip
CDI
    Children's Depression Inventory
CDIS
    continuous distention irrigation
    system
cDNA
    complementary DNA
CEA
    carcinoembryonic antigen
CEA-125
    carcinoembryonic antigen-125
ceasmic
cebocephalus

cebocephaly
cecal carcinoma
Ceclor
cecocolic intussusception
Cecon
Cedilanid
    C.-D
Cedocard-SR
cefaclor
cefadroxil
Cefadyl
cefamandole
cefazolin
    c. sodium
Cefixime
Cefizox
Cefobid
cefonicid
cefoperazone
    c. sodium
ceforanide
Cefotan
cefotaxime
    c. sodium
cefotetan
    c. disodium
cefoxitin sodium
cefpodoxime
    c. proxetil
cefprozil
ceftazidime
Ceftin
ceftizoxime
ceftriaxone
    c. sodium
cefuroxime
    c. axetil
celery stalking
Celestone
celiac
    c. disease
    c. infantilism
    c. sprue
celibacy
celibate
celiohysterectomy
celiohysterotomy

celiomyomectomy
celiomyomotomy
celioparacentesis
celiosalpingectomy
celiosalpingotomy
celiotomy
    vaginal c.
cell
    c. adhesion factor (CAF)
    c. adhesion molecule (CAM)
    amniogenic c.'s
    antigen-sensitive c.
    atypical c.
    B c.
    c. block analysis
    CD_4 c.
    CD_8 c.
    c. collector
    committed c.
    corona radiata c.
    c. culture
    cumulus c.
    c. cycle
    c. cycling in chemotherapy
    cytotoxic c.
    daughter c.
    decidual c.
    c. determination
    diploid c.
    dome c.
    double c.
    dysplastic c.
    effector c.
    egg c.
    endodermal c.'s
    endothelial c.
    extragonadal germ c.
    fetal c.
    fetouterine c.
    frozen red c.'s
    c. generation time
    germ c.
    glandular c.'s
    granulosa c.
    granulosa lutein c.
    c. growth inhibitor
    haploid c.

NOTES

cell *(continued)*
    HeLa c.'s
    helper T c.
    hematopoietic stem c.
      (HSC)
    hobnail c.
    Hofbauer c.
    human endothelial c. (HEC)
    immunocompetent c.
    c. interaction gene
    interstitial c.
    K c.
    c. kill
    killer c.'s
    c. kinetics
    koilocytotic c.
    Langhans c.'s
    Leydig c.'s
    lipid c.
    luteal c.
    lutein c.
    lymphoblastoid c.
    lymphoid c.
    lymphokine-activated
      killer c. (LAK)
    maturation of c.'s
    memory c.
    mutant c.
    myoepithelial c.
    natural killer c.'s (NK cells)
    osteoblast-like c.
    owl's eye c.'s
    packed c.'s
    packed red blood c.'s
    peripheral blood
      mononuclear c. (PBMC)
    pituitary c.
    placental giant c.
    pregnancy c.
    pregranulosa c.'s
    primary embryonic c.
    primordial germ c.
    Purkinje c.'s
    Raji c.
    red blood c.
    Sertoli c.
    Sertoli-Leydig c.'s
    sex c.
    sickle c.
    silver c.
    somatic c.
    somatic c.'s
    squamous c.
    steroid c.
    stromal c.
    suppressor c.
    suppressor T c.
    c. surface antigen
    T c.
    target c.
    theca c.
    thecal/interstitial c.
    theca lutein c.
    totipotent c.
    totipotential c.
    trophoblastic c.
    tuboendometrial c.
    Vero c.
    Vignal c.'s
    white blood c.
    WI-38 c.'s
    yolk c.'s
cell-extracellular matrix adhesion
cell-mediated immunity (CMI)
cellular
    c. cytotoxic mechanism
    c. division
    c. immunity
    c. migration
cellulicidal
cellulitic phlegmasia
cellulitis
    pelvic c.
Cell-VU disposable semen analysis
   chamber
Celontin
celosomia
Cemill
cenadelphus
Cenafed
Cena-K
center
    birth care c.
    C.'s for Disease Control
      (CDC)
    epiphyseal ossification c.
    Huntington Reproduction C.
    lower limb ossification c.
    Poison Control C. (PCC)
    X inactivation c. (XIC)
centigray (cGy)
centimeter
    cubic c.'s (cc)
Centocor CA 125
   radioimmunoassay kit

central
- c. axis depth dose
- c. defect
- c. hyperalimentation
- c. jaundice
- c. line
- c. nervous system (CNS)
- c. nervous system differentiation
- c. nervous system disease
- c. nervous system tumor
- c. placenta previa
- c. type neurofibromatosis
- c. venous catheter (CVC)
- c. venous line (CVL)
- c. venous pressure (CVP)
- c. venous pressure catheter
- c. venous pressure line

centralis
- placenta previa c.

central Recklinghausen disease type 2
centrifuge
centromere
centromeric banding
Century urodynamics chair
Ceo-Two
cephalexin
cephalhematoma
- c. deformans

cephalhydrocele
cephalic
- c. cry
- c. forceps
- c. pole
- c. presentation
- c. replacement
- c. version

cephalization
cephalocele
cephalocentesis
cephalodactyly
- Vogt c.

cephalodiprosopus
cephalohematoma
cephalomelus

cephalometry
- ultrasonic c.

cephalonia
cephalopagus
cephalopelvic
- c. disproportion (CPD)

cephalopelvimetry
cephalosporin
cephalothin
- c. sodium

cephalothoracopagus
cephalotome
cephalotomy
cephalotribe
cephapirin
cephradine
Cephulac
Ceporex
Ceptaz
cercaria, pl. cercariae
- schistosomal cercariae

cerclage
- Barnes c.
- cervical c.
- Mann isthmic c.
- McDonald cervical c.
- Shirodkar cervical c.
- transabdominal cervicoisthmic c.

cerebellar
- c. ataxia
- c. degeneration

cerebral
- c. angioma
- c. blood flow
- c. dysfunction
- c. edema
- c. embolism
- c. gigantism
- c. infarction
- c. leukodystrophy
- c. palsy (CP)
- c. palsy antecedent
- c. thrombosis

cerebrale
- cranium c.

cerebral-placental ratio

NOTES

cerebri
    pseudotumor c.
cerebroatrophic hyperammonemia
cerebrocostomandibular syndrome
cerebrohepatorenal syndrome
cerebromacular degeneration
cerebrospinal
    c. fluid (CSF)
cerebrovascular
    c. accident (CVA)
    c. disease
Cerespan
Cerrobend
    C. blocks
    C. castings
certificate
    birth c.
Certified
    C. Nurse-Midwife (CNM)
    C. Registered Nurse
        Anesthetist (CRNA)
Cerubidine
cerulean cataract
ceruloplasmin
cerumen
Cervex-Brush
    C.-B. cervical cell sampler
cervical
    c. abnormality
    c. adenitis
    c. adenopathy
    c. amputation
    c. anomaly
    c. artery
    c. canal
    c. cancer
    c. cannula
    c. cap
    c. carcinoma
    c. carcinoma stimulation
    c. cerclage
    c. clamp
    c. clear cell adenocarcinoma
    c. cockscomb
    c. combing
    c. condyloma
    c. cone biopsy
    c. conization
    c. culture
    c. cytology
    c. dilation
    c. dysplasia
    c. dystocia

    c. ectropion
    c. effacement
    c. epithelial neoplasia
    c. epithelium
    c. erosion
    c. eversion
    c. factor
    c. GIFT
    c. incision
    c. incompetence (CI)
    c. infection
    c. insemination
    c. intraepithelial neoplasia
      (CIN)
    c. isthmus
    c. laceration
    c. leiomyoma
    c. lesion
    c. motion tenderness (CMT)
    c. mucorrhea
    c. mucus
    c. myoma
    c. neoplasia
    c. os
    c. polyp
    c. pregnancy
    c. priming
    c. prolapse
    c. ripening
    c. sarcoma
    c. score
    c. smear
    c. stenosis
    c. stroma
    c. stump cancer
    c. stump tumor
    c. tenaculum
    c. tissue impedance range
    c. transformation zone
    c. zone
cervicectomy
cervices (*pl. of* cervix)
cervicitis
    chlamydial c.
    gonorrheal c.
    mucopurulent c.
    nongonococcal c.
cervicography
cervicoplasty
cervicotomy
cervicovaginal
    c. fistula

c. infection
c. ridge
cervigram
Cervilaxin
Cerviprost
C. gel
cervix, pl. **cervices**
atretic c.
barrel-shaped c.
carcinoma of c.
collared c.
cone biopsy of c.
conization of c.
dilation of c.
effacement of c.
fish-mouth c.
incompetent c.
international classification of cancer of c.
malignant tumor of c.
multiple c.
strawberry c.
cesarean
c. delivery
c. hysterectomy
low transverse c. (LTC)
c. operation
c. section (C-section)
vaginal birth after c.
cesarean section (C-section)
extraperitoneal c. s.
Latzko c. s.
low cervical c. s.
transperitoneal c. s.
cesium
c.-137 (^{137}Cs)
c. applicator
c. candle
c. cylinder
c. implant
c. irradiation
c. source
cesium-137 level
cessation
Cetamide
Cetane

Cetus trial
Cevalin
Cevi-Bid
Ce-Vi-Sol
Cevita
CF
cystic fibrosis
^{252}**Cf**
californium-252
c-fms proto-oncogene
CFUC
colony-forming unit in culture
CG
chorionic gonadotropin
cGy
centigray
Chadwick sign
Chagas disease
chain
β c., beta chain
c. cystourethrography
heavy c.
K c.
kappa c.
light c.
chair
birthing c.
Century urodynamics c.
Midmark 413 power female procedure c.
chalasia
chalazion
challenge
intravenous glucose c.
progestational c.
chamber
Cell-VU disposable semen analysis c.
face c.
hyperbaric c.
Makler reusable semen analysis c.
Chamberlen forceps
Champetier de Ribes bag
chancre
hunterian c.

NOTES

chancroid
chancroidal bubo
chandelier sign
change
    atrophic c.
    breast c.
    concomitant c.
    fibrocystic breast c.
    focal c.
    glomerular c.
    harlequin color c.
    hematological c.
    hormone-stimulated
      endometrial c.
    immunohistochemical c.
    immunologic c.
    libidinal c.
    c. of life
    ovarian cycle c.
    polyneuropathy,
      organomegaly,
      endocrinopathy, M protein,
      skin c.'s (POEMS)
    retinal c.
    Rias-Stella c.
    sensorineural c.
    visual c.
channel
    surface epithelium
      vascular c.
    vascular c.
Chapple syndrome
character
    classifiable c.
    denumerable c.
    discrete c.
    Y-linked c.
characteristic
    epidemiological c.
    morphological c.
    secondary sex c.
characterization
    immunohistochemical
      stromal leukocyte c.
Charcot-Marie-Tooth (CMT)
    C.-M.-T. disease
Charcot-Marie-Tooth-Hoffmann
  syndrome
CHARGE
    coloboma, heart anomaly,
      choanal atresia, retardation,
      and genital and ear anomalies
      CHARGE syndrome

Charlson score
chart
    Babson c.
    Ballard c.
    basal body temperature c.
    Genentech growth c.
    Liley three-zone c.
    pedigree c.
    POMARD anthropomorphic
      measurement reference c.
    Ross growth c.
    Walker c.
Chassar
    C. Moir-Sims procedure
    C. Moir sling procedure
chaste
chastity
chat
    cri du c.
CHD
    congenital hip dislocation
Cheadle disease
Checklist
    Child Behavior C. (CBCL)
Chédiak-Higashi
    C.-H. anomaly
    C.-H. syndrome
cheek
    chipmunk c.'s
cheese-wiring
cheesy discharge
cheilognathopalatoschisis
cheilognathoprosoposchisis
cheilognathoschisis
cheilognathouranoschisis
cheiloschisis
chemical
    c. carcinogen
    c. diabetes
    c. pneumonia
    c. pneumonitis
    c. pregnancy
    c. sampling
chemiluminescence
chemiluminescent immunoassay
  (CIA)
chemoimmunotherapy
chemoprophylaxis
chemoreceptor
chemotactic factor
chemotaxis
chemotherapeutic agent

chemotherapy
adjuvant c.
alkylating c.
cancer c.
cell cycling in c.
combination c.
high-dose c.
intraperitoneal c.
intraperitoneal cisplatin c.
Karnofsky performance
status of c.
metabolism in
intraperitoneal c.
c. phase trial
postoperative c.
prophylactic c.
chemstrip
C. bG
Micral c.
C. 4 The OB
C. 10 with SG
Cherney incision
cherubism
cherub sign
chest
c. examination
funnel c.
keel c.
c. percussion and
auscultation
c. physical therapy
c. radiography
c. x-ray (CXR)
Cheyne-Stokes respiration
Chiari anomaly
Chiari-Arnold syndrome
Chiari-Frommel syndrome
chiasma, pl. **chiasmata**
c. formation
Chiba needle
Chicago classification
Chicco breast pump
chickenpox
c. pneumonia
Chid breast pump
Chilaiditi syndrome

CHILD
congenital hemidysplasia with
icthyosiform erythroderma and
limb defects
CHILD syndrome
child
c. abuse
C. Behavior Checklist
(CBCL)
C. Protective Services (CPS)
term birth, living c. (TBLC)
unborn c.
child-adult mist (CAM)
childbearing
c. age
childbed fever
childbirth
Bradley method of
prepared c.
Kitzinger method of c.
natural c.
physiologic c.
childhood
c. breast
erythroblastic anemia of c.
c. fibromyalgia
c. genital trauma
papular acrodermatitis of c.
(PAC)
childlessness
children
C.'s Cancer Study Group
(CCSG)
C.'s Depression Inventory
(CDI)
C.'s Depression Inventory
test
Kaufman Assessment
Battery for C.
living c. (LC)
Children-Revised
Wechsler Intelligence Scale
for C.-R. (WISC-R)
chimera
chimeric
c. gene

NOTES

chimerism
blood c.
chin
galoche c.
c. position
CHIP
Coping Health Inventory for
Parents
chipmunk cheeks
CHL
crown-heel length
Chlamydia
C. *psittaci*
C. sepsis
C. *trachomatis*
chlamydial
c. cervicitis
c. conjunctivitis
c. infection
c. pneumonia
c. urethritis
c. vaginitis
Chlamydiazyme
C. immunoassay
C. test
Chlo-Amine
chloasma
Chlor-100
chloral hydrate
chlorambucil
chloramphenicol
chlorcyclizine hydrochloride
chlordecone
chlordiazepoxide
chloride
acetylcholine c.
ammonium c.
bethanechol c.
doxacurium c.
oxybutynin c.
potassium c.
pralidoxime c.
sodium c.
tubocurarine c.
chloridorrhea
chlormethiazole
Chlor-Niramine
Chlorohist-LA
Chloromycetin
chlorophyllin copper complex
Chloroptic
chloroquine
chlorothiazide

chlorotrianisene
chlorpheniramine
Chlor-Pro
Chlorpromanyl
chlorpromazine
chlorpropamide
chlorprothixene
Chlortab
chlortetracycline
c. fluorescence test
chlorthalidone
Chlor-Trimeton
Chlor-Tripolon
chlorzoxazone
choanal atresia
chocolate cyst
cholangiogram
operative c.
cholangiopancreatography
endoscopic retrograde c.
(ERCP)
Cholebrine
cholecalciferol
cholecystectomy
cholecystitis
cholecystokinin
choledochal cyst
choledochojejunostomy
Roux-en-Y c.
Choledyl
cholelithiasis
cholera
c. infantum
c. vaccine
cholestasis
maternal c.
cholestatic
c. hepatosis of pregnancy
c. jaundice
cholesterol
c. 20,22 desmolase
c. ester storage disease
cholesterolemia
familial c.
cholestyramine
choline
c. salicylate
c. theophyllinate
cholinergic
c. agonist
c. drug
cholinesterase
c. inhibitor

Choloxin
chondrodysplasia
    c. punctata
chondrodystrophia
    c. calcificans congenita
    c. congenita punctata
    c. fetalis calcificans
chondrodystrophy
    hereditary deforming c.
chondroectodermal dysplasia
chondromalacia fetalis
chondromere
chondroosteodystrophy
chondroplastic dwarfism
chondrosarcoma
    uterine c.
chondrosome
Chooz
chorda, pl. chordae
    c. umbilicalis
chordablastoma
chordamesoderm
chordate
chordee
chorea
    c. gravidarum
    Huntington c.
    Sydenham c.
Chorex
chorioadenoma
    c. destruens
chorioallantoic
    c. membrane (CAM)
    c. placenta
    c. vessel
chorioamnionic
    c. infection
    c. placenta
chorioamnionitis
    Gardnerella vaginalis c.
chorioamniotic bands
chorioangioma
chorioangiomatosis
chorioangiosis
chorioblastoma
choriocarcinoma

chorioepithelioma
choriogonadotropin
choriomeningitis
    lymphocytic c.
chorion
    c. frondosum
    c. laeve
    c. sampling
chorionic
    c. adrenocorticotropin
    c. cyst
    c. gonadotropic hormone
    c. gonadotropin (CG)
    c. growth hormone
    c. sac
    c. somamammotropin
    c. thyrotropin
    c. vascularization
    c. vesicle
    c. villi
    c. villus biopsy (CVB)
    c. villus sampling (CVS)
chorioretinitis
choriovitelline placenta
choroid plexus papilloma
Choron
Chotzen syndrome
Christian-Opitz syndrome
Christmas
    C. disease
    C. factor
    C. tree pattern
Christ-Siemens-Touraine syndrome
chromaffinoma
Chromagen
    C. OB
chromatid
    sister c.
chromatin
    sex c.
    X c.
    Y c.
chromatography
    thin-layer c.
chromatophore nevus of Naegeli

NOTES

chromic
  c. gut pelviscopic loop ligature
  c. phosphate
chromogene
chromohydrotubation
chromopertubation
chromophobic adenoma
chromosomal
  c. aberration
  c. abnormality
  c. analysis
  c. anomaly
  c. banding
  c. deletion
  c. mosaicism
  c. pattern
  c. sex
  c. structural abnormality
  c. translocation
chromosome
  c. 21
  accessory c.
  acentric c.
  acrocentric c.
  arm of c.
  c. arm
  B c.
  c. band
  c. banding
  bivalent c.
  c. breakage
  11p13 c. deletion
  c. complement
  daughter c.
  derivative c.
  dicentric c.
  founder c.
  fractured c.'s
  fragile X c.
  gametic c.
  giant c.
  heterotropic c.
  heterotypical c.
  homologous c.'s
  insertion of c.
  inversion of c.'s
  iso-X c.
  lampbrush c.
  late replicating c.
  long arm of c.
  c. map
  marker c.

  marker X c.
  metacentric c.
  mitochondrial c.
  mitotic c.
  nonhomologous c.'s
  nucleolar c.
  odd c.
  4p+ c.
  c. pair
  c. 9p disorder
  Ph c.
      Philadelphia chromosome
  Philadelphia c. (Ph chromosome)
  polytene c.
  c. 15q23-24
  c. reduction
  ring c.
  ring 18 c.
  ring 22 c.
  c. sequencing
  sex c.
  sex-linked c.
  short arm of c.
  small c.
  somatic c.
  submetacentric c.
  supernumerary c.
  telocentric c.
  translocation c.
  unpaired c.
  W c.
  c. walking
  X c.
  XO c.
  XX c.
  Y c.
  Z c.
chromospermism
chromotubation
chronic
  c. atrophic vulvitis
  c. bullous dermatitis
  c. cystic mastitis
  c. hepatitis
  c. hypertension
  c. hypertrophic vulvitis
  c. interstitial salpingitis
  c. lung disease (CLD)
  c. obstructive bronchitis
  c. pelvic pain (CPP)
  c. scrotal hypothermia
  c. vascular disease

Chronulac
Chvostek sign
chyle (*var. of* chylus)
chylomicron
chylothorax
chylous ascites
chylus, chyle
CI
    cervical incompetence
Ci
    curie
CIA
    chemiluminescent immunoassay
ciclopirox
Cidex soak
CI Direct Blue #53
Cidomycin
CIE
    counterimmunoelectrophoresis
CI Food Blue #1
cilastatin
cilia, sing. cilium
    immotile c.
ciliated
    c. cell endometrial
      adenocarcinoma
    c. metaplasia
Ciloxan
cimetidine
CIN
    cervical intraepithelial neoplasia
cineangiography
    biplane c.
Cineloop
    C. image review ultrasound
      system
    C. Ultrasound
cinnarizine
Cinobac
cinoxacin
Cin-Quin
Cipro
ciprofloxacin
    c. hydrochloride
circadian
    c. cycle
    c. rhythm

circle
    Baudelocque uterine c.
    Carus c.
    Huguier c.
Circon-ACMI
    C.-A. cannula
    C.-A. hysteroscope
    C.-A. trocar
circulating
    c. hormone
    c. platelet antibody
circulation
    ductal-dependent
      pulmonary c.
    extracorporeal c. (ECC)
    fetal c.
    fetoplacental c.
    hypophyseal portal c.
    hypothalamic-hypophyseal
      portal c.
    persistent fetal c. (PFC)
    c. time
    umbilical c.
circulatory arrest
circumcise
circumcision
    c. clamp
circumference
    abdominal c. (AC)
    fetal abdominal c.
    head c. (HC)
    midarm c.
circumflexa
    ichthyosis linearis c.
circumflex artery
circummarginate placenta
circumscribed mass
circumscriptum
    angiokeratoma c.
    lymphangioma c.
circumscriptus
    albinismus c.
Circumstraint
circumvalate placenta
circumvallata
    placenta c.
cirrhonosus

NOTES

cirrhosis
    biliary c.
    hypertrophic c.
    c. of liver
cirsomphalos
cirumscripta
    myositis ossificans c.
CIS
    carcinoma in situ
cisplatin
    intraperitoneal c.
    vinblastine, bleomycin, c.
      (VBP)
cis-platinum, cyclophosphamide,
    Eldesine (PCE)
cisplatin, vinblastine, and
    bleomycin
cissa, citta, cittosis
cisternal puncture
cisternography
    isotope c.
Citracal
citrate
    calcium c.
    clomiphene c.
    fentanyl c.
    magnesium c.
    oral transmucosal
      fentanyl c.
    potassium c.
    sufentanil c.
    tamoxifen c.
citrovorum
    c. factor
citrulline
citrullinemia
citrullinuria
citta (*var. of* cissa)
cittosis (*var. of* cissa)
CK
    creatine kinase
CL
    capacity of lung
    cleft lip
    compliance of lung
Clado anastomosis
Claforan
clamp
    Allis c.
    Babcock c.
    Backhaus c.
    Ballentine c.
    cervical c.

    circumcision c.
    DeBakey c.
    Gomco circumcision c.
    Heaney c.
    Kelly c.
    Kocher c.
    Lem-Blay circumcision c.
    Mogen c.
    pediatric bulldog c.
    pediatric vascular c.
    pedicle c.
    Pennington c.
    Sztehlo umbilical c.
    thoracic c.
    umbilical c.
    vulsellum c.
    Willett c.
    Winston cervical c.
    Yellen c.
clamped down
clarithromycin
Clark classification of vulvar
    melanoma
Clarke
    C. Hadfield syndrome
    C. ligator scissor forceps
Clarus model 5169 peristaltic
    pump
CLAS
    congenital localized absence of
    skin
classic abdominal Semm
    hysterectomy (CASH)
classical
    c. genetics
    c. transverse incision
classifiable character
classification
    Acosta c.
    American Society of
      Anesthesiologists c.
    Astler-Coller modification of
      Dukes c.
    Bethesda Pap smear c.
    Caldwell-Moloy c.
    Chicago c.
    Cori c.
    Denver c.
    Dripps–American Society of
      Anesthesiologists c.
    Dukes c.
    FAB c.

Federation of Gynecology
and Obstetrics c.
HIV c.
International Federation of
Gynecology and
Obstetrics c.
Jansky c.
Jewett c.
Kajava c.
microinvasive carcinoma c.
Moss c.
Pulec and Freedman c.
Schuknecht c.
TNM c.
tumor, node, metastasis c.
Wassel c.
White c.
Wolfe c. of breast cancer
class I, II receptor
clastogenic
clathrin
clavulanic acid
clawfoot
clawhand
CLD
chronic lung disease
clean-catch
c.-c. urinalysis
c.-c. urine specimen
cleaner
Sklar aseptic germicidal c.
**clean intermittent self-
catheterization**
clear
c. cell adenocarcinoma
c. cell endometrial
carcinoma
c. cell sarcoma
c. cell vaginal cancer
clearance
creatinine c.
immune c.
urate c.
urea c.
Clearblue
C. Easy
C. Improved

Clearplan
C. Easy
C. Easy ovulation predictor
Clearview
C. hCG
C. hCG pregnancy test
cleavage
embryonic c.
cleft
branchial c.
c. face
hyobranchial c.
c. jaw
laryngeal c.
c. lip (CL)
natal c.
c. palate (CP)
c. spine
Stillman c.
visceral c.
clefting
ectrodactyly, ectodermal
dysplasia, c. (EEC)
cleidocranial
c. dysostosis
c. dysplasia
c. dysplasia syndrome
c. dystosis
cleidorrhexis
cleidotomy
cleidotripsy
clemastine
Cleocin
C. HCl
C. Phosphate
C. T
C. vaginal cream
**Clevedan positive pressure
respirator**
click
hip c.
Ortolani c.
pulmonary ejection c.'s
clidinium
clidoic
Clifford syndrome

NOTES

climacteric
 grand c.
 c. psychosis
 c. syndrome
climacterium
climatic bubo
clinch knot
clindamycin
 c. phosphate
 c. phosphate topical
  solution
clinical
 c. crib
 c. finding
 c. prognosis
 c. staging
clinicopathological analysis
Clinistix
Clinitest
clinocephaly
clinodactyly
Clinoril
clip
 Bleier c.
 Filshie c.
 Hulka c.
 Hulka-Clemens c.
 Liga c.
 c. technique
 towel c.
Clistin
clitoral
 c. hood
 c. hypertrophy
clitoridectomy
clitoridis
 phimosis c.
clitoriditis
clitoris
 c. crisis
 c. enlargement
clitorism
clitoritis
clitoromegaly
clitoroplasty
cloaca
 congenital c.
cloacal
 c. duct
 c. membrane
clobetasol
 c. propionate
clofibrate

Clomid
clomiphene
 c. citrate
 c. fetal malformation
clomiphene-resistant polycystic ovary syndrome
clomipramine
clomocycline
clonality
clonal selection theory
clonazepam
clone
 molecular c.
clonidine
cloning
 DNA c.
 embryo c.
 gene c.
clonogenic
 c. technique
clonus
 ankle c.
Clopra
Cloquet node
clorazepate
Clorpactin
closed
 c. chest massage
 c. drainage
closing
 c. coagulum
 c. ring of Winkler-Waldeyer
 c. volume
Clostridium
 C. difficile
 C. perfringens
clostridium, pl. clostridia
closure
 incision c.
 premature airway c.
 premature ductus
  arteriosis c.
 Smead-Jones c.
 Steri-Strip skin c.
 Tom Jones c.
clot
 retroplacental c.
clotrimazole
Clouston syndrome
cloven spine
cloverleaf
 c. skull

c. skull deformity
c. skull syndrome
cloxacillin
Cloxapen
clubbing
hereditary c.
clubfeet
clubfoot
Turco posteromedial release of c.
club foot
clubhand
radial c.
clue cell
Clutton joints
Clyman endometrial curette
CMF
cyclophosphamide, methotrexate, 5-fluorouracil
CMFP
cyclophosphamide, methotrexate, 5-fluorouracil, and prednisone
CMFVP
cyclophosphamide, methotrexate, 5-fluorouracil, vincristine, and prednisone
CMI
cell-mediated immunity
CMP
cow's milk protein
CMT
cervical motion tenderness
Charcot-Marie-Tooth
CMV
controlled mechanical ventilation
cytomegalovirus
c-*myc* gene
CNAP
continuous negative airway pressure
CNM
Certified Nurse-Midwife
CNS
central nervous system
CNS development

CO$_2$
carbon dioxide
CO$_2$ laser
^{60}Co
cobalt-60
Coactin
coagulation
cold c.
c. defect
diffuse intravascular c. (DIC)
c. disorder
disseminated intravascular c. (DIC)
c. factor
c. profile
c. test
coagulator
argon beam c.
cold c.
Elmed BC 50 M/M digital bipolar c.
coagulopathy
consumption c.
maternal c.
coagulum
closing c.
coaptation
urethral c.
coarctation
c. of aorta
juxtaductal c.
coarse
c. calcification
c. rales
Coats disease
cobalt
c.-60 (^{60}Co)
c. megavoltage machine
radioactive c.
cobalt-60 moving strip technique
Coban dressing
Cobantril
Cobb-Ragde needle
Cobe gun
cocaine
c. addiction

NOTES

cocaine *(continued)*
 c. baby
 crack c.
 perinatal c.
cocci *(pl. of* coccus)
coccidioidomycosis
coccidiomycosis
coccus, pl. **cocci**
 Gram-negative cocci
 Gram-positive cocci
coccygeus muscle
coccygodynia
coccyx
Cockayne syndrome
cockscomb
 cervical c.
cocktail
 Brompton c.
 GI c.
 pediatric c.
code
 genetic c.
codeine
Codman Accu-Flow shunt
codominant
 c. gene
 c. inheritance
codon
coefficient
 bone attenuation c.
 c. of inbreeding
 c. of variation (CV)
coelom
coelomic
 c. epithelium
 c. metaplasia
coelosomy
coexistent fetus
Coffey suspension
Coffin-Lowry syndrome
Coffin-Siris syndrome
Cogentin
Cohen uterine cannula
Cohnheim theory
coil
 Margulies c.
 metal c.
coiled artery
coin biopsy
coital
 c. age
 c. factor
coitarche

coition
coitus
 c. incompletus
 c. interruptus
 c. la vache
 c. reservatus
 c. Saxonius
Colace
cola-colored neonate
colarium
Colax
colchicine
cold
 c. biopsy forceps
 c. coagulation
 c. coagulator
 c. conization
 c. knife method
 c. potassium cardioplegia
cold-knife conization
Cole
 C. endotracheal tube
 C. intubation procedure
 C. orotracheal tube
coleitis
coleocele
coleotomy
colfosceril palmitate
coli
 Escherichia c.
 pterygium c.
colic
 c. artery
 infantile c.
 meconial c.
 menstrual c.
 ovarian c.
 renal c.
 tubal c.
 uterine c.
colicky
colistimethate sodium
colistin
colitis
 amoebic c.
 granulomatous c.
 infectious c.
 pseudomembranous c.
 tuberculous c.
 ulcerative c.
collagen
 bovine dermal c.
 GAX c.

microfibrillar c.
c. vascular disease
collagenosis
mediastinal c.
collapse
cardiopulmonary c.
collapsed subpectoral implant
collar
c. of pearls
venereal c.
c. of Venus
collared cervix
collateral
venous c.
collector
cell c.
Cytobrush cell c.
Cytobrush-Plus cell c.
Cytopick endocervical and uterovaginal cell c.
Endocell endometrial cell c.
Leukotrap red cell c.
Papette cervical c.
Uterobrush endometrial sample c.
Wallach-Papette disposable cervical cell c.
Colles
C. fascia
C. fracture
colli
pterygium c.
collimator
collodion
c. baby
c. skin
colloid
c. carcinoma
c. cyst
c. infusion
c. osmotic pressure (COP)
radioactive c.
coloboma
coloboma, heart anomaly, choanal atresia, retardation, and genital and ear anomalies (CHARGE)
colocolic intussusception

colocolponeopoiesis
colocolpopoiesis
Kun c.
colon
c. carcinoma
rectosigmoid c.
sigmoid c.
colonic
c. obstruction
c. polyp
c. polyposis
colonization
stool c.
colonoscopy
colony-forming unit in culture (CFUC)
colony-stimulating
c.-s. activity (CSA)
c.-s. factor (CSF)
Colorado tick fever
color echocardiogram
colorectal
c. anastomosis
c. cancer
c. tumor
color-flow Doppler
colostomy
diverting c.
fecal diversion c.
temporary diverting c.
colostration
colostric
colostrorrhea
colostrous
colostrum
colovaginal fistula
colpatresia
colpectasis, colpectasia
colpectomy
skinning c.
colpitis
c. mycotica
colpocele
colpocleisis
Latzko c.
LeFort partial c.
colpocystitis

NOTES

colpocystocele
colpocystoplasty
colpocystotomy
colpocystoureterotomy
colpocystourethropexy (CCUP)
colpodynia
colpohyperplasia
    c. cystica
    c. emphysematosa
colpohysterectomy
colpohysteropexy
colpohysterotomy
colpomicrohysteroscope
    Hamou c.
colpomicroscopy
colpomycosis
colpomyomectomy
colpopathy
colpoperineoplasty
colpoperineorrhaphy
colpopexy
colpoplasty
colpopoiesis
colpoptosis, colpoptosia
colporectopexy
colporrhagia
colporrhaphy
    Goffe c.
colporrhexis
colposcope
    Accuscope c.
    Leisegang c.
    OMPI c.
    Zeiss c.
    Zoomscope c.
colposcopic
    c. diagnosis
    c. screening
colposcopically-directed
colposcopy
    digital imaging c.
    endocervical canal c.
    estrogen-assisted c.
colpospasm
colpostat
    afterload c.
    Henschke c.
colpostenosis
colpostenotomy
colposuspension
    Burch c.
colpotomy
    c. incision

colpoureterotomy
colpourethrocystopexy
    retropubic c.
colpourethropexy
    Burch c.
colpoxerosis
columnar
    c. epithelium
    c. epithelium papilla
Coly-Mycin
    C.-M. M
    C.-M. S
Colyte
coma
    diabetic c.
    hyperosmolar c.
combination
    c. chemotherapy
    estrogen-progestogen c.
    norgestrel/ethinyl estradiol c.
    c. oral contraceptive
combined
    c. birth control pill
    c. immunodeficiency
    c. pregnancy
    c. version
combing
    cervical c.
Comby sign
comedocarcinoma
Comfort
    C. personal lubricant
    C. personal lubricant gel
commissure
    anterior c.
    posterior c.
commissurotomy
    mitral c.
committed cell
communicable disease
communicating uterus
communication
    autocrine c.
    fetal-maternal c.
    paracrine c.
    vascular c.
compacta
Companion 318 Nasal CPAP System
comparative embryology
compatibility
    maternal-fetal HLA c.
Compazine

complement
    chromosome c.
    c. fixation
    c. value
complemental inheritance
complementary
    c. DNA (cDNA)
    c. genes
complete
    c. abortion
    c. atrioventricular block
    c. breech presentation
    c. heart block
    c. hydatidiform mole
    c. precocious puberty
    c. remission
complete/complete/+ station
complex
    Adam c.
    AIDS dementia c. (ADC)
    AIDS-related c. (ARC)
    antigen-antibody c.
    chlorophyllin copper c.
    Diana c.
    Eisenmenger c.
    Electra c.
    gene c.
    Ghon c.
    Jocasta c.
    Lear c.
    nipple-areola c.
    Oedipus c.
    Phaedra c.
    tuboovarian c.
    vitamin B c.
complexion
    florid c.
compliance
    lung c.
    c. of lung (CL)
complication
    cardiovascular c.
    intraoperative c.
    neurologic c.
    obstetrical c.
    operative site c.
    postoperative c.

    pregnancy c.
    pulmonary c.
    respiratory c.
    vascular c.
component
    blood c.
    buffy coat c.
    extensive intraductal c.
    (EIC)
    extracellular matrix c.
compound
    nitroimidazole c.
    c. pregnancy
    c. presentation
compressibility
    vein c.
compression
    cord c.
    external pneumatic calf c.
    (EPC)
    c. force
    head c.
    intermittent pneumatic c.
    pneumatic c.
    spot c.
    tracheal c.
    c. ultrasonography
    uterine c.
compressus
    fetus c.
Compton effect
computed
    c. axial tomography (CAT)
    c. tomographic pelvimetry
    c. tomography (CT)
concealed hemorrhage
Conceive
    C. Ovulation Predictor
concentrate
    factor c.
    platelet c.
concentration
    ambient oxygen c.
    blood alcohol c. (BAC)
    fetal steroid c.
    inhibin c.
    lipoprotein c.

NOTES

concentration *(continued)*
    maternal steroid c.
    mean hemoglobin c.
    mean plasma iron c.
    minimum inhibitory c.
     (MIC)
    plasma iron c.
    serum c.
    serum lithium c.
    steroid c.
concepti (*pl. of* conceptus)
conception
    assisted c.
    estimated date of c. (EDC)
    natural c.
    products of c. (POC)
    wrongful c.
Conceptrol
conceptus, pl. concepti
Concise Plus hCG urine test
concomitant change
concussion
condition
    fetal c.
    local ovarian c.
    maternal c.
    neonatal c.
    orthopaedic c.
    X-linked dominant c.
    X-linked recessive c.
conditional probability
condom
    female c.
    intravaginal c.
    vaginal c.
conductance
    airway c.
conduction
    abbreviated
     atrioventricular c.
    c. analgesia
    c. anesthesia
conduit
    ileal c.
    intestinal c.
    urinary c.
conduplicato corpore
condyloma, pl. condylomata
    c. acuminatum
    cervical c.
    c. latum
Condylox

cone
    c. biopsy
    c. biopsy of cervix
    transvaginal c.
    vaginal c.
confidence limits
confinement
    estimated date of c. (EDC)
    expected date of c. (EDC)
congenita
    aglossia c.
    amaurosis c.
    amyoplasia c.
    amyotonia c.
    aplasia axialis
     extracorticalis c.
    aplasia cutis c.
    arthrochalasis multiplex c.
    arthrogryposis multiplex c.
    chondrodystrophia
     calcificans c.
    dyskeratosis c.
    pachyonychia c.
    Thomsen myotonia c.
congenital
    c. abducens facial paralysis
    c. abnormality
    c. adrenal hyperplasia
     (CAH)
    c. adrenal hypoplasia
    c. afibrinogenemia
    c. aleukia
    c. alveolar dysplasia
    c. amputation
    c. anemia
    c. anemia of newborn
    c. anomaly
    c. atelectasis
    c. atheosis
    c. bullous urticaria
     pigmentosa
    c. cloaca
    c. contractural
     arachnodactyly (CCA)
    c. cystic adenomatoid
     malformation (CCAM)
    c. defect
    c. dislocated hip (CDH)
    c. ectodermic scalp defect
    c. ectropion
    c. elephantiasis
    c. elevation of the scapula
    c. epulis

c. epulis of the newborn
c. erythropoietic porphyria
c. folate malabsorption
c. glaucoma
c. heart block
c. heart defect
c. heart disease
c. hemidysplasia with icthyosiform erythroderma and limb defects (CHILD)
c. hemolytic jaundice
c. hip dislocation (CHD)
c. hypofibrinogenemia
c. hypogammaglobulinemia
c. hypoplastic anemia
c. hypothyroidism
c. hypothyroidism syndrome
c. ichthyosis
c. injury
c. lobar emphysema
c. localized absence of skin (CLAS)
c. macular degeneration
c. malformation
c. megacolon
c. myotonic dystrophy
c. nephrosis
c. nonhemolytic jaundice
c. nonregenerative anemia
c. nonspherocytic hemolytic anemia
c. obliterative jaundice
c. oculofacial paralysis
c. photosensitive porphyria
c. pneumonia
c. postural deformity
c. pterygium
c. pulmonary lymphangiectasia
c. rubella
c. rubella syndrome
c. spastic paraplegia
c. syphilis
c. toxoplasmosis

congenitalis
alopecia c.

congestion
pelvic vein c.
congestive heart failure
conglobata
acne c.
conglutination
conization
cautery c.
cervical c.
c. of cervix
cold c.
cold-knife c.
hot-knife c.
laser cervical c.
loop diathermy cervical c.
conjoined twins
conjugata diagonalis
conjugate
c. axis
diagonal c.
c. diameter of the pelvic inlet
c. diameter of pelvic inlet
effective c.
external c.
false c.
c. of inlet
internal c.
obstetric c. of outlet
c. of outlet
c. of pelvic outlet
true c.
urinary steroid c.
conjugated
c. antibody
c. equine estrogen
c. estrogen and meprobamate
c. estrogens
conjunctiva, pl. conjunctivae
xerosis c.
conjunctivitis
chlamydial c.
gonococcal c.
infantile purulent c.
neonatal c.
silver nitrate c.

NOTES

conjunctivitis *(continued)*
    trachoma inclusion c.
      (TRIC)
connection
    anomalous pulmonary
      venous c.
    decidua-macrophage c.
    total cavopulmonary c.
connective
    c. tissue
    c. tissue disorder
Conners Scale
Conn syndrome
conotruncus
Conradi
    C. disease
    C. syndrome
Conradi-Hünermann syndrome
consanguinity
consent
    informed c.
conservative
    c. drug use
    c. surgery
consideration
    adrenal morphologic c.
constant
    association c.
    dissociation c.
    pulmonary time c.
constipation
constitutional
    c. delay
    c. dwarfism
    c. hirsutism
    c. precocious puberty
    c. short stature
constriction ring
construction
    Abbe vaginal c.
consumption
    c. coagulopathy
    maternal alcohol c.
    oxygen c.
contagiosa
    impetigo c.
contagiosum
    molluscum c.
contaminant
contaminate
contamination
    bacterial c.

content
    aspiration of gastric c.'s
    bone mineral c.
    evacuation of uterine c.'s
Contigen glutaraldehyde cross-
linked collagen implant
contiguous gene syndrome
Contin
    MS C.
continence
continent
    c. ileostomy
    c. supravesical bowel
      urinary diversion
    c. urinary pouch
continua
    epilepsia partialis c.
continuous
    c. ambulatory peritoneal
      dialysis (CAPD)
    c. arteriovenous
      hemofiltration (CAVH)
    c. distending airway
      pressure (CDAP)
    c. distention irrigation
      system (CDIS)
    c. epidural analgesia
    c. murmur
    c. negative airway pressure
      (CNAP)
    c. positive airway pressure
      (CPAP)
    c. random variable
    c. running monofilament
      suture
    c. subcutaneous insulin
      infusion
    c. subcutaneous insulin
      injection
    c. variable
continuous/combined treatment
continuous-wave ultrasound imaging
contour
    cranial c.
contraception
    barrier c.
    hormonal c.
    long-acting c.
    oral c.
    postcoital c. (PCC)
    vaginal ring c.
contraceptive
    barrier c.

combination oral c.
c. device
c. diaphragm
estrogen-progestin c.
c. failure
c. foam
injectable c.
intrauterine c. device
 (IUCD)
intravaginal c.
c. jelly
long-acting c.
low-dose oral c.
low steroid content
 combined oral c.
c. method
monophasic oral c.
oral c. (OC)
oral steroid c.
ParaGard T380A
 intrauterine copper c.
progestin oral c.
c. ring
sequential oral c.
c. sponge
steroid c.
c. technique
triphasic oral c.
vaginal c.
contracted pelvis
contractility
detrusor hyperactivity with
 impaired c.
contraction
atrial c.
Braxton Hicks c.
myometrial c.
pelvic c.
premature ventricular c.
 (PVC)
smooth muscle c.
c. stress test (CST)
uterine c.
Z,Z,'Z" degree of c.'s
contractural
c. arachnodactyly disease
c. arachnodactyly syndrome

contralateral
c. ovulation
c. synchronous carcinoma
control
birth c.
Centers for Disease C.
 (CDC)
glycemic c.
seizure c.
controlled
c. mechanical ventilation
 (CMV)
c. vaginal delivery
controversy
transfusion c.
conversion
extraglandular c.
convex probe
convulsion
benign familial neonatal c.'s
 (BFNC)
benign infantile familial c.'s
 (BIFC)
febrile c.
puerperal c.'s
Cooley anemia
Coombs test
Cooper
C. fascia
C. Surgical Monopolor
 ELSG LEEP System
C. suspensory ligaments
cooperativity
theca-granulosa cell c.
Coopernail sign
COP
colloid osmotic pressure
**Coping Health Inventory for
 Parents (CHIP)**
Copper-7
C. intrauterine device
Copper T intrauterine device
copulating pouch
copulation
c. plug
copy
DNA c.

NOTES

cor
- c. biloculare
- c. pulmonale
- c. triatriatum
- c. triatriatum dexter
- c. triloculare biatriatum

cord
- c. abnormality
- c. blood
- c. blood gas (CBG)
- c. compression
- genital c.
- kinked c.
- medullary c.
- nephrogenic c.
- nuchal c.
- omphalomesenteric c.
- palpable c.
- c. of Pflüger
- presentation of c.
- prolapse of umbilical c.
- rete c.'s
- sex c.
- spermatic c.
- spinal c.
- three-vessel c.
- umbilical c.
- vitelline c.

Cordarone
cordate pelvis
Cordguard umbilical cord sampler
cordiform
- c. pelvis
- c. uterus

cordis
- accretio c.
- ectopia c.

cordocentesis
cordotomy
core
- C. Dynamics disposable cannula
- C. Dynamics disposable trocar
- c. temperature

Corey ovum forceps
Corgard
Cori
- C. classification
- C. disease
- C. enzyme deficiency

Coricidin

coring biopsy gun
corkscrew
- c. maneuver
- c. vessel

cornea
- xerosis c.

corneal opacity
Cornelia de Lange syndrome
Corner-Allen test
Corning method
Cornoy solution
cornu, pl. cornua
- c. uteri

cornual
- c. anastomosis
- c. pregnancy

Corometrics
- C. fetal monitor
- C. Gold Quik Connect Spiral electrode tip
- C. Model 900SC in-office mammography
- C. Quik Connect Spiral electrode tip

corona
- c. of penis
- c. radiata
- c. radiata cell

coronal suture line of skull
coronary
- c. artery disease
- c. heart disease
- c. thrombosis

Coronex
corporis
- pediculosis c.
- tinea c.

corpus, pl. corpora
- c. albicans cyst
- c. fibrosum
- c. luteum
- c. luteum cyst
- c. luteum deficiency syndrome
- c. luteum dysfunction
- c. luteum function
- c. luteum insufficiency
- c. luteum size
- c. luteum spurium
- c. luteum verum
- uterine c.
- c. uterus

corpuscle
	Bennett small c.'s
	genital c.
	meconium c.
	Nunn engorged c.'s
corrodens
	Bacteroides c.
	Eikenella c.
Corson myoma forceps
Cortenema enema
cortex, pl. cortices
	adrenal c.
	renal c.
cortical
	c. granule
	c. granule exocytosis
	c. implantation
	c. mass
	c. necrosis
	c. nephron
	c. reaction
	c. supremacy stage
corticalis
	agenesia c.
cortices (*pl. of* cortex)
corticoid
corticosteroid
	fluorinated c.
corticosteroid-binding
	c.-b. globulin (CBG)
	c.-b. globulin-binding
	capacity (CBG-BC)
corticosterone
corticotrope
corticotropin-like intermediate lobe
	peptide
corticotropin-releasing
	c.-r. factor
	c.-r. hormone (CRH)
	c.-r. inhibitor
cortisol
	24-hour urinary free c.
	c. level
	c. response
cortisone
cortol
Cortone

Cortrosyn
	C. stimulation test
Corynebacterium
	C. parvum
	C. vaginitis
coryza
Cosmegen
costovertebral angle tenderness
	(CVAT)
cosyntropin
	c. stimulation test
cot
	finger c.
Cotazym
co-trimoxazole
Cotte operation
Cottle-Neivert retractor
co-twin
cotyledon
	fetal c.
	maternal c.
	placental c.
cotyledonary placenta
coudé catheter
cough
	barking c.
	croupy c.
	Pedituss C.
	staccato c.
	uterine c.
	whooping c.
cough-pressure transmission ratio
Cough-X lozenge
Coulter
	C. Channelyser cell analyzer
	C. counter
Coumadin
coumarin
	c. derivative
Council on Resident Education in
	Obstetrics and Gynecology
	(CREOG)
counseling
	genetic c.
Counsellor-Davis artificial vagina
	operation

NOTES

Counsellor-Flor modification of McIndoe technique
Counsellor vaginal mold
count
    bacterial c.
    blood c.
    differential cell c.
    erythrocyte c.
    hemolysis, elevated liver enzymes, and low platelet c. (HELLP)
    kick c.
    leukocyte c.
    platelet c.
    reticulocyte c.
    sperm c.
counter
    Coulter c.
counterimmunoelectrophoresis (CIE)
coupling
    receptor c.
court-ordered obstetrical intervention
couvade
Couvelaire uterus
covariance
    analysis of c. (ANCOVA)
cover
    Sheathes ultrasound probe c.
    Ultra Cover transducer c.
Cowper gland
cowperian duct
cow's milk protein (CMP)
coxa vara
coxsackievirus
    C. B
    c. infection
CP
    cerebral palsy
    cleft palate
CPAP
    continuous positive airway pressure
    nasal CPAP
    CPAP ventilator
CPD
    cephalopelvic disproportion
C-peptide
CPK
    creatine phosphokinase
CPP
    chronic pelvic pain

CPR
    cardiopulmonary resuscitation
C_{21} progestin
CPS
    Child Protective Services
cps
    cycles per second
crab louse
crack
    c. baby
    c. cocaine
cracked pot sound
crackling rales
cradle cap
cramp
    leg c.
cramping
    uterine c.
cranial
    c. contour
    c. duplication
    c. meningocele
    c. suture
    c. synostosis
    c. ultrasound
craniocarpotarsal
    c. dystrophy
    c. syndrome
craniocaudal view
cranioclasia, cranioclasis
cranioclast
    Zweifel-DeLee c.
craniodiaphyseal dysplasia
craniodidymus
craniofacial
    c. dysostosis
    c. dystosis
craniofenestria
craniolacunia
craniomalacia
craniomeningocele
craniometaphyseal dysplasia
craniopagus
craniopharyngioma
craniorrhachischisis
cranioschisis
craniostenosis
craniostosis
craniosynostosis
craniosynostosis-radial aplasia syndrome
craniotabes
craniotome

craniotomy
cranium
    c. bifidum
    c. bifidum occultum
    c. cerebrale
    c. viscerale
Cranley Maternal-Fetal Attachment
  Scale
C-reactive protein (CRP)
cream, creme
    Amino-Cerv pH 5.5
    cervical C.'s
    Cleocin vaginal c.
    Emla c.
    Estrace vaginal c.
    estradiol vaginal c.
    intravaginal c.
    Nupercainal c.
    nystatin and
      triamcinolone c.
    Ogden vaginal c.
    PEN-Kera moisturizing c.
    Preparation-H hydrocortisone
      1% c.
    Sklar c.
    Terazol 3 vaginal c.
    Terazol 7 vaginal c.
    Triple Sulfa vaginal c.
    vaginal antibiotic c.
creamy vulvitis
crease
    palmar c.
    plantar c.
    simian c.
    sole c.
creatine
    c. kinase (CK)
    c. phosphokinase (CPK)
creatinine
    c. clearance
Credé
    C. maneuver
    C. maneuver of eyes
    C. maneuver of uterus
creeping

cremasteric fascia
creme (*var. of* cream)
cremnocele
crenation sign
CREOG
    Council on Resident Education
      in Obstetrics and Gynecology
Creon
crepitant rales
crepitation
crepitus
crescent cell anemia
Crescormon
CREST
    calcinosis cutis, Raynaud
      phenomenon, esophageal
      motility disorders,
      sclerodactyly, telangiectasia
      CREST syndrome
cretin dwarfism
cretinism
    athyreotic c.
cretinoid dysplasia
Creutzfeldt-Jakob syndrome
CR-gram
    cardiorespirogram
CRH
    corticotropin-releasing hormone
crib
    clinical c.
    c. death
    open c.
    tongue c.
cribogram
cribriform hymen
cricoid split
cri du chat
cri-du-chat syndrome
Crigler-Najjar syndrome
Crile
    C. forceps
    C. hemostat
Crile-Wood needle holder
criminal abortion
crisis, pl. crises
    addisonian c.

NOTES

crisis *(continued)*
    adrenal c.
    aplastic c.
    clitoris c.
    hypercalcemic c.
    lupus c.
    sickle cell c.
    thyroid c.
crisscross heart
crista dividens
criteria, sing. **criterion**
    Bell staging c.
    Friedrich c.
    Jones c.
    Kass c.
    Norris-Carrol c.
    Spiegelberg c.
critical
    c. care monitoring
    c. temperature
    c. weight hypothesis
CRL
    crown-rump length
CRNA
    Certified Registered Nurse
    Anesthetist
crocodile
    c. skin
    c. tongue
Crohn disease
cromolyn
    c. sodium
    c. sodium inhalation aerosol
Crosby-Kugler pediatric capsule
crossed
    c. adductor reflex
    c. extension reflex
cross-linking
Cross-McKusick-Breen syndrome
cross-over
cross-reaction
cross-sectional
Cross syndrome
croup
croupette
croupy cough
Crouzon
    C. disease
    C. syndrome
crowding
    fetal c.
crown-heel length (CHL)

crowning
crown-rump length (CRL)
CRP
    C-reactive protein
CRS
    caudal regression syndrome
CRST
    calcinosis cutis, Raynaud
    phenomenon, sclerodactyly,
    telangiectasia
    CRST syndrome
Cruiser hip abduction brace
cruris
    tinea c.
crusta lactea
cry
    cat c.
    cephalic c.
    high-pitched c.
    uterine c.
cryocautery
cryoconization
CryoGenetics CryoPrism
cryogun
    Wallach LL100
    cryosurgical c.
Cryomedics
    C. disposable LLETZ
    electrode
    C. electrosurgery system
cryoprecipitate
cryopreservation
    oocyte c.
CryoPrism
    CryoGenetics C.
cryosurgery
cryotherapy
cryovial
cryptic hyperandrogenism
cryptocephalus
cryptococcal meningitis
cryptococcosis
cryptodidymus
cryptomenorrhea
cryptomerorachischisis
cryptophthalmia
    c. syndrome
cryptophthalmia-syndactyly
    syndrome
cryptophthalmos
    c. syndrome
cryptorchid
cryptorchidism

cryptotia
crystallina
    miliaria c.
crystallization
    fern-leaf c.
crystalloid
    Reinke c.'s
crystal violet
Crystapen
Crysticillin AS
Crystodigin
CS
    Poly-Histine C.
C&S
    culture and sensitivity
^{137}Cs
    cesium-137
CSA
    colony-stimulating activity
Csapo abortion
C-section
    cesarean section
        LUST C.-s.
            lower uterine segment
            transverse cesarean
            section
CSF
    cerebrospinal fluid
    colony-stimulating factor
Csillag disease
CST
    contraction stress test
C_{19}-steroid
CT
    computed tomography
        CT pelvimetry
C-thalassemia
CTP
    carboxyl terminal peptide
Cu 7
cube pessary
cubic
    c. centimeters (cc)
    c. centimeters per hour
      (cc/hr)
    c. centimeters per kilogram
      per day (cc/kg/d)

cuff
    Ethox c.
cuirass respirator
Culcher-Sussman technique
cul-de-sac
    Douglas c.-d.-s.
    c.-d.-s. of Douglas
    rectouterine c.-d.-s.
culdocentesis
    nondiagnostic c.
    Wiegernick c.
culdoplasty
    Halban c.
    Marion-Moschcowitz c.
    McCall c.
culdoscope
culdoscopy
culdotomy
Cullen sign
Culpolase laser
culture
    amniotic fluid cell c.
    blood c.
    cell c.
    cervical c.
    colony-forming unit in c.
      (CFUC)
    gonorrhea c.
    oocyte c.
    c. and sensitivity (C&S)
    sputum c.
    tracheal-aspirate c.
    Ureaplasma c.
    urine c.
cumulative gene
cumulus cell
cumulus oophorus
cup
    c. ear
    c. insemination
    Malström c.
    Milex cervical c.
    Mityvac obstetric vacuum
      extractor c.
    Tender-Touch vacuum
      birthing c.
Cuprimine

NOTES

curage
curetment (*var. of* curettement)
curettage
    dilatation and c. (D & C)
    dilation and c. (D & C)
    endocervical c. (ECC)
    fractional dilation and c.
    repeat c.
    suction c.
curette, curet
    Accurette endometrial
      suction c.
    Bumm c.
    Clyman endometrial c.
    Duncan c.
    Green uterine c.
    Heaney c.
    Helix endocervical c.
    Helix uterine biopsy c.
    Kelly-Gray c.
    Kevorkian c.
    Kevorkian-Younge c.
    Mi-Mark disposable
      endocervical c.
    Novak c.
    Pipelle endometrial
      suction c.
    Randall suction c.
    Ridpath c.
    Shapleigh c.
    Sims c.
    St. Clair-Thompson c.
    Tabb c.
    Thomas c.
    uterine c.
    Z-Sampler endometrial
      suction c.
curettement, curetment
curie (Ci)
Curling ulcer
currant jelly stool
Currarino triad
currens
    larva c.
current
    diathermy c.
Curretab
curse
    Ondine c.
    c. of Ondine
Curtis syndrome
curve
    Barnes c.

    Carus c.
    Friedman c.
    isodose c.
    Kaplan-Meier survival c.
    Liley c.
    oxygen dissociation c.
    sexual response c.
    standard c.
curved hemostat
CUSALap
    C. ultrasonic accessory
      needle
Cushing
    C. disease
    C. syndrome
cushingoid
    c. appearance
    c. facies
    c. syndrome
Cushing-Rokitansky ulcer
cushion
    c. defect of heart
    sucking c.
cutaneomastocystosis
cutaneous
    c. albinism
    c. anthrax
    c. blood flow
    c. hepatic porphyria
    c. larva migrans
    c. leishmaniasis
    c. lesion
    c. melanoma
    c. mucormycosis
    c. nevi
    c. vasculitis
cutis
    c. elastica
    c. hyperelastica
    c. laxa
    c. marmorata
    c. navel
    c. verticis gyrata
    xanthosis c.
cutter
    endoscopic linear c.
    Polaris reusable c.'s
cutting loop
CV
    cardiovascular
    coefficient of variation
CVA
    cerebrovascular accident

CVAT
costovertebral angle tenderness
CVB
chorionic villus biopsy
CVC
central venous catheter
CVL
central venous line
CVP
central venous pressure
CVP line
CVS
chorionic villus sampling
CXR
chest x-ray
cyanocobalamin
cyanosis
perioral c.
cyanotic
c. congenital heart disease
(CCHD)
cybernin
cyclacillin
cyclamate
calcium c.
sodium c.
cyclandelate
cyclase
adenylate c.
cyclazocine
cycle
battering c.
cell c.
circadian c.
endometrial c.
estrogen-progestin
artificial c.
fertility c.
genesial c.
glutamate c.
intrauterine pressure c.
itch-scratch c.
menstrual c.
menstrual-ovarian c.
ovarian c.
ovulatory c.
postmenarchal c.

reproductive c.
sexual response c.
spontaneous menstrual c.
cyclencephalus
cycle-nonspecific agent
cycle-specific agent
cycles per second (cps)
cyclic
c. adenosine monophosphate
(cAMP)
c. adenosine
3',5'-monophosphate
c. guanosine
3',5'-monophosphate
c. proliferative endometrium
cyclicity
postmenarchal c.
cyclizine lactate
cycloheximide
cyclopentanoperhydrophenanthrene
cyclopenthiazide
cyclopentolate
c. hydrochloride
cyclophosphamide
cyclophosphamide, doxorubicin,
cisplatin (CAP)
cyclophosphamide, doxorubicin, and
5-fluorouracil (CAF)
cyclophosphamide, methotrexate,
5-fluorouracil (CMF)
cyclophosphamide, methotrexate,
5-fluorouracil, and prednisone
(CMFP)
cyclophosphamide, methotrexate,
5-fluorouracil, vincristine, and
prednisone (CMFVP)
cyclopia
cyclopropane
Cyclo-Provera
cyclops
c. hypognathus
C. procedure
cycloserine
Cyclospasmol
Cyclosporin A
cyclosporine
cyclothiazide

NOTES

cycrimine hydrochloride
Cycrin
cyesis
cylinder
    cesium c.
    Delclos c.
cylindrical embryo
cyllosoma
cymbocephaly
CYP21A
CYP11B1
CYP11B2
CYP21B
cypionate
    estradiol c.
    testosterone c.
cyproheptadine
    c. hydrochloride
    c. receptor blocker
cyproterone acetate
cyst
    adnexal c.
    allantoic c.
    apocrine c.
    c. aspiration
    Bartholin c.
    benign c.
    blue dome c.
    branchial c.
    breast c.
    chocolate c.
    choledochal c.
    chorionic c.
    colloid c.
    corpora lutea c.'s
    corpus albicans c.
    corpus luteum c.
    Dandy-Walker c.
    dermoid c.
    dermoid c. of ovary
    dysontogenetic c.
    echinococcal c.
    endometrial c.
    epidermal inclusion c.
    epithelial c.
    fetal ovarian c.
    follicular c.
    functional ovarian c.
    Gartner c.
    gartnerian c.
    hydatid c.
    inclusion c.
    involution c.

    keratin c.
    lacteal c.
    luteal ovarian c.
    massive ovarian c.
    milk c.
    müllerian c.
    multilocular c.
    multiple c.
    nabothian c.
    oil c.
    omental c.
    omphalomesenteric c.
    oophoritic c.
    ovarian c.
    paraovarian c.
    paratubal c.
    perimesonephric c.
    pilonidal c.
    popliteal c.
    porencephalic c.
    posterior fossa c.
    rete c. of ovary
    Sampson c.
    sebaceous c.
    siderophagic c.
    simple c.
    tarry c.
    tension c.
    theca lutein c.
    umbilical c.
    urachal c.
    vaginal c.
    vaginal dysontogenetic c.
    vaginal embryonic c.
    vaginal inclusion c.
    vestibular c.
    vitelline duct c.
    vitellointestinal c.
    vulvar c.
    vulvar inclusion c.
cystadenocarcinoma
    mucinous c.
    ovarian c.
    papillary serous c.
cystadenofibroma
cystadenoma
    ovarian c.
    ovarian proliferative c.
    serous c.
cystathionine
cystathioninuria
cystectomy
    Bartholin c.

ovarian c.
vulvovaginal c.
cystencephalus
cystic
    c. adenomatous
      malformation (CAM)
    c. adnexal mass
    c. disease of the breast
    c. fibrosis (CF)
    c. glandular hyperplasia
    c. hygroma
    c. hyperplasia
    c. hyperplasia of the breast
    c. kidney
    c. lymphangioma
    c. mole
    c. myoma degeneration
cystica
    osteogenesis imperfecta c.
    spina bifida c.
cysticum
    epithelioma adenoides c.
    lymphangioma c.
cystinosis
cystinuria
cystitis
    acute c.
    bacterial c.
    hemorrhagic c.
    honeymoon c.
    Hunner interstitial c.
    irradiation c.
    postoperative c.
    postradiation c.
    radiation c.
cystoblast
Cystocath catheter
cystocele
    c. repair
cystography
cystological
cystometer
    Lewis recording c.
cystometric capacity
cystometrics
    office c.

cystometrogram
    multichannel c.
cystometry
cystosarcoma
    c. phyllodes
cystoscopy
Cystospaz
cystotomy
    suprapubic c.
cystourethrocele
cystourethrogram
    voiding c. (VCU, VCUG)
cystourethrography
    chain c.
    metallic bead-chain c.
cystourethropexy
    vaginal c.
cystourethroscopy
Cytadren
cytarabine
cytidine
    c. diphosphate-choline
    c. diphosphate-diacylglycerol
    c. monophosphate
    c. triphosphate-
      phosphocholine
      cytidyltransferase
cytidyltransferase
    cytidine triphosphate-
      phosphocholine c.
Cytobrush
    C. cell collector
    C. Plus endocervical cell
      sampler
    C. spatula
Cytobrush-Plus cell collector
cytochrome
    c. *c* oxidase deficiency
    c. P450scc
cytogenetics
cytogenetic study
cytogenic analysis
cytokine
cytologic screening
cytology
    c. brush
    brush c.

NOTES

cytology *(continued)*
    cervical c.
    peritoneal c.
    sputum c.
    urine c.
    vaginal c.
cytomegalic inclusion disease
cytomegalovirus (CMV)
    c. disease
    c. infection
Cytomel
cytopathogenesis
cytophagocytosis
cytophilic antibody
Cytopick endocervical and uterovaginal cell collector
cytopipette
cytoplasm
cytoplasmic
    c. inheritance

cytoreduction
cytoreductive surgery
Cytosar
    C.-U
cytosine
    c. arabinoside
cytoskeleton
Cytospray
Cytotec
cytotoxic
    c. agent
    c. cell
    c. effect
    c. factor
cytotoxicity
cytotrophoblast
    malignant c.
Cytoxan
Czerny anemia

D

2-D
> 2-D Doppler
> 2-D echocardiogram

D920
> Audio Doppler D.

DA
> developmental age
> ductus arteriosus

dacarbazine
Dacron fiber
dacryoadenitis
dacryocystitis
dacryocystostenosis
dacryostenosis
dactinomycin
dactylitis
> sickle cell d.
> tuberculous d.

dactylomegaly
Dagenan
daily fetal movement record
Dalacin C
Dale abdominal binder
Dalkon shield
Dalmane
Dalrymple sign
damage
> brain d.
> hepatocellular d.
> obstetrical d.
> obturator nerve d.

D-amino acid
dAMP
> deoxyadenylic acid

danazol
> low-dose d.

dance
> St. Vitus d.

Dandy-Walker
> D.-W. cyst
> D.-W. deformity
> D.-W. syndrome

Danforth sign
danger
> radiation d.

Danlos
> D. disease
> D. syndrome

Dann respirator

Danocrine
danthron
D-antigen isoimmunization
dantrolene
Danus-Fontan procedure
Danus-Stanzel repair
DAP
> direct agglutination pregnancy
> DAP test

Dapa
Daranide
Darbid
Daricon
dark-field
> d.-f. examination
> d.-f. microscopy

Darrier sign
Darrow-Gamble syndrome
Dartal
Darvocet-N
Darvon
> D.-N

Darwin
> D. ear
> D. theory of evolution

darwinian
> d. evolution
> d. reflex

dashboard perineum
data
> mortality d.

date of birth (DOB)
dating
> biopsy d.
> endometrial d.
> pregnancy d.

Datril
daughter
> d. cell
> d. chromosome
> DES d.

daunomycin
daunorubicin
DAV
> dibromodulcitol with
> doxorubicin and vincristine

Davis
> D. bladder catheter

Davydov procedure
dawn phenomenon

Dawson
- D. disease
- D. encephalitis

day
- calories per kilogram per d. (cal/kg/day)
- cubic centimeters per kilogram per d. (cc/kg/d)

dazzle reflex

dB
- decibel

DBCP
- dibromochloropropane

D & C
- dilatation and curettage
- dilation and curettage

dCMP
- deoxycytidylic acid

DCYS
- Department of Children and Youth Services

DDAVP
- desmopressin acetate
    - DDAVP nasal spray

DDP
- *cis*-diamminedichloroplatinum

DDST
- Denver Developmental Screening Test

D & E
- dilatation and evacuation
- dilation and evacuation

de
- D. Crecchio syndrome
- d. la Chapelle dysplasia
- d. Lange syndrome
- d. Morsier-Gauthier syndrome
- D. Sanctis-Cacchione syndrome
- d. Toni-Fanconi-Debré syndrome
- d. Toni-Fanconi syndrome
- D. Vaal syndrome

dead
- d. fetus syndrome
- full term, born d. (FTBD)

DEAE
- diethylaminoethyl
    - DEAE beads

deafness, onycho-osteodystrophy, mental retardation (DOOR)

death
- brain d.
- crib d.
- early embryonic d.
- fetal d.
- fetal brain d.
- infant d.
- intrauterine d.
- maternal d.
- neonatal d.
- nonmaternal d.
- perinatal d.
- single intrauterine d.
- sudden infant d. (SID)

Deaver retractor

DeBakey
- D. clamp
- D. tissue forceps

debendox

Debetrol

debrancher enzyme deficiency

Debré-Fibiger syndrome

Debré-Sémélaigne syndrome

debulking
- ovarian carcinoma d.
- d. of tumor

Decadron

Deca-Durabolin

decamethonium bromide

decannulate

Decanoate
- Hybolin D.

decapitate

decapitation

decarboxylase
- ornithine d.
- pyruvate d.

Decaspray

decay
- bottle tooth d.

deceleration
- abnormal d.'s
- early d.'s
- fetal heart rate d.
- late d.'s
- variable d.'s

decibel (dB)

decidua
- d. basalis
- d. capsularis
- d. compacta
- ectopic d.
- d. menstrualis

d. parietalis
d. polyposa
tuberous subchorial
  hematoma of the d.
d. vera
decidual
d. cast
d. cell
d. endometritis
d. prolactin synthesis
d. reaction
decidualized endometrium
decidua-macrophage connection
deciduate placenta
deciduation
deciduitis
deciduoma
Loeb d.
decline
recurrent premenstrual
  lithium serum
  concentration d.
Declomycin
decompensation
decomposition
decompression
small intestine d.
uterine d.
decondensation
sperm chromatin d.
decongestant
decreased libido
decubitus position
deep
d. circumflex iliac artery
d. tendon reflex (DTR)
d. vein thrombophlebitis
d. vein thrombosis (DVT)
d. venous thrombosis
  (DVT)
defecography
defect
atrial septal d. (ASD)
atrioventricular septal d.
biosynthetic d.
birth d.
central d.

coagulation d.
congenital d.
congenital ectodermic
  scalp d.
congenital heart d.
congenital hemidysplasia
  with icthyosiform
  erythroderma and
  limb d.'s (CHILD)
endocardial cushion d.
  (ECD)
genetic d.
genitourinary d.
iodide trap d.
luteal phase d.
neural tube d. (NTD)
ostium primum d.
ostium secundum d.
ovulatory d.
perineal d.
single-gene d.
sinus venosus d.
ventricular septal d. (VSD)
vertebral defects,
  imperforate anus,
  tracheoesophageal fistula,
  renal d.'s (VATER)
defeminization
defensive obstetrics
deferens
vas d.
deferoxamine
defibrillator
LifePak d.
deficiency
abdominal muscle d.
ACTH d.
arginase d.
brancher d.
carnitine d.
Cori enzyme d.
cytochrome *c* oxidase d.
debrancher enzyme d.
3β-dehydrogenase d.
disaccharidase d.
enterokinase d.
enzyme d.

NOTES

deficiency *(continued)*
    erythrocyte enzyme d.
    erythrocyte glutathione
      peroxidase d.
    factor I d.
    factor II d.
    factor III d.
    factor IV d.
    factor V d.
    factor VI d.
    factor VII d.
    factor VIII d.
    factor IX d.
    factor X d.
    factor XI d.
    factor XII d.
    factor XIII d.
    factor D d.
    factor H d.
    fibrinogen d.
    folic acid d.
    fructose galactokinase d.
    glucose-6-phosphate
      dehydrogenase d.
    gonadotropic d.
    hexosaminidase A d.
    17-hydroxylase d.
    IgA d.
    IgE d.
    IgM d.
    immune d.
    immunoglobulin d.
    intrinsic sphincter d. (IDS)
    nonclassic 21-hydroxylase d.
    phosphorylase kinase d.
    placental sulfatase d.
    prostacyclin d.
    proximal femoral focal d.
    pyruvate kinase d.
    red cell enzyme d.
    riboflavin d.
    skeletal calcium d.
    steroid sulfatase d.
    thymic-dependent d.
    thyroid d.
    transcobalamine d.
    xylulose dehydrogenase d.
deficit
    base d.
    focal neurological d.
    sensory d.
deflazacortum

deflexion
    d. abnormality
defloration
deformans
    cephalhematoma d.
    dystonia musculorum d.
    osteochondrodystrophia d.
deformation
deformity
    Arnold-Chiari d.
    cloverleaf skull d.
    congenital postural d.
    Dandy-Walker d.
    gibbous d.
    gooseneck d.
    hip d.
    joint d.
    lobster-claw d.
    Michel d.
    postural d.
    sabre shin d.
    spinning-top d.
    Sprengel d.
    Volkmann d.
degenerated fibroadenolipoma
degenerating myoma
degeneration
    carneous d.
    cerebellar d.
    cerebromacular d.
    congenital macular d.
    cystic myoma d.
    hepatolenticular d.
    hyaline myoma d.
    malignant d.
    molar d.
    mucoid myoma d.
    red d.
    sarcomatous myoma d.
    vitelliform d.
degradation
degree of kindred
dehiscence
    wound d.
dehydration
    d. fever
    hypernatremia d.
dehydroepiandrosterone (DHEA)
    d. sulfate (DHEAS)
    d. sulfate loading test
dehydrogenase
    3β-d. deficiency
    20α-dihydroprogestin d.

17β-estradiol d.
glucose-6-phosphate d.
  (G6PD)
15-hydroxyprostaglandin d.
3β-hydroxysteroid d.
  (3βHSD)
18-hydroxysteroid d.
lactate d. (LDH)
lactic acid d.
dehydroisoandrosterone
  d. sulfate
Dejerine disease
Dejerine-Klumpke syndrome
Dejerine-Sottas
  D.-S. atrophy
  D.-S. disease
Deladroxate
Deladumone
Delalutin
Delaprem
Delatest
Delatestryl
delay
  atrioventricular
    conduction d.
  constitutional d.
  developmental d.
delayed
  d. first stage
  d. hypersensitivity
  d. menarche
  d. menstruation
  d. puberty
del Castillo syndrome
Delclos
  D. cylinder
  D. ovoid
DeLee
  D. forceps
  D. instrumentation
  D. maneuver
  D. suctioning
  D. Universal retractor
Delestrogen
deletion
  autosomal d.
  chromosomal d.

13-q d. syndrome
gene d.
21-hydroxylase gene d.
interstitial d.
11p13 chromosome d.
terminal d.
Delfen
delinquency
delirium
delivered
  pregnancy, uterine, not d.
    (PUND)
delivery
  abdominal d.
  assisted breech d.
  assisted cephalic d.
  breech d.
  cesarean d.
  controlled vaginal d.
  Duncan mechanism of
    placental d.
  en caul d.
  failed forceps d.
  forceps d. (FD)
  high forceps d.
  labor and d. (L&D)
  low forceps d.
  midforceps d.
  d. mode
  outlet forceps d.
  oxygen d.
  perimortem d.
  postmortem d.
  precipitate labor and d.
  precipitous d.
  premature d.
  preterm d.
  rotational d.
  spontaneous cephalic d.
  spontaneous preterm d.
  sterile, spontaneous,
    controlled vaginal d.
    (SSCVD)
  sterile, spontaneous
    vaginal d. (SSVD)
  sunny-side up d.
  term d.

NOTES

delivery *(continued)*
 twin d.
 vacuum-assisted d.
 vacuum extractor d.
 vaginal d.
 vertex d.
Dellepiane hysterectomy
delta
 d. agent
 d. hepatitis
Deltalin
demecarium
demeclocycline
demedroxyprogesterone acetate (DMPA)
Demerol
4-demethyl-epipodophyllotoxin
demise
 fetal d.
Demons-Meigs syndrome
Demser
Demulen
 D. 1/35
 D. 1/50
demyelinating encephalopathy
dengue
Denhardt solution
denidation
Denis
Denis Browne
 D. B. bar
 D. B. clubfoot splint
 D. B. splint
Denman spontaneous evolution
Dennett diet
Dennie-Marfan syndrome
Dennis-Brown pouch
de novo
dense body
densitometer
 Expert bone d.
 Hologic 1000 QDR d.
density
 arterial linear d.
 bone mineral d. (BMD)
 fat d.
 hip bone d.
 hypoechoic d.
 optical d.
dental caries
dentatorubral-pallidoluysian atrophy
dentia precox
denticulate hymen

denumerable character
Denver
 D. classification
 D. Developmental Screening
 D. Developmental Screening Test (DDST)
 D. hydrocephalus shunt
deodorant artifact
deoxyadenylic acid (dAMP)
deoxycorticosterone (DOC)
deoxycytidylic acid (dCMP)
deoxyguanylic acid (dGMP)
deoxyribonuclease (DNase)
deoxyribonucleic
 d. acid (DNA)
 d. acid index
deoxythymidylic acid (dTMP)
Depakene
Department of Children and Youth Services (DCYS)
Depen
depGynogen
depigmentation
depigmentosus
 nevus d.
depletion
 juvenile spermatogonial d.
Depo-Estradiol
Depogen
depolarization
 ectopic ventricular d.
Depo-Medrol
depo-medroxyprogesterone
Depo-Provera
depot
 fat d.
 Lupron D.
Depotest
Depo-Testosterone
depression
 agitated d.
 fetal skull d.
 narcotic d.
 postpartum d.
 respiratory d.
deprivation
 antagonist-induced gonadotropin d.
 estrogen d.
depth dose
depth-dose distribution
Dercum disease
derepressed gene

derivation
  sexual d.
derivative
  acetoxyprogesterone d.
  17-alpha-
    acetoxyprogesterone d.
  d. chromosome
  coumarin d.
  19-nortestosterone d.
dermatitis, pl. dermatitides
  allergic d.
  atopic d.
  candidal diaper d.
  chronic bullous d.
  diaper d.
  d. excoriativa infantum
  d. exfoliativa infantum
  d. gangrenosa infantum
  d. herpetiformis
  irradiation d.
  Jacquet d.
  juvenile plantar d.
  nickel d.
  papular d. of pregnancy
  progesterone d.
  seborrheic d.
  d. venenata
  vulvar contact d.
  vulvar seborrheic d.
dermatofibroma
dermatomyositis
  primary idiopathic d.
dermatophytosis
dermatosis
  bullous d.
  dermolytic bullous d.
  plantar d.
dermocyma
dermoid
  d. cyst
  d. cyst of ovary
dermolytic bullous dermatosis
Deronil
DES
  diethylstilbestrol
  DES daughter
  DES exposure

DESAD
  National Collaborative
    Diethylstilbestrol Adenosis
    Project
desaturation
Descemet membrane
descending aorta
descensus
  d. uteri
descent
  fetal d.
  rapid d.
  rotation and d.
Deschamps ligature
descriptive embryology
desensitization
  pituitary d.
Desferal
desferrioxamine mesylate
designated donor blood
desipramine
desire
  inhibited sexual d.
Desitin
deslanoside
desmins
desmiognathus
desmocranium
desmolase
  cholesterol 20,22 d.
desmopressin
  desmopressin acetate
    (DDAVP)
desmosome
Desogen
desogestrel
  ethinyl estradiol and d.
  d. and ethinyl estradiol
DeSouza exercises
desoxycorticosterone (DOC)
Desoxyn
desquamation
desquamative inflammatory vaginitis
desquamativum
  erythroderma d.
desultory labor
Desyrel

NOTES

105

detachment
retinal d.
detection
d. bias
mammographic d.
prenatal d.
determinant
antigen d.
d. group
determination
blood gas d.
cell d.
emesis pH d.
gender d.
hemoglobin A_{Ic} d.
parentage d.
prenatal sex d.
scalp pH d.
sex d.
sweat chloride d.
testis d.
Dethyrona
Dethyrone
detrusor
d. hyperactivity with
impaired contractility
d. instability
d. muscle
d. sphincter dyssynergia
development
abnormal fetal d.
arrested d.
Bayley Scale of Infant D.
(BSID)
Briggance Diagnostic
Inventory of Early D.
CNS d.
early follicular d.
endometrial d.
excretory system d.
fetal d.
genital d.
goiter d.
male genital duct d.
mental d.
National Institute of Child
Health and Human D.
(NICHD)
neurologic d.
reproductive system d.
stromal d.
Tanner stages of d.

developmental
d. age (DA)
d. delay
d. diapause
d. level
d. stages
Deventer pelvis
deviation
sexual d.
standard d. (SD)
device
barium-impregnated plastic
intrauterine d.
Cameco syringe pistol
aspiration d.
contraceptive d.
Copper-7 intrauterine d.
Copper T intrauterine d.
double-umbrella d.
Hollister collecting d.
intrauterine d. (IUD)
intrauterine contraceptive
device (IUCD)
Lippes-type intrauterine d.
Makler insemination d.
Mucat cervical sampling d.
Multiload Cu-375
intrauterine d.
Nite Train-R enuresis
conditioning d.
Poly CS d.
Progestasert intrauterine d.
progesterone-releasing T-
shaped d.
Shug male contraceptive d.
Venodyne pneumatic
compressive d.
Wallach Endocell
collection d.
DeWeese axis traction forceps
Dewey obstetrical forceps
DEXA
dual-energy x-ray absorptiometry
Dex-A-Diet
dexamethasone
d. suppression test
Dexamfetamine
Dexatrim
dexbrompheniramine
dexchlorpheniramine
Dexedrine

Dexide
    D. disposable cannula
    D. disposable trocar
Dexone
Dexon suture
dexpanthenol
dexter
    cor triatriatum d.
dextran
    d. 40
    high molecular weight d.
    low molecular weight d.
Dextran-70 barrier material
dextroamphetamine
dextrocardia
dextro formula
dextrose
    d. in water
Dextrostix (D-stix)
dextrosuria
dextrothyroxine
dextrotransposition (D-transposition)
dextroversion
DFA
    direct fluorescent antigen
    DFA test
D-fenfluramine
D-galactose
dGMP
    deoxyguanylic acid
DHE
    dihydroergotamine
DHEA
    dehydroepiandrosterone
    DHEA sulfate
DHEAS
    dehydroepiandrosterone sulfate
DHT
    dihydrotestosterone
Diabeta
diabetes
    borderline d.
    brittle d.
    bronze d.
    chemical d.
    drug-induced d.

    gestational d.
    d. insipidus
    insulin-dependent d. mellitus
    (IDDM)
    juvenile d.
    juvenile-onset d.
    ketosis-prone d.
    ketosis-resistant d.
    latent d.
    maternal d.
    d. mellitus
    d. neonatorum
    non-insulin-dependent d.
    mellitus (NIDDM)
    overt insulin-dependent d.
    mellitus
diabetic
    d. acidosis
    d. coma
    d. embryopathy
    d. fetopathy
    insulin-dependent d.
    d. ketoacidosis (DKA)
    d. mother
    d. nephropathy
    non-insulin-dependent d.
    pregnant d.
    d. retinopathy
Diabinese
diacetate
    ethinyl estradiol and
    ethynodiol d.
    ethynodiol d.
diacylglycerol
diadochokinesis
diagnosis, pl. diagnoses
    antenatal d.
    colposcopic d.
    fetal d.
    genetic d.
    histologic d.
    histopathological d.
    neonatal d.
    prenatal d.
    prenatal genetic d.
    Prospective Investigation of d.

NOTES

diagnosis *(continued)*
    Pulmonary Embolus D.
    (PIOPED)
    ultrasound d.
diagnostic
    d. accuracy
    d. hysteroscope
    d. imaging
    d. procedure
    d. radiation
diagnostics
    Amplicor PCR d.
    DNA d.
    Franklin D.
    Roche D.
    Vivigen d.
diagonal conjugate
diakinesis
    d. stage
    d. stage of oocyte meiosis
Dialose
dialysate
dialysis, pl. dialyses
    continuous ambulatory
      peritoneal d. (CAPD)
    kidney d.
    peritoneal d.
dialytic parabiosis
diameter
    anteroposterior d. of the
      pelvic inlet
    aortic root d.
    Baudelocque d.
    biischial d.
    biparietal d. (BPD)
    bitemporal d.
    conjugate d. of the pelvic
      inlet
    fetal biparietal d.
    gestational sac mean d.
    internal d.
    intertuberous d.
    Loehlein d.
    d. mediana
    d. medianus
    oblique d., d. obliqua
    occipitofrontal d.
    occipitomental d.
    posterior sagittal d.
    suboccipitobregmatic d.
    trachelobregmatic d.
    transverse d., d. transversa

diamine oxidase
cis-**diamminedichloroplatinum**
    (DDP)
    c.-d. II
diamniotic
Diamond-Blackfan
    D.-B. congenital hypoplastic
      anemia
    D.-B. juvenile pernicious
      anemia
    D.-B. syndrome
diamond-shaped murmur
Diamox
Dianabol
Diana complex
Dianeal dialysis solution
diapause
    developmental d.
    embryonic d.
diaper
    d. dermatitis
    double d.'s
    triple d.'s
diaphanography
diaphragm
    contraceptive d.
    intrauterine d.
    Ortho All-Flex d.
    pelvic d.
    d. pessary
    urogenital d.
diaphragmatic
    d. agenesis
    d. hernia
diaphyseal
    d. aclasis
    d. dysplasia
Diapid
diarrhea
diastasis
    d. recti
diastematomyelia
diastolic murmur
diastrophic
    d. dwarfism
    d. dysplasia
diathermy
    d. current
    electrocoagulation d.
diathesis, pl. diatheses
    bleeding d.
    familial d.
    gouty d.

diatrizoate
diazepam
diazoxide
Dibbell
    D. cleft lip-nasal
      reconstruction
    D. cleft lip-nasal revision
Dibenzyline
dibrachia
dibromochloropropane (DBCP)
dibromodulcitol
    d. with doxorubicin and
      vincristine (DAV)
DIC
    diffuse intravascular coagulation
    disseminated intravascular
      coagulation
Dicarbosil
dicentric chromosome
dicephalus
dicheilia
dicheiria
dichloroacetic acid
dichlorphenamide
dichorial, dichorionic
    d. twins
dichorionic-diamniotic (di-di)
    d.-d. placenta
    d.-d. twins
diclofenac sodium
dicloxacillin sodium
dictyate
    d. stage
    d. stage of oocyte meiosis
dicumarol
    d. resistance
dicyclomine
didanosine
Diday law
didelphic uterus
didelphys
di-di
    dichorionic-diamniotic
didymus
Dieckmann intraosseous needle
diembryony

diencephalic syndrome
Dienestrol
    Ortho D.
dienestrol
Dienst test
diet
    ADA d.
    BRAT d.
    Dennett d.
    gluten-free d.
    high-calorie d.
    high-fiber d.
    low-cholesterol d.
    low-fat d.
    low-residue d.
    low-salt d.
    low-sodium d.
    Moro-Heisler d.
    Pulmocare d.
    vegetarian d.
dietary
    d. amenorrhea
    d. fat
    d. fiber
    d. problem
diethylamide
    lysergic acid d. (LSD)
diethylaminoethyl (DEAE)
diethylenetriamine pentaacetic acid
  (DPTA)
diethylpropion
diethylstilbestrol (DES)
difference
    alveolar-arterial pressure d.
      $(p(A\text{-}a)O_2)$
    arteriovenous oxygen d.
    d. in partial pressures of
      oxygen in mixed alveolar
      gas and mixed arterial
      blood $((A\text{-}a)D_{O2})$
    racial d.
differential
    d. cell count
    d. effect
    d. vascular resistance

NOTES

differentiation
central nervous system d.
fetal sexual d.
genital d.
male sex d.
sexual d.
testicular d.
difficile
Clostridium d.
diffuse
d. fasciitis
d. fibrocystic disease
d. intravascular coagulation (DIC)
Diflucan
DiGeorge syndrome
digestive system
Dighton-Adair syndrome
digit
supernumerary d.
digital
d. imaging colposcopy
d. radiography
digitalis
digitata
Laminaria d.
digitoxin
dignathus
digoxin
digoxin-like immunoreactive factor (DLIF)
dihydrate
azithromycin d.
dihydrocodeine bitartrate
dihydrocodeinone
dihydroergotamine (DHE)
d. mesylate
dihydrofolate
d. reductase
d. reductase inhibitor
dihydromorphinone hydrochloride
5α-dihydroprogesterone
20α-dihydroprogestin dehydrogenase
dihydrotachysterol
dihydrotestosterone (DHT)
dihydroxyphenylalanine (dopa, DOPA, Dopa)
dihydroxyprogesterone acetophenide
1,25-dihydroxyvitamin D_3
diiodohydroxyquin
diiodohydroxyquinoline
diiodothyronine (T_2)
d. test

diisopropyl fluorophosphate
diisopropyl-iminodiacetic acid (DISIDA)
Dilantin
Dilapan
D. hygroscopic cervical dilator
D. laminaria
dilatation
d. and curettage (D & C)
esophageal d.
d. and evacuation (D & E)
dilated
d. collateral vein
fingertip d.
dilation
cervical d.
d. of cervix
d. and curettage (D & C)
d. and evacuation (D & E)
Frank technique of d.
d. of ventricle
dilator
Dilapan hygroscopic cervical d.
Goodell d.
Hanks d.
Hegar d.
Hurtig d.
laminaria cervical d.
Lucite d.
Pharmaseal disposable cervical d.
Pratt d.
vaginal d.
Walther d.
Dilaudid
dildo, dildoe
dimelia
Dimelor
dimenhydrinate
dimension
left atrial d. (LAD)
dimercaptosuccinic acid
Dimetabs
Dimetane
dimethindene maleate
dimethothiazine mesylate
dimethylsulfoxide (DMSO)
dimethyl-triazeno-imidazole carboxamide (DTIC)
dimethylxanthine
dimetria

dimidiate
dimorphism
    sexual d.
dimple
    pilonidal d.
    sacral d.
    vaginal d.
Dinamap blood pressure monitor
dinitrate
    isosorbide d.
dinitrochlorobenzene
dinitrofluorobenzene
dinoprost
    d. tromethamine
dinoprostone
    d. cervical gel
Diocto
Diodoquin
Dioeze
3α-diol-G
    5α-androstane-3α,17β-diol
    glucuronide
diosgenin
Diosuccin
Dio-Sul
Dioval
diovular twins
dioxide
    carbon d. (CO_2)
    fraction of alveolar
      carbon d. ($FACO_2$)
    fraction in expired gas of
      carbon d. ($FECO_2$)
    partial pressure of arterial
      carbon d. ($PaCO_2$)
    partial pressure of
      carbon d. (PCO_2)
dioxin
dioxyline
dipalmitoylphosphatidylcholine
diphallus
diphemanil methylsulfate
diphenadione
Diphenadryl
Diphenatol
diphenhydramine
Diphenylan Sodium

diphenylhydantoin
diphenylthiourea
diphosphate
    menadiol sodium d.
diphosphate-choline
    cytidine d.-c.
diphosphate-diacylglycerol
    cytidine d.-d.
diphosphoglycerate
diphtheria
diphtheria, pertussis, tetanus
    (DPT)
diphyllobothriasis
Diphyllobothrium latum
diplegia
    atonic-astatic d.
    facial d.
    infantile d.
    spastic d.
Diplococcus pneumoniae
diplogenesis
diploid
    d. cell
    d. distribution
    d. merogony
diploidy
diplomyelia
diplopagus
diplopia
diplosomatia
diplosome
diplotene
    d. phase of meiosis
diploteratology
dipodia
diproprionate
    beclomethasone d.
dipstick
dipus
dipygus parasiticus
dipyridamole
direct
    d. agglutination pregnancy
    (DAP)
    d. fluorescent antigen
    (DFA)

NOTES

direct *(continued)*
    d. fluorescent antigen test (DFA test)
    d. intraperitoneal insemination
    d. oocyte sperm transfer (DOST)
    d. oocyte transfer (DOT)
direction
    pelvic d.
disability
    neurodevelopmental d.
disaccharidase deficiency
Disalcid
disappearance
    fetal d.
disaturated
    d. lecithin
    d. phosphatidylcholine
disc *(var. of* disk)
discharge
    cheesy d.
    gleety d.
    mucous d.
    nipple d.
    pulsatile d.
    urethral d.
    vaginal d.
discoplacenta
discordance
    atrioventricular d.
discordancy
    growth d.
discordant artery flow velocity waveform
discrepancy
    size-date d.
discrete
    d. character
    d. random variable
    d. variable
discus proligerus
disease
    ABO hemolytic d. of the newborn
    acute fatty liver d.
    Addison d.
    adhesive d.
    Albright d.
    Alexander d.
    allogeneic d.
    Alpers d.
    Andersen d.

    antiglomerular basement membrane antibody d.
    aortic valve d.
    Apert d.
    Apert-Crouzon d.
    Aran-Duchenne d.
    arterial occlusive d.
    arterial vascular d.
    autoimmune d.
    Azorean d.
    Barlow d.
    Bassen-Kornzweig d.
    Batten-Mayou d.
    Beck d.
    Béguez César d.
    benign breast d.
    Berger renal d.
    Best d.
    Bielschowsky-Jansky d.
    Bloodgood d.
    Blount d.
    Bornholm d.
    Bourneville d.
    breast d.
    Brown-Symmers d.
    Bruton d.
    bubble boy d.
    Buhl d.
    Byler d.
    Caffey d.
    Caffey-Kenny d.
    Canavan d.
    Caroli d.
    cat-scratch d.
    celiac d.
    central nervous system d.
    cerebrovascular d.
    Chagas d.
    Charcot-Marie-Tooth d.
    Cheadle d.
    cholesterol ester storage d.
    Christmas d.
    chronic lung d. (CLD)
    chronic vascular d.
    Coats d.
    collagen vascular d.
    communicable d.
    congenital heart d.
    Conradi d.
    contractural arachnodactyly d.
    Cori d.
    coronary artery d.

coronary heart d.
Crohn d.
Crouzon d.
Csillag d.
Cushing d.
cyanotic congenital heart d.
  (CCHD)
cystic d. of the breast
cytomegalic inclusion d.
cytomegalovirus d.
Danlos d.
Dawson d.
Dejerine d.
Dejerine-Sottas d.
Dercum d.
diffuse fibrocystic d.
distal tubal d.
Dukes d.
Duroziez d.
end-stage kidney d.
Erb-Goldflam d.
ethanolaminosis in glycogen-
  storage d.
extramammary Paget d.
Fabry d.
Farber d.
Feer d.
fetal heart d.
fibrocystic d.
fifth d.
fifth venereal d.
Filatov-Dukes d.
Folling d.
Forbes d.
Fordyce d.
fourth venereal d.
Fox-Fordyce d.
Freiberg d.
gallbladder d.
ganglioside storage d.
Gaucher d.
Gee d.
Gee-Herter d.
Gee-Herter-Heubner d.
genetic d.
genetotrophic d.

gestational trophoblastic d.
  (GTD)
Gierke d.
Gilbert d.
Glanzmann d.
Glenard d.
glycogen-storage d.
Goldstein d.
graft-versus-host d. (GVHD)
Graves d.
Greenfield d.
Günther d.
Hailey-Hailey d.
Hallervorden-Spatz d.
Hand-Schüller-Christian d.
Hansen d.
Hartnup d.
heart d.
Heller-Döhle d.
helminthic d.
hemoglobin C d.
hemoglobin H d.
hemoglobin M d.
hemolytic d. of the
  newborn (HDN)
hemorrhagic d.
Henoch d.
hereditary d.
heredoconstitutional d.
heredodegenerative d.
Hers d.
Hirschsprung d.
Hodgkin d.
homologous d.
Hünermann d.
Huntington d.
Hutinel d.
hyaline membrane d.
  (HMD)
hydatid d.
hydrocephaloid d.
hypothalamic d.
I-cell d.
infantile celiac d.
infantile polycystic
  kidney d. (IPKD)
infectious d.

NOTES

disease *(continued)*
    inflammatory bowel d.
    International Society for the
      Study of Vulvar D.'s
      (ISSVD)
    intraperitoneal endometrial
      metastatic d.
    ischemic heart d.
    Jaksch d.
    Jeune d.
    Joseph d.
    Kashin-Beck d.
    Kawasaki d. (KD)
    kidney d.
    Kikuchi d.
    Kimmelstiel-Wilson d. (KW)
    kinky hair d.
    Kohdschnetter d.
    Köhler bone d.
    Kozlowski d.
    Krabbe d.
    Kramer d.
    Krause d.
    Kufs d.
    Kugelberg-Welander d.
    kwashiorkor d.
    kyphoscoliotic heart d.
    Lafora body d.
    Langdon Down d.
    Leber d.
    Legg-Calvé-Perthes d.
    Legionnaire d.
    Leigh d.
    Leiner d.
    Letterer-Siwe d.
    Little d.
    liver d.
    Lobstein d.
    Luft d.
    Lyell d.
    Lyme d.
    lyosomal storage d.
    Machado-Joseph d.
    Maher d.
    maple syrup urine d.
      (MSUD)
    Marion d.
    maternal cyanotic heart d.
    McArdle d.
    medullary cystic d.
    Melnick-Needles d.
    Menkes d.
    Merzbacher-Pelizaeus d.

Milroy d.
Minamata d.
Minot d.
mixed connective-tissue d.
Moeller-Barlow d.
Mondor d.
Morquio d.
moyamoya d.
neoplastic trophoblastic d.
New York Heart
  Association classification of
  heart d.
Nicolas-Favre d.
Niemann-Pick d.
nonmetastatic gestational
  trophoblastic d. (NMGTD)
Norrie d.
Oppenheim d.
Osgood-Schlatter d.
Osler-Weber-Rendu d.
Owren d.
oxygen toxicity lung d.
Paas d.
Paget d.
Panner d.
parathyroid d.
Parkinson d.
Pelizaeus-Merzbacher d.
pelvic adhesive d. (PAD)
pelvic inflammatory d.
  (PID)
peptic ulcer d.
Peyronie d.
Phocas d.
phytanic acid storage d.
pink d.
placental site gestational
  trophoblastic d.
polycystic kidney d. (PKD)
polycystic ovarian d.
polycystic renal d.
Pompe d.
Portuguese d.
postpartum pleuropulmonary
  and cardiac d.
Potter d.
preinvasive cervical d.
premalignant d.
psychosomatic d.
pulmonary d.
pulmonary parenchymal d.
pulseless d.
Raussly d.

reactive airway d. (RAD)
Recklinghausen d.
Recklinghausen d. type 1
Reclus d.
Refsum d.
renal d.
Rh d.
rhesus D d.
rhesus hemolytic d.
rheumatic d.
rheumatic heart d.
Rh hemolytic d.
Riga-Fede d.
Ritter d.
runt d.
Sandhoff d.
Saunders d.
S-C d.
Scheuermann d.
Schilder d.
Schimmelbusch d.
Scholz d.
sclerocystic d. of the ovary
S-D d.
    sickle cell-hemoglobin D
    disease
secretory d.
Seitelberger d.
severe combined
  immunodeficiency d.
  (SCID)
sexually transmitted d.
  (STD)
sickle cell d.
sickle cell-hemoglobin C d.
  (S-C disease)
sickle cell-hemoglobin D d.
  (S-D disease, S-D disease)
sickle cell-hemoglobin S d.
sickle cell-thalassemia d.
sickle cell-β-thalassemia d.
silent pelvic
  inflammatory d.
Simmonds d.
Siver d.
sixth d.
skin d.

Sly d.
Spielmeyer-Vogt d.
spinocerebellar
  degenerative d.
Stargardt d.
startle d.
Steinert d.
Sticker d.
Still d.
Strumpell-Lorrain d.
Swift d.
Tangier d.
Taussig-Bing d.
Tay-Sachs d.
Thiemann d.
third d.
Thomsen d.
Thomson d.
thromboembolic d. (TED)
thyroid d.
Tillaux d.
Trevor d.
trophoblastic d.
trophoblastic neoplastic d.
tubulointerstitial d.
underlying renal d.
Underwood d.
Unverricht d.
valvular heart d.
van Bogaert d.
vascular d.
venereal d.
Vogt-Spielmeyer d.
Volkmann d.
Voltolini d.
von Gierke d.
von Hippel-Lindau d.
von Recklinghausen d.
von Willebrand d.
Vrolik d.
Wegner d.
Weil d.
Werdnig-Hoffmann d.
Werlhof d.
Whipple d.
Wilkins d.
Williams d.

NOTES

disease *(continued)*
    Wilson d.
    Winckel d.
    Wolman d.
    wooly-hair d.
    X-linked d.
    X-linked dominant d.
    X-linked recessive d.
disengagement
disgerminoma
dish
    d. face
    insemination d.
DISIDA
    diisopropyl-iminodiacetic acid
disiens
    Prevotella d.
disinfectant
    Sklar asceptic germicidal d.
    Sklarsoak d.
disintegrin
Disipal
disk, disc
    AccuPoint hCG Pregnancy
      Test D.
    embryonic d.
dislocation
    congenital hip d. (CHD)
disodium
    cefotetan d.
    etidronate d.
    intermittent cyclical
      etidronate d.
    moxalactam d.
    ticarcillin d.
D isoimmunization
disomus
disomy
    uniparental d.
Disonate
disopyramide
disorder
    affective d.
    alpha-chain d.
    arrest d.
    attention deficit d. (ADD)
    attention deficit
      hyperactivity d. (ADHD)
    autosomal chromosome d.
    autosomal dominant d.
    autosomal recessive d.
    brain d.

    carnitine transferase
      enzyme d.
    chromosome 9p d.
    coagulation d.
    connective tissue d.
    eating d.
    endocrine d.
    familial bipolar mood d.
    gamma-chain d.
    gamma-loop d.
    gastrointestinal d.
    genetic d.
    hematologic d.
    hematopoietic d.
    heme metabolism d.
    hepatic d.
    hypothalamic-pituitary d.
    inherited d.
    lipid metabolism d.
    lysosomal enzyme d.
    mendelian genetic d.
    metabolic d.
    metal metabolism d.
    musculoskeletal d.
    neurologic d.
    ovarian d.
    parathyroid d.
    pervasive developmental d.
      (PDD)
    pituitary d.
    platelet d.
    polygenic d.
    porphyrin metabolism d.
    premenstrual dysphoric d.
      (PMDD)
    pulmonary d.
    purine metabolism d.
    recessive d.
    reproductive d.
    rheumatologic d.
    seizure d.
    transport d.
    urinary tract d.
    X-linked d.
dispermy
disperse placenta
displacement implantation
display
    M-mode d.
disproportion
    cephalopelvic d. (CPD)
    fetopelvic d.
disputed maternity

disruption
    anal sphincter d.
    perineal sphincter d.
dissecans
    osteochondritis d.
dissecting aortic aneurysm
dissection
    gauze d.
    groin d.
    inguinal-femoral node d.
    partial zona d.
    pelvic node d.
    selective inguinal node d.
dissector
    ENDO-ASSIST cutting d.
    Kitner d.
    Polaris reusable d.
disseminated
    d. gonococcal infection
    d. gonorrhea
    d. infection
    d. intravascular coagulation
    (DIC)
dissemination
    iatrogenic d.
disseminatus
    lupus erythematosus d.
dissimilar twins
dissociation
    d. constant
    hemoglobin-oxygen d.
distal
    d. occlusion
    d. tubal disease
    d. tubal microsurgery
    d. tubal obstruction
distance
    source-to-axis d. (SAD)
    source-to-skin d. (SSD)
distasonis
    Bacteroides d.
distention
    abdominal d.
distigmine bromide
distress
    fetal d.
    iatrogenic fetal d.

    neonatal d.
    respiratory d.
    transient fetal d.
distribution
    binomial d.
    depth-dose d.
    diploid d.
    tetraploid d.
disturbance
    architectural d.
    mental d.
    ovulatory d.
    visual d.
disulfiram
Ditropan
Diucardin
Diuchlor H
Diulo
Diurese-R
diuresis, pl. diureses
diuretic
    thiazide d.
Diuril
diurnus
    pavor d.
diversion
    continent supravesical bowel
    urinary d.
    ileal d.
    urinary d.
diverticula (*pl. of* diverticulum)
diverticulitis
diverticulosis
diverticulum, pl. diverticula
    Meckel d.
    Nuck d.
    pharyngeal d.
    tubal d.
    urethral d.
diverting colostomy
diving reflex
division
    cellular d.
    equatorial d.
    meiotic d.
    miotic d.

NOTES

division *(continued)*
    premature centromere d.
    transcervical d.
dizygotic twin
dizygous
DKA
    diabetic ketoacidosis
DLIF
    digoxin-like immunoreactive
    factor
DM
    Poly-Histine DM
6-DMAP
DMPA
    demedroxyprogesterone acetate
DMSO
    dimethylsulfoxide
DNA
    deoxyribonucleic acid
    DNA amplification
    DNA cloning
    complementary DNA
     (cDNA)
    DNA copy
    DNA diagnostics
    DNA fingerprinting
    genome DNA
    DNA hybridization
    DNA index
    DNA library
    DNA ligase
    DNA marker
    mitochondrial DNA
    DNA
     nucleotidylexotransferase
    DNA nucleotidyltransferase
    plasmid DNA
    DNA polymerase
    DNA probe
    recombinant DNA
    DNA sequence
    Y-specific DNA
DNA-directed
    DNA-d. polymerase
    DNA-d. RNA polymerase
DNase
    deoxyribonuclease
DOB
    date of birth
dobutamine
    d. hydrochloride
Dobutrex

DOC
    deoxycorticosterone
    desoxycorticosterone
docusate
    d. calcium
    d. sodium
Döderlein
    D. bacillus
    D. method
    D. method of vaginal
     hysterectomy
    D. roll-flap operation
dog-like facies
Döhle body
Dolacet
Dolanex
Dolene
dolichocephalic
    d. head
dolichopellic, dolichopelvic
doll
    d. eye reflex
    d. head maneuver
Dolophine
dome cell
dominance
    thromboxane d.
dominant
    autosomal d. (AD)
    d. follicle
    d. gene
    d. inheritance
    d. lethal trait
Donahue-Uchida syndrome
Donald-Fothergill operation
Donald procedure
donation
    autologous blood d.
    embryo d.
    oocyte d.
    sperm d.
Donohue syndrome
donor
    artificial insemination d.
    artificial insemination by d.
    (AID)
    embryo d.
    oocyte d.
    sperm d.
    d. sperm
donor-specific blood
Donovan body
donovanosis

DOOR
deafness, onycho-
osteodystrophy, mental
retardation
DOOR syndrome
dopa, DOPA, Dopa
dihydroxyphenylalanine
L-**dopa**
levodopa
Dopamet
dopamine
d. agonist
d. hydrochloride
d. receptor agonist
dopaminergic agonist
Dopar
Dopcord recorder
Doppler
color-flow D.
2-D D.
D. effect
D. evaluation
D. flow
D. flow-velocity wave form
IMEX Pocket-Dop OB D.
D. principle
range-gated D. (RGD)
D. shift
D. shift spectra
spectral D.
D. ultrasonography
D. ultrasound
D. velocimetry
D. waveform
Dopplex
Fetal D.
Dopram
Doptone fetal stethoscope
dornase alfa
dorsal
d. birthing position
d. lithotomy position
d. penile nerve block
Doryx
dose, dosage
average radiation d.
central axis depth d.

depth d.
HypRho-D Mini D.
maximal permissible d.
minimum lethal d. (MLD)
physiologic replacement d.
radiation d.
radiation-absorbed d. (rad)
DOST
direct oocyte sperm transfer
DOT
direct oocyte transfer
dot
Schuffner d.'s
dot-blot
d.-b. hybridization
d.-b. procedure
d.-b. technique
dothiepin
double
d. cell
d. diapers
d. gloving
d. helix
d. ring
d. ureter
double-balloon catheter
double-bank bili lights
double-breech presentation
double-bubble
d.-b. flushing reservoir
d.-b. isolette
d.-b. sign
double-focus tube
double-footling presentation
double-freeze technique
double-inlet
d.-i. left ventricle
d.-i. right ventricle
double-J stent
double-mouthed uterus
double-tooth tenaculum
double-umbrella device
double-volume exchange transfusion
double-walled
d.-w. bubble isolette
d.-w. incubator
doubling time

NOTES

douche, douching
 fan d.
 Fritsch d.
 iodine d.
 Massengill d.
 maternal d.
 povidone-iodine d.
 vaginal d.
 yogurt d.
doughnut pessary
Douglas
 D. abscess
 cul-de-sac of D.
 D. cul-de-sac
 D. mechanism
 D. method
 D. pouch
 D. spontaneous evolution
douglascele
dovetail sign
dowager's hump
down
 clamped d.
 D. syndrome
 testes d.
doxacurium chloride
doxapram hydrochloride
doxepin
doxorubicin
 d. hydrochloride
Doxy
 doxycycline
 Doxy-Caps
Doxychel
doxycycline (Doxy)
 d. hyclate
 d. monohydrate
doxylamine
Doyen vaginal hysterectomy
Doyle operation
D^u-positive mother
DPT
 diphtheria, pertussis, tetanus
 DPT vaccine
DPTA
 diethylenetriamine pentaacetic
 acid
DR
 human lymphocyte antigen-
 locus DR
dragon
 d. pyelogram
 d. sign

drain
 butterfly d.
 fluted d.
 Freyer suprapubic d.
 Hysto-vac d.
 Jackson-Pratt suction d.
 Penrose d.
 retroperitoneal d.
drainage
 closed d.
 hematoma d.
 lymphatic d.
 lymph node d.
 percutaneous d.
 pulmonary venous d.
 suction d.
 waterseal d.
Dramamine
Dramilin
Dramocen
Dramoject
drape
 Barrier laparoscopy d.
 Ioban d.
 OPMI d.
 Steri-Drape d.
Drash syndrome
dressing
 Biobrane/HF d.
 Coban d.
 d. forceps
Drew-Smythe catheter
Dri-Dot
 Prognosticon D.-D.
drift
 genetic d.
 pure random d.
drill
 bladder d.
drilling
 zona d.
Drinker respirator
Dripps–American Society of
 Anesthesiologists classification
Drisdol
Drize
dromedary hump
drooling
droperidol
drops
 Ayr saline d.
 Phazyme infant d.

drug
    d. addiction
    adrenergic d.
    anticholinergic d.
    anticonvulsant d.
    antihypertensive d.
    antimalarial d.
    antineoplastic d.
    antipsychotic d.
    antithyroid d.
    beta-adrenergic d.
    cholinergic d.
    d. fever
    intravenous d.
    nonestrogen d.
    nonsteroidal anti-
      inflammatory d. (NSAID)
    psychiatric d.
    psychoactive d.
    psychotropic d.
    recreational d.
    social d.
drug-depressed infant
drug-induced diabetes
dry
    d. birth
    d. labor
    d. vagina
DS
    Septra D.
D-stix
    Dextrostix
DTIC
    dimethyl-triazeno-imidazole
      carboxamide
    DTIC -Dome
dTMP
    deoxythymidylic acid
DTR
    deep tendon reflex
D-transposition
    dextrotransposition
dual-energy
    d.-e. photon absorptiometry
    d.-e. x-ray absorptiometry
      (DEXA)
dual-photon absorptiometry

Duane
    D. anomaly
    D. syndrome
DUB
    dysfunctional uterine bleeding
Dubin-Johnson syndrome
Dubois abscess
Dubowitz
    D. evaluation
    D. examination
    D. Neurological Assessment
    D. score
Duchenne
    D. muscular dystrophy
    D. paralysis
duckbill speculum
Duckett procedure
Duckey nipple
Ducrey bacillus
duct
    allantoic d.
    Bartholin d.
    branchial d.'s
    cloacal d.
    cowperian d.
    focally dilated d.
    Gartner d.
    gartnerian d.
    genital d.
    lactiferous d.
    male genital d.
    mesonephric d.
    metanephric d.
    müllerian d.
    nasolacrimal d.
    omphalomesenteric d.
    paramesonephric d.
    paraurethral d.
    Reichel cloacal d.
    Skene d.
    solitary dilated d.
    Stensen d.
    vestibular d.
    vitelline d.
    vitello-intestinal d.
    wolffian d.

NOTES

ductal
  d. adenoma
  d. carcinoma
  d. ectasia
  d. hyperplasia
  d. papilloma
ductal-dependent
  d.-d. lesion
  d.-d. pulmonary circulation
ductule
ductuli efferentia
ductus
  d. arteriosus (DA)
  d. venosus
Duffy system
Dufourmentel technique
Dukes
  D. classification
  D. disease
Dulbecco phosphate buffered saline
Dulcolax
dullness
  absolute cardiac d.
  area of cardiac d. (ACD)
dummy
  d. source
  d. spacer
Dumontpallier pessary
Duncan
  D. curette
  D. folds
  D. mechanism
  D. mechanism of placental
    delivery
  D. placenta
  D. position
  D. presentation
duodenal
  d. atresia
  d. duplication
  d. ileus
  d. obstruction
  d. ulcer
Duosol
Duotrate
Duphalac
duplex
  d. scanning
  d. ultrasound
  d. uterus
duplication
  caudal d.
  cranial d.

duodenal d.
fetal d.
gene d.
d. of ileum
renal d.
ureteral d.
duplication-deficiency syndrome
duplicitas
  d. anterior
  d. symmetros
Durabolin
Duracillin AS
Dura-Estrin
Duragen
Duralon-UV nylon membrane
dural spinal angioma
Duralutin
Duramorph
Dura Neb portable nebulizer
DuraPrep surgical solution
Duraquin
Duratest
Durathate
Duretic
Duroziez disease
duskiness
dusky skin
Dutch
  D. cap
  D. pessary
Duverney gland
Duvoid
DVT
  deep vein thrombosis
  deep venous thrombosis
dwarf
  achrondoplastic d.
  d. pelvis
  d. syndrome
dwarfism
  achondroplastic d.
  Amsterdam d.
  asexual d.
  ateliotic d.
  bird-headed d.
  Brissaud d.
  chondroplastic d.
  constitutional d.
  cretin d.
  diastrophic d.
  geleophysic d.
  hypophysial d.
  hypothyroid d.

infantile d.
Kniest d.
Langer mesomelic d.
Laron-type d.
lethal d.
Levi-Lorain d.
micromelic d.
nanocephalic d.
pituitary d.
primordial d.
rhizomelic d.
Robinow d.
Russell-Silver d.
Saldino-Noonan d.
Seckel d.
sexual d.
short-limb d.
short-rib d.
Silver d.
thanatophoric d.
Walt Disney d.
Dyadic Adjustment Scale
Dyazide
Dyban technique
Dycill
Dyclone
dydrogesterone
dye
  azo d.
  Evans blue d.
  indigo carmine d.
  triple d.
Dyflos
Dyggve-Melchior-Clausen syndrome
dying
Dyke-Davidoff syndrome
Dymelor
Dymenate
dynamic image on ultrasound
dynamics
  androgen d.
Dynapen
dynorphin
Dynothel
Dyonic DyoBride 300 illuminator
dyphylline
Dyrenium

dysadrenalism
dysautonomia
  familial d.
dysbetalipoproteinemia
dyscephaly
dyschezia
dyschondroplasia
dyscrasia
  blood d.
dysdiadochokinesis
dysembryoma
dysembryoplasia
dysencephalia splanchnocystica
dysentery
  amebic d.
  bacillary d.
dysfibrinogenemia
dysfunction
  bladder d.
  cerebral d.
  corpus luteum d.
  family d.
  hypertonic uterine d.
  hypothalamic d.
  hypothalamic-pituitary
    axis d.
  hypotonic uterine d.
  lymphocyte d.
  placental d.
  postoperative bladder d.
  postoperative voiding d.
  sexual d.
  thyroid d.
  urinary bladder d.
  uterine d.
  voiding d.
dysfunctional
  d. family
  d. labor pattern
  d. uterine bleeding (DUB)
dysgammaglobulinemia
dysgenesia
dysgenesis
  gonadal d.
  mixed gonadal d.
  ovarian d.
  pure gonadal d.

NOTES

123

dysgenesis *(continued)*
    renal d.
    X-linked recessive d.
    XY gonadal d.
dysgenitalism
dysgerminoma
    ovarian d.
dyshepatia
    lipogenic d.
dyshidrosis
dyshidrotic eczema
dyshormonogenesis
dyskaryosis
dyskeratosis congenita
dyskinesia
dyslexia
dysmature
dysmaturity
    d. syndrome
dysmenorrhea
    essential d.
    functional d.
    intrinsic d.
    mechanical d.
    membranous d.
    obstructive d.
    ovarian d.
    primary d.
    secondary d.
    spasmodic d.
    tubal d.
    ureteral d.
    uterine d.
    vaginal d.
dysmenorrheal membrane
dysmorphic
dysmorphism
dysmorphology
dysmotility
dysmyelinisatus
    status d.
dysnomia
dysontogenesis
dysontogenetic cyst
dysorganoplasia
dysosteogenesis
dysosteoses (*pl. of* dystosis)
dysostosis
    acrofacial d.
    cleidocranial d.
    craniofacial d.
    epiphyseal d.
    mandibulofacial d.

    metaphyseal d.
    d. multiplex
    Nager acrofacial d.
    orodigitofacial d.
dyspareunia
    Friedrich criteria for d.
dysplasia
    anhidrotic ectodermal d.
    arteriohepatic d.
    asphyxiating thoracic d.
    bronchopulmonary d. (BPD)
    camptomelic d.
    cervical d.
    chondroectodermal d.
    cleidocranial d.
    congenital alveolar d.
    craniodiaphyseal d.
    craniometaphyseal d.
    cretinoid d.
    de la Chapelle d.
    diaphyseal d.
    diastrophic d.
    ectodermal d.
    endocervical glandular d.
    d. epiphysealis hemimelia
    d. epiphysealis punctata
    faciogenital d.
    fetal skeletal d.
    frontometaphyseal d.
    hereditary bone d.
    hidrotic ectodermal d.
    high-grade cervical d.
    Holt-Oram atriodigital d.
    hydrocephalus, agyria,
      retinal d. (HARD)
    intraepithelial cervical d.
    Kniest d.
    Langer d.
    mammary d.
    mesomelic d.
    metaphoric d.
    metaphyseal d.
    metatropic d.
    oculoauricular d.
    oculoauriculovertebral d.
    oculodentodigital d.
    ophthalmomandibulomelic d.
    polycystic fibrous d.
    polyostotic fibrous d.
    punctate epiphyseal d.
    radiation d.
    renal d.
    Robinow mesomelic d.

skeletal d.
spondyloepiphyseal d.
spondylometaphyseal d.
Streeter d.
thanatophoric d.
thymic d.
trichorhinophalangeal d.
dysplasia-clefting
ankyloblepharon-
ectodermal d.-c. (AEC)
dysplastic
d. cell
dyspnea
paroxysmal nocturnal d.
(PND)
dyspraxia
dysraphia of spine
dysraphism
dysrhythmia
cardiac d.
gastric d.
dysspermia
dyssynergia
detrusor sphincter d.
dystaxia cerebralis infantilis
dysthymic
dysthyroidal infantilism
dystocia
cervical d.
fetal d.
maternal d.
placental d.
shoulder d.
dystocia-dystrophia syndrome
dystonia
d. musculorum deformans
torsion d.
dystosis, pl. dysostoses
cleidocranial d.

craniofacial d.
mandibulofacial d.
metaphyseal d.
orodigitofacial d.
dystrophic calcification
dystrophin gene
dystrophy
asphyxiating thoracic d.
Becker muscular d.
congenital myotonic d.
craniocarpotarsal d.
Duchenne muscular d.
Erb juvenile muscular d.
facioscapulohumeral
muscular d.
infantile neuroaxonal d.
juvenile epithelial corneal d.
Landouzy-Dejerine
muscular d.
Leyden-Möbius muscular d.
limb-girdle d.
limb-girdle muscular d.
macular d.
Meesman d.
muscular d.
myotonic d.
oculocerebrorenal d.
oculopharyngeal muscular d.
reflex sympathetic d. (RSD)
severe childhood autosomal
recessive muscular d.
(SCARMD)
short-limb d.
Steinert myotonic d.
twenty-nail d.
vulvar d.
dysuria
dysuria-sterile pyuria syndrome
dyszoospermia

NOTES

E₁
  estrone
E₂
  estradiol
E₃
  estriol
EA
  early amniocentesis
EACA
  ε-aminocaproic acid
  epsilon-aminocaproic acid
Eagle-Barrett syndrome
Eagle test
ear
  Aztec e.
  bat e.
  cup e.
  Darwin e.
  lop e.
  low-set e.'s
  Morel e.
  Mozart e.
  satyr e.
  scroll e.
  Wildermuth e.
early
  e. amniocentesis (EA)
  e. cardiac motion
  e. deceleration
  e. embryonic death
  e. embryonic loss
  e. follicular development
  e. neonate
  E. and Periodic Screening, Diagnosis, and Treatment program (EPSDT)
  e. pregnancy factor
  e. pregnancy loss
  e. pregnancy test (EPT)
  e. pregnancy wastage
  e. stromal invasion
early-onset preeclampsia
Eastern
  E. blot
  E. blot test
Easy
  Clearblue E.
  Clearplan E.

eating
  e. disorder
  e. habits
EBNS
  endoscopic bladder neck suspension
Ebola hemorrhagic fever
Ebstein anomaly
EBV
  Epstein-Barr virus
ECBI
  Eyberg Child Behavior Inventory
ecbolic
ECC
  endocervical curettage
  extracorporeal circulation
eccentrochondroplasia
ecchymosis
eccouchement forcé
eccrine gland
eccyesis
ECD
  endocardial cushion defect
ECG
  electrocardiogram
echinococcal cyst
echinocyte
ECHO
  enteric cytopathogenic human orphan
    ECHO virus
echo
  echocardiogram
  e. formation
  scattered e.
  specular e.
echocardiogram (echo)
  color e.
  2-D e.
  M-mode e.
  two-dimensional e.
echocardiography
echodensity
echoencephalogram
echoencephalography
echogenic
  e. tissue
echogenicity
echogram
  M-mode e.

echolucency
echolucent
echoplanar magnetic resonance
  imaging
echothiophate iodide
eclampsia
    puerperal e.
    superimposed e.
eclamptic
    e. retinopathy
    e. seizure
eclamptogenic, eclamptogenous
ECM
    erythema chronicum migrans
    ECM rash
ECMO
    extracorporeal membrane
    oxygenation
ECOR
    extracorporeal CO_2 removal
Ecotrin
ectasia, ectasis
    ductal e.
    familial aortic e.
    mammary duct e.
ecthyma
ectocervical
ectocervix
ectoderm
ectodermal dysplasia
ectolecithal
ectomere
ectomesoblast
ectopagus
ectoparasite
ectopia
    e. cordis
    e. lentis
    renal e.
    ureteral e.
ectopic
    e. anus
    e. decidua
    e. endometrial tissue
    e. pregnancy
    e. ureter
    e. ventricular depolarization
ectrodactyly
    e., ectodermal dysplasia,
      clefting (EEC)
    e., ectodermal dysplasia,
      clefting syndrome
ectromelia

ectrometacarpia
ectrometatarsia
ectrophalangia
ectropion
    cervical e.
    congenital e.
ectrosyndactyly
eczema
    dyshidrotic e.
    e. herpeticum
    infantile e.
    e. marginatum
    e. neonatorum
    nummular e.
    e. vaccinatum
eczematoid
EDC
    estimated date of conception
    estimated date of confinement
    expected date of confinement
Eddowes syndrome
Edebohl position
Edecrin
edema
    angioneurotic e.
    brawny e.
    cerebral e.
    gestational e.
    hereditary e.
    leg e.
    lung e.
    menstrual e.
    e. neonatorum
    premenstrual e.
    pulmonary e.
    vulvar e.
Eden-Lawson hysterectomy
EdenTec 2000W in-home
    cardiorespiratory monitor
edge effect
EDRF
    endothelium-derived relaxing
    factor
edrophonium chloride
EDTA
Edwards syndrome
EEA stapler
EEC
    ectrodactyly, ectodermal
    dysplasia, clefting
      EEC syndrome
EEG
    electroencephalogram

eelworm
EEP
   end-expiratory phase
   end-expiratory pressure
E.E.S.
EFE
   endocardial fibroelastosis
efface
effacement
   cervical e.
   e. of cervix
effect
   adverse e.
   anemic e.
   antiestrogenic e.
   Arias-Stella e.
   Bohr e.
   cardioprotective e.
   cardiovascular e.
   Compton e.
   cytotoxic e.
   differential e.
   Doppler e.
   edge e.
   estrogen e.
   fetal alcohol e. (FAE)
   Hawthorne e.
   hormonal e.
   hypnotic e.
   iatrogenic e.
   Mach band e.
   marijuana e.
   neurologic adverse e.
   perinatal e.
   pituitary gonadotropin e.
   Posiero e.
   psychological e.
   returning-soldier e.
   salutary e.
   sedative e.
   social factor e.
   star e.
   teratogenic e.
effective
   e. conjugate
   e. refractory period
effector cell

efferentia
   ductuli e.
efficacy
   oral contraceptive e.
efficiency
   female fertility e.
effluvium
   telogen e.
efflux
Effortil
effusion
   malignant e.
   malignant pleural e.
   pleural e.
EFM
   electronic fetal monitoring
   external fetal monitoring
Efroxine
Efudex
EFW
   estimated fetal weight
EGA
   estimated gestational age
EG/BUS
   external genitalia/Bartholin,
      urethral, and Skene glands
EGF
   epidermal growth factor
egg
   e. activation
   e. cell
   frozen e.
   e. membrane
   e. transport
   e. yolk extender
Egnell breast pump
EH
   endometrial hyperplasia
Ehlers-Danlos syndrome
Ehrlich catheter
EIA
   enzyme immunoassay
EIC
   extensive intraductal component
eicosanoid
EIFT
   embryo intrafallopian transfer

NOTES

eight-cell embryo
Eikenella corrodens
EIN
    endometrial intraepithelial
      neoplasia
Einthoven equilateral triangle
Eisenmenger
    E. complex
    E. syndrome
ejaculate
    sperm-free e.
ejaculation
    premature e.
ejecta
    laser e.
ejection
    milk e.
EKG
    electrocardiogram
Eklund technique
elastic
    e. recoil of the bronchus
    e. stocking
elastica
    cutis e.
elastin
elastosis performans serpiginosa
Elavil
elderly
    e. primigravida
elective abortion
Electra complex
electrocardiogram (ECG, EKG)
electrocardiography
    abdominal fetal e.
    fetal e.
electrocautery
    AmpErase e.
    bipolar e.
    Endoclip monopolar e.
    laparoscopic e.
    transurethral e.
electrocoagulation diathermy
electrode
    Aspen laparoscopy e.
    ball e.
    bipolar e.
    Cryomedics disposable
      LLETZ e.
    fetal scalp e.
    Kontron e.
    Littmann ECG e.
    LLETZ-LEEP active loop e.

    loop e.
    Medi-Trace e.
    Megadyne/Fann E-Z clean
      laparoscopic e.
    REM PolyHesive II patient
      return e.
    rollerball e.
    roller-bar e.
    spiral e.
    unipolar e.
    Valleylab ball e.
    Valleylab loop e.
electrodesiccation
electroencephalogram (EEG)
electroencephalography
Electro-Gel conductivity gel
electrohysterograph
electrolysis
electrolyte
    e. balance
    e. imbalance
electromagnetic
    e. radiation
    e. spectrum
electrometrogram
electrometrography
electromyelogram (EMG)
electromyogram (EMG)
electromyography
electron
electronic fetal monitoring (EFM)
electron-volt (eV, ev)
electrophoresis
    e. gel
electroshock therapy
electrosurgical plume
Elema angiocardiogram
element
    transposable e.
elemental iron
elephantiasis
    congenital e.
    genital e.
    e. vulvae
elephant pelvis
elevated
    e. enzyme activity
    e. liver enzymes
elevation
    alpha-fetoprotein e.
    fetus growth e.
elevator
    lemon-squeezer obstetrical e.

Somer uterine e.
uterine e.
Wadia e.
elfin
e. facies
e. facies syndrome
Elimite
ELISA
enzyme-linked immunosorbent
assay
Elispot test
Elixicon
Elixomin
Elixophyllin
Elliot
E. forceps
E. sign
elliptical uterine incision
elliptocytic anemia
elliptocytosis
Ellis-van Creveld syndrome
Elmed
E. BC 50 M/M digital
bipolar coagulator
E. peristaltic irrigation
pump
Elmiron
elongation
Elscint ESI-3000 ultrasound
Eltroxin
E-Mac
English MacIntosh
E-Mac laryngoscope blade
Embden-Meyerhof pathway
Embolex
emboli (*pl. of* embolus)
embolism
amniotic fluid e.
cerebral e.
pulmonary e.
embolization
e. therapy
transcatheter e.
embolus, pl. emboli
amniotic fluid e.
gas e.
Gianturco spring e.

pulmonary emboli
trophoblastic e.
embrace reflex
embroscopy
embryatrics
embryectomy
embryo
abnormal e.
e. biopsy
e. carrier
e. cloning
cylindrical e.
e. donation
e. donor
eight-cell e.
e. encapsulation
four-cell e.
frozen e.
e. intrafallopian transfer
(EIFT)
Janosik e.
nodular e.
preimplantation e. (PIE)
presomite e.
previllous e.
e. reduction
somite e.
Spee e.
e. splitting
stunted e.
e. transfer (ET)
embryoblast
embryocardia
embryocide
embryoctony
embryogenesis
embryography
embryoid
embryology
breast e.
causal e.
comparative e.
descriptive e.
experimental e.
genital tract e.
Leydig cell e.
reproductive tract e.

NOTES

embryoma
embryomorphous
embryonal
    e. carcinoma
    e. rhabdomyosarcoma
    e. sarcoma
embryonate
embryonic
    e. anideus
    e. axis
    e. blastoderm
    e. cleavage
    e. diapause
    e. disk
    e. loss
    e. neural tube
    e. period
    e. sac
    e. testicular regression
      syndrome
embryoniform
embryonization
embryonum
    smegma e.
embryony
embryopathology
embryopathy
    diabetic e.
    rubella e.
    warfarin e.
embryoplastic
embryoscope
embryoscopy
embryotome
embryotomy
embryotrophy
Emcyt
Emerson respirator
emesis
    e. pH determination
    salivation, lacrimation,
      urination, defecation,
      gastrointestinal distress
      and e. (SLUDGE)
emetic
EMG
    electromyelogram
    electromyogram
    exomphalos, macroglossia, and
      gigantism
    MyoTrac EMG
    EMG syndrome

eminence
    median e.
Emko
EMLA
    eutectic mixture of local
      anesthetics
Emla cream
emmenagogic
emmenagogue
emmenia
emmenic
emmeniopathy
emmenology
Emmert-Gelhorn pessary
Emmet operation
Emmett cervical tenaculum
emotional amenorrhea
emphysema
    congenital lobar e.
    perivascular e.
    pulmonary interstitial e.
      (PIE)
Empirin
emprosthotonos
emptying
    gastric e.
empty scrotum syndrome
empty-sella syndrome
empyema
    epidural e.
emulsion
    Pusey e.
    Soyacal IV fat e.
    Travamulsion IV fat e.
E-Mycin
en
    e. bloc
    e. bloc resection
    e. caul delivery
    e. face position
enalapril
enanthate
    estradiol e.
    norethindrone e. (NET-EN)
    testosterone e.
encainide
encapsulation
    embryo e.
Encare
enceinte
encelitis, enceliitis
encephalitis
    Dawson e.

neonatal HSV-1 e.
neonatal HSV-2 e.
Rasmussen e.
Schilder e.
St. Louis e.
viral e.
encephalocele
encephalofacial angiomatosis
encephalomeningocele
encephalomere
encephalomyelitis
postinfectious e. (PIE)
encephalomyelocele
encephalomyopathy of Leigh
encephalopathy
anoxic-ischemic e.
bilirubin e.
demyelinating e.
hypertensive e.
hypoxic-ischemic e. (HIE)
neonatal e.
spongiform e.
e. with prolinemia
encephalotomy
encephalotrigeminal angiomatosis
enchondroma
enchondromatosis
encode
encopresis
encranius
encu method
encyesis
endadelphos
end bud
Endcaps
Glucolet E.
Endep
end-expiratory
e.-e. phase (EEP)
e.-e. pressure (EEP)
ENDO-ASSIST
E.-A. cutting dissector
E.-A. endoscopic forceps
E.-A. endoscopic knot
pusher
E.-A. endoscopic ligature
carrier

E.-A. endoscopic needle
holder
E.-A. retractable blade
E.-A. retractable scalpel
E.-A. sponge aspirator
Endo-Avitene
E.-A. microfibrillar collagen
hemostat
endocardial
e. cushion defect (ECD)
e. fibroelastosis (EFE)
endocarditis
bacterial e.
infective e.
subacute bacterial e. (SBE)
endocavitary radiation therapy
Endocell endometrial cell collector
endocervical
e. aspirator
e. canal
e. canal colposcopy
e. curettage (ECC)
e. glandular dysplasia
e. mucosa
e. polyp
e. sampling
e. sampling brush
e. sinus tumor
endocervicitis
endocervix
endochondroma
endochorion
Endoclip
E. cautery
E. monopolar electrocautery
endocolpitis
endocrine
e. disorder
e. factor
e. gland
e. system
endocrinologic sex
endocrinology
reproductive e.
endocrinopathy
endocytosis
receptor-mediated e.

NOTES

endoderm
endodermal
    e. cells
    e. sinus tumor
endodermatosis
endogenous
    e. catecholamines
    e. estrogen
    e. gonadotropin activity
      suppression
    e. hormone
    e. opiate
    e. opiate receptor
    e. opioid peptide
    e. pyrogen
    e. steroid
Endo-GIA30 suture stapler
Endo-GIA stapler
Endoloop suture
EndoMax advanced laparoscopic
    instrument
EndoMed LSS laparoscopy system
endometria (*pl. of* endometrium)
endometrial
    e. ablation
    e. ablator
    e. adenoacanthoma
    e. adenocarcinoma
    e. aspirator
    e. atrophy
    e. biopsy
    e. breakdown
    e. cancer
    e. cannula
    e. carcinoma
    e. clear cell adenocarcinoma
    e. cycle
    e. cycling activity
    e. cyst
    e. dating
    e. development
    e. histology
    e. hyperplasia (EH)
    e. implant
    e. intraepithelial neoplasia
    (EIN)
    e. metastasizing leiomyoma
    e. morphology
    e. neoplasia
    e. polyp
    e. protein
    e. receptor
    e. resection

    e. sampling
    e. sarcoma
    e. secretory adenocarcinoma
    e. shedding
    e. spiral artery
    e. stimulation
    e. stromal sarcoma (ESS)
    e. thickness
    e. tuberculosis
endometrioid
    e. carcinoma
    e. tumor
endometrioma
    large e.
endometriosis
    adhesive e.
    asymptomatic mild e.
    e. interna
    internal e.
    ovarian e.
    rectosigmoid colon e.
    retroperitoneal e.
    small bowel e.
    stromal e.
    tubal e.
    urinary tract e.
    vulvar e.
endometriosis-associated infertility
endometriotic focus
endometritis
    decidual e.
    e. dissecans
endometrium, pl. endometria
    cyclic proliferative e.
    decidualized e.
    hyperechoic e.
    inactive e.
    menstrual e.
    nonpregnant e.
    Swiss cheese e.
    tubal e.
endometropic
endomyometritis
endonuclease
    e. analysis
    restriction e.
endoparametritis
Endopath
    E. endoscopic articulating
      stapler
    E. needle tip electrosurgery
      probe
endopelvic fascia

endoperoxide
endophytic
endoplasmic
Endopouch
endorectal flap
endorphin
β-endorphin (*var. of* beta-endorphin)
endorphin, dopamine, and prostaglandin theory
endosalpingiosis
endosalpingitis
endosalpingoblastosis
endoscope
  Storz e.
endoscopic
  e. bladder neck suspension (EBNS)
  e. linear cutter
  e. retrograde cholangiopancreatography (ERCP)
endoscopy
Endotek
  E. OM-3 Urodata monitor
  E. UDS-1000 monitor
  E. urodynamics system
endothelial cell
endothelin-1, -2, -3
endothelin plasma level
endotheliochorial placenta
endothelio-endothelial placenta
endotheliosis
  glomerular capillary e.
endothelium-derived relaxing factor (EDRF)
endotoxic shock
endotoxin
  lipopolysaccharide e.
endotracheal (ET)
  e. intubation
  e. tube
endotrachelitis
endovaginal
  e. finding
  e. imaging

  e. probe
  e. transducer
endovasculitis
  hemorrhagic e.
end-stage kidney disease
end-tidal CO2 monitoring
Enduron
enema
  barium e.
  Cortenema e.
  Fleet e.
  lactulose e.
  oil e.
  soapsuds e.
energy expenditure
Enfamil
  E. human milk fortifier
  E. Next Step toddler formula
  E. Premature 20 Formula
enflurane
engaged head
engagement
Engerix-B hepatitis B vaccine
engineering
  genetic e.
English
  E. lock
  E. MacIntosh (E-Mac)
  E. position
  E. yew
engorged breast
engorgement
  breast e.
  vascular e.
engraftment
  fetal e.
Engstrom respirator
enhancement
  acoustic e.
  e. factor
  immunologic e.
enhancer
  XP Xcelerator ultrasound e.
Enkaid
enkephalin

NOTES

135

enlargement
    abdominal e.
    clitoris e.
    parotid e.
    pelvis e.
    sellar e.
enolase
    neuron-specific e. (NSE)
Enovid
enoxacin
Enseals
    potassium iodide E.
ensu method
Ensure
Entamoeba histolytica
enteral feeding
enteric
    e. cytopathogenic human
      orphan (ECHO)
    e. cytopathogenic human
      orphan virus
    e. feeding
enteritis
    bacterial e.
    regional e.
Enterobacter
enterobiasis
Enterobius vermicularis
enterocele
enterococcus, pl. enterococci
enterocolic
enterocolitica
    Yersinia e.
enterocolitis
    necrotizing e. (NEC)
    pseudomembranous e.
enterokinase deficiency
enteromenia
enteropathica
    acrodermatitis e.
enteropathy
enterostomal therapy
enterostomy
enterotoxin F
enterovaginal fistula
enteroviral
Enterovirus
enuresis
envelope
    peritoneal e.
Environment
    Home Observation for the

Measurement of the E.
    (HOME)
environmental toxin
Envision endocavity probe
enzmatic
enzygotic twins
enzyme
    e. activity
    angiotensin-converting e.
    (ACE)
    e. assay
    e. deficiency
    elevated liver e.'s
    e. immunoassay (EIA)
    proteolytic e.
enzyme-linked
    e.-l. antiglobulin test
    e.-l. immunosorbent assay
    (ELISA)
enzymopathy
eosinophilia
    pulmonary e.
    pulmonary infiltrate with e.
    (PIE)
eosinophilic
    e. fasciitis
    e. gastroenteritis
    e. leukemia
    e. pneumonia
EP
    etoposide
EPC
    external pneumatic calf
    compression
ependymoma
ephebiatrics
ephebic
ephebogenesis
ephebogenic
ephebology
ephedrine
    racemic e.
    e. sulfate
ephelis, pl. ephelides
ephemeral
    e. fever
    e. temperature
epicanthal
    e. fold
epicanthus
epidemic
    e. capillary bronchitis

epidemiological
   e. characteristic
   e. feature
   e. genetics
epidemiology
epidermal
   e. growth factor (EGF)
   e. inclusion cyst
   e. nevus syndrome
epidermides (*pl. of* epididymis)
epidermidis
   Staphylococcus e.
epidermis
epidermodysplasia verruciformis
epidermolysis
   e. bullosa
epidermolytic hyperkeratosis
epidermophytosis
epididymal sperm
epididymis, pl. epidermides
epididymitis
epidural
   e. abscess
   e. analgesia
   e. anesthesia
   e. empyema
   e. hemangioma
   e. hemorrhage
   e. morphine
Epifrin
epigaster
epigastric
   e. artery
   e. hernia
   e. pain
epigastrius
epignathus
epilepsia partialis continua
epilepsy
   abdominal e.
   focal e.
   grand mal e.
   jacksonian e.
   e. management
   myoclonus e.
   nocturnal e.
   petit mal e.

   photosensitive e.
   psychomotor e.
   rolandic e.
   temporal lobe e.
epileptic
   e. seizure
epilepticus
   status e.
epileptiform
epiloia
epimenorrhagia
epimenorrhea
Epinal
epinephrine
   racemic e.
EpiPen
   E. Jr.
epiphyseal
   e. dysostosis
   e. growth
   e. ossification center
   e. syndrome
epiphysis, pl. epiphyses
epipygus
episioperineoplasty
episioperineorrhaphy
episioplasty
episiorrhaphy
episiostenosis
episiotomy
   median e.
   mediolateral e.
   e. repair
   ruptured e.
episome
epispadias
epistaxis
epistemology
episthotonos
epitarsus
17-epitestosterone
epithelial
   e. autoantibody localization
   e. cancer
   e. cyst
   e. hyperplasia
   e. ovarian carcinoma

NOTES

epithelial *(continued)*
    e. plug
    e. stromal ovarian neoplasm
    e. stromal tumor
    e. tumor
epithelialization
epitheliochorial placenta
epithelioma
    e. adenoides cysticum
    basal cell e.
epithelium
    acetowhite e.
    atypical e.
    cervical e.
    coelomic e.
    columnar e.
    germinal e.
    luminal e.
    native squamous e.
    ovarian germinal e.
    papilla of columnar e.
    squamous e.
    stratified squamous e.
    surface e.
    uterine e.
    white e.
epitope
epituberculosis
Epo
    erythropoietin
epoophorectomy
epoophoron
Eppendorfer
    E. biopsy forceps
    E. biopsy punch
Eppy/N
Eprolin
EPSDT
    Early and Periodic Screening,
    Diagnosis, and Treatment
    program
epsilon-aminocaproic acid (EACA)
Epstein-Barr virus (EBV)
Epstein pearls
EPT
    early pregnancy test
epulis
    congenital e.
    e. gravidarum
    e. of newborn
    e. of pregnancy
Equagesic
equal conjoined twins

Equanil
equation
    Bohn e.
    Hadlock e.
    Henderson-Hasselbalch e.
    Kučera e.
    Rose e.
    Shepard e.
    Starling e.
equatorial
    e. division
    e. plane
Equilet
equilibrium
    acid-base e.
    genetic e.
    Hardy-Weinberg e.
    Starling e.
equinovalgus
    talipes e.
equinovarus
    talipes e.
equinus
    talipes e.
equivalent
    lethal e.
E-R
    Betachron E.-R.
Erb
    E. juvenile muscular
    dystrophy
    E. palsy
Erb-Duchenne paralysis
Erb-Goldflam
    E.-G. disease
    E.-G. syndrome
ERCP
    endoscopic retrograde
    cholangiopancreatography
erection
    capillary e.
ergocalciferol
ergonovine
    e. maleate
ergot
ergotamine
    e. tartrate
Ergotrate
Erhardt Developmental Prehension Assessment
erigentes
    nervi e.
Erlacher-Blount syndrome

Ernst radium applicator
E-rosette receptor
erosion
 cervical e.
erosive
 e. adenomatosis of nipple
 e. vulvitis
error
 alpha e.
 beta e.
 e. of the first kind
 metabolic e.
 e. of the second kind
ERT
 estrogen replacement therapy
eruption
 Kaposi varicelliform e.
eruptive
 e. fever
 e. temperature
Er:YAG laser
Eryc
EryPed
erysipelas
 e. internum
Ery-Tab
erythema
 e. chronicum migrans
  (ECM)
 e. infectiosum
 Jacquet e.
 e. marginatum
 e. multiforme exudativum
 e. neonatorum
 e. neonatorum toxicum
 e. nodosum
 e. nodosum leprosum
 palmar e.
 e. streptogenes
 e. toxicum neonatorum
erythematosus
 lupus e. (LE)
 neonatal lupus e.
 systemic lupus e. (SLE)
erythredema polyneuropathy
erythrityl tetranitrate

erythroblastic
 e. anemia
 e. anemia of childhood
erythroblastopenia
erythroblastosis
 ABO e.
 e. fetalis
 e. neonatorum
Erythrocin
erythrocyte
 e. count
 e. enzyme deficiency
 e. glutathione peroxidase
  deficiency
 e. membrane
 e. mosaicism
 packed e.
 e. sedimentation rate (ESR)
 e. transfusion
erythrocytosis
erythroderma
 atopic e.
 bullous congenital
  ichthyosiform e.
 e. desquamativum
erythrohepatic porphyria
erythrokeratodermia
 e. variabilis
erythroleukoblastosis
Erythromid
erythromycin
erythron
erythrophagocytic
 lymphohistiocytosis
erythroplasia
 Queyrat e.
 Zoon e.
erythropoiesis
erythropoietic porphyria
erythropoietin (Epo)
escape beats
Escherichia
 E. coli
 E. coli sepsis
 E. coli vaccine
escutcheon
Eserine

NOTES

Esidrix
Eskalith
esmolol hydrochloride
esophageal
    e. atresia
    e. dilatation
    e. pressure
    e. reflux
    e. sphincter
    e. stenosis
    e. varix
esophagitis
    infectious e.
    monilial e.
    reflux e.
esophagoscope
    Holinger infant e.
esophagus
ESR
    erythrocyte sedimentation rate
ESS
    endometrial stromal sarcoma
essential dysmenorrhea
ester
    phorbol e.
esterified
    e. estrogens
Estes
    E. operation
    E. procedure
estetrol
esthesioneuroblastoma
esthiomene
estimated
    e. date of conception
    (EDC)
    e. date of confinement
    (EDC)
    e. fetal weight (EFW)
    e. gestational age (EGA)
estimation
    gestational age e.
estimator
    least squares e.
    maximum likelihood e.
Estinyl
Estrace
    E. vaginal cream
Estra-D
Estraderm
    E. Transdermal
    E. transdermal system
estradiol (E_2)

e. assay
bound e.
e. cypionate
desogestrel and ethinyl e.
e. enanthate
ethinyl e.
ethynodiol diacetate and e.
free e.
e. level
levonorgestrel and ethinyl e.
micronized e.
norethindrone acetate and
    ethinyl e.
norethindrone and ethinyl e.
norgestimate and ethinyl e.
e. receptor
e. suppression
e. transdermal system
e. vaginal cream
e. valerate
estradiol-17β, 17β-estradiol
Estradurin
Estra-L
estramustine phosphate sodium
estrane
Estratab
Estratest
    E.-H.S.
    E. Oral
Estraval
estriol (E_3)
    e. level
Estro-Cyp
estrogen
    e. breakthrough bleeding
    catechol e.
    conjugated e.'s
    conjugated equine e.
    e. deprivation
    e. effect
    endogenous e.
    esterified e.'s
    e. excess
    e. level
    e. loss
    e. metabolism
    oral conjugated e.
    orally-administered e.
    postcoital e.
    e. receptor
    e. receptor localization
    e. replacement

e. replacement therapy (ERT)
serum e.
e. sulfotransferase
e. surge
e. synthesis
e. therapy
transdermal e.
uninterrupted e.
unopposed e.
e. window etiologic hypothesis
e. withdrawal
e. withdrawal bleeding
e.'s with methyltestosterone
estrogen-assisted colposcopy
estrogen-dependent neoplasia
estrogenic
estrogen-induced prolactinoma
estrogen/progesterone ratio
estrogen-progesterone withdrawal bleeding
estrogen-progestin
    e.-p. artificial cycle
    e.-p. contraceptive
    e.-p. replacement therapy
    e.-p. test
estrogen-progestogen combination
Estroject
    E.-L.A.
estrone (E_1)
    oral e.
    e. sulfate
estropipate
Estrovis
estrus
ET
    embryo transfer
    endotracheal
ethacrynic acid
Ethamide
ethanol, ethyl alcohol
    blood e.
ethanolaminosis in glycogen-storage disease
ethanol, ethyl alcohol (EtOH)

ethchlorvynol
ether
Ethicon
    E. disposable cannula
    E. disposable trocar
ethinamate
ethinyl
    e. estradiol
    e. estradiol and desogestrel
    e. estradiol and ethynodiol diacetate
    e. estradiol and levonorgestrel
    e. estradiol and norethindrone
    e. estradiol and norgestimate
    e. estradiol and norgestrel
    e. testosterone
ethiodized oil
Ethiodol
ethionamide
ethisterone
ethmocephalus
ethmocephaly syndrome
ethnicity
ethoheptazine citrate
ethopropazine hydrochloride
ethosuximide
ethotoin
Ethox cuff
ethoxzolamide
Ethrane
ethyl alcohol (*var. of* ethanol)
ethyl biscoumacetate
ethylenediaminetetraacetic acid
ethylnorepinephrine
ethylphenylephrine
ethynodiol
    e. diacetate
    e. diacetate and estradiol
Etibi
etidronate disodium
etiocholanolone
etiology
    fever of unknown e. (FUE)

NOTES

EtOH
  ethanol, ethyl alcohol
etoposide (EP)
etretinate
ETV8 CCD ColorMicro video camera
EUB-405
  E. ultrasound scanner
  E. ultrasound system
Eubacterium
eugonadotropic
  e. amenorrhea
  e. hypogonadism
eukaryote
Eulipos
eunuch
eunuchoid gigantism
eunuchoidism
  female e.
  hypergonadotropic e.
  hypogonadotropic e.
euploid
  e. abortion
  e. pregnancy
eupnea
eupneic
euprolactinemic woman
Euro-Med FNA-21 aspiration needle
europium
eustachian tube
eutectic mixture of local anesthetics (EMLA)
Euthroid
euthyroid
Eutonyl
eV, ev
  electron-volt
evacuation
  dilatation and e. (D & E)
  dilation and e. (D & E)
  fimbrial e.
  e. proctography
  e. of uterine contents
evacuator
  smoke e.
  uterine e.
evaluation
  Doppler e.
  Dubowitz e.
  infertility e.
  mental status e.

quantity not sufficient for e. (QNS)
  urological e.
  uterine e.
Evans blue dye
Evans-Steptoe procedure
evaporated
  e. milk
  e. milk formula
evaporation
event
  apparent life-threatening e. (ALTE)
  iatrogenic e.
  life e.
eventration
Everard Williams procedure
Everone
Evershears
  E. bipolar laparoscopic forceps
  E. bipolar laparoscopic scissors
eversion
  cervical e.
evidence
  rape e.
  sexual assault forensic e. (SAFE)
evisceration
evoked potential technique
evolution
  darwinian e.
  Darwin theory of e.
  Denman spontaneous e.
  Douglas spontaneous e.
  spontaneous e.
Ewing
  E. sarcoma
  E. tumor
ex
  e. lap
    exploratory laparotomy
  e. vivo
  e. vivo fertilization
exaggerated craniocaudal view
examination
  abdominal e.
  Allen and Capute neonatal neurodevelopmental e.
  Ballard e.
  bimanual pelvic e.
  chest e.

dark-field e.
Dubowitz e.
eye e.
neonate e.
neurologic e.
newborn e.
Pediatric Early Elemental E.
  (PEEX)
pelvic e.
radiological e.
rectal e.
rectovaginal e.
self-breast e.
speculum e.
sterile vaginal e. (SVE)
stool e.
vaginal e.
excavator
Merlis obstetrical e.
excavatum
pectus e.
excess
androgen e.
e. androgen
base e.
estrogen e.
glucocorticoid e.
soluble antigen e.
excessive blood loss
exchange
fetal-maternal e.
sister chromatid e.
Starling law of
  transcapillary e.
e. transfusion
excision
local e.
radical e.
excisional biopsy
excitation
exclusion
allelic e.
excretion
sodium e.
water e.
excretory system development
exencephaly

exenteration
anterior pelvic e.
pelvic e.
posterior pelvic e.
pyelonephritis in e.
stress reaction in e.
total pelvic e.
exercise
DeSouza e.'s
Kegel e.'s
maternal e.
pelvic e.
exercise-induced
e.-i. amenorrhea
e.-i. incontinence
exfoliation
lamellar e.
exhaustion
ovarian follicle e.
Exna
exocelomic
e. cavity
e. membrane
exocervix
exocytosis
cortical granule e.
exogenous
e. gonadotropin
e. gonadotropin stimulation
e. hormone
e. obesity
exomphalos
e., macroglossia, and
  gigantism (EMG)
e., macroglossia, and
  gigantism syndrome
exon
exophthalmos
exophytic
exostosis, pl. exostoses
multiple exostoses
pelvic e.
Exosurf
E. Neonatal
exotoxin
e. C
Pseudomonas e.

NOTES

Expander
    Meshgraft Skin E.
expansion
    plasma volume e.
    volume e.
expectancy
    life e.
expectant management
expected date of confinement (EDC)
expenditure
    energy e.
experimental
    e. embryology
    e. obesity
Expert bone densitometer
exploratory laparotomy (ex lap, ex lap)
exposure
    anesthetic gas e.
    DES e.
    maternal mercury e.
    methamphetamine e.
    prenatal diethylstilbestrol e.
    in utero e.
expression
    oncogene e.
expressivity
expulsion
expulsive
    e. force
    e. pains
exsanguination
    fetal e.
exstrophy
extended
    e. field irradiation therapy
    e. radical mastectomy
    e. rubella syndrome
extender
    egg yolk e.
extension
extensive intraductal component (EIC)
externa
    otitis e.
external
    e. beam irradiation
    e. conjugate
    e. fetal monitoring (EFM)
    e. genitalia
    e. genitalia/Bartholin,

urethral, and Skene glands (EG/BUS)
    e. hemorrhage
    e. os
    e. pneumatic calf compression (EPC)
    e. radiation therapy
    e. rotation
    e. version
    e. x-ray therapy
exterogestate
extirpation
    Amreich vaginal e.
extraamniotic pregnancy
extracellular
    e. fluid
    e. matrix
    e. matrix component
extrachorial pregnancy
extrachromosomal inheritance
extracorporeal
    e. circulation (ECC)
    e. CO_2 removal (ECOR)
    e. membrane oxygenation (ECMO)
extract
extraction
    breech e.
    Marshall-Taylor vacuum e.
    menstrual e.
    partial breech e.
    podalic e.
    spontaneous breech e.
    total breech e.
    vacuum e.
extractor
    Bird vacuum e.
    Kobayashi vacuum e.
    Malmström vacuum e.
    Mityvac vacuum e.
    M-type e.
    mucus e.
    Murless head e.
    plastic cup vacuum e.
    Silastic cup e.
    Silc e.
    Tender-Touch e.
    vacuum e.
    Vantos vacuum e.
extradural
    e. anesthesia
    e. block
    e. hematoma

extraembryonic
    e. fetal membrane
    e. mesoderm
extrafascial hysterectomy
extraglandular conversion
extragonadal
    e. germ cell
extrahepatic
extramammary Paget disease
extramedullary hematopoiesis
extramembranous pregnancy
extramural upper airway
  obstruction
extraovular
extrapelvic malignancy
extraperitoneal cesarean section
extrapulmonary
extrapyramidal
extrarenal
extrasystole
extrathoracic tuberculosis
extrauterine
    e. pregnancy

extremity
    flaccid e.
extrusion
    oocyte e.
    placental e.
extubation
exudativum
    erythema multiforme e.
Eyberg Child Behavior Inventory
  (ECBI)
eye
    Credé maneuver of e.'s
    e. examination
eyelids
    fusion of e.
E-Z-EM
    E-Z-EM BioGun automated
      biopsy system
    E-Z-EM PercuSet
      amniocentesis tray

NOTES

FA
- Nestabs FA
- Pramet FA
- Pramilet FA

F.A.
- Mission Prenatal F.A.

FAB
- French-American-British
- F. classification
- F. staging of carcinoma

Fabricius
- bursa of F.

Fabry disease

face
- asymmetry of f.
- bovine f.
- f. chamber
- cleft f.
- dish f.
- f. presentation

face/chin presentation

FACES-III
- Family Adaptability and Cohesion Scale-III

face-to-pubes position

facial
- f. asymmetry
- f. diplegia
- f. nerve
- f. nerve palsy
- f. nerve paralysis
- f. paralysis

facies
- adenoid f.
- f. bovina
- bovine f.
- cushingoid f.
- dog-like f.
- elfin f.
- leonine f.
- leprechaun f.
- Marshall Hall f.
- Potter f.

faciodigitogenital syndrome
faciogenital dysplasia
facioscapulohumeral
- f. muscular dystrophy
- f. syndrome of Landouzy-Dejerine

faciotelencephalic malformation

faciotelencephalopathy
FACO₂
- fraction of alveolar carbon dioxide

FACS
- fluorescence-activated cell sorter

factitious precocious puberty
factor
- f. I (fibrinogen)
- f. II (prothrombin)
- f. III (thromboplastin)
- f. IV (calcium ions)
- f. V (proaccelerin)
- f. VI (factor VI - cannot be identified)
- f. VII (proconvertin)
- f. VIII (antihemophilic f.)
- f. VIII:C (von Willebrand f.)
- f. IX (Christmas f.)
- f. X (Stuart f. or Stuart-Prower f.)
- f. XI (plasma thromboplastin antecedent f.)
- f. XII (Hageman f.)
- f. XIII (fibrin stabilizing f.)
- f. Xa
- acidic fibroblast growth f. (FGFa)
- alloimmune f.
- angiogenic growth f.
- antihemophilic f.
- atrial natriuretic f. (ANF)
- autocrine motility f. (AMF)
- autoimmune f.
- blocking f.
- cell adhesion f. (CAF)
- cervical f.
- chemotactic f.
- Christmas f.
- citrovorum f.
- coagulation f.
- coital f.
- colony-stimulating f. (CSF)
- f. concentrate
- corticotropin-releasing f.
- cytotoxic f.
- f. D deficiency

factor *(continued)*
digoxin-like
immunoreactive f. (DLIF)
early pregnancy f.
endocrine f.
endothelium-derived
relaxing f. (EDRF)
enhancement f.
epidermal growth f. (EGF)
fetal f.
fibrin stabilizing f.
fibroblast growth f.
fibroblast pneumocyte f.
follicular f.
glass f.
granulocyte colony-
stimulating f. (G-CSF)
granulocyte-macrophage
colony-stimulating f.
(GM-CSF)
growth f. (GF)
growth-like f.
Hageman f.
f. H deficiency
helper f.
HG f.
humoral f.
f. I deficiency
f. II deficiency
f. III deficiency
immune f.
infertility f.
insulin-like growth f. (IGF)
f. IV deficiency
f. IX deficiency
kidney-derived growth f.
lymphocyte-activating f.
macrophage-activating f.
(MAF)
macrophage colony-
stimulating f.
macrophage-inhibition f.
male f.
maternal f.
maturation-promoting f.
(MPF)
microbial f.
migration-inhibitory f. (MIF)
mixed lymphocyte reaction
blocking f.
mortality risk f.
M-phase-promoting f.
müllerian duct inhibitory f.

müllerian inhibiting f.
(MIF)
nerve growth f. (NGF)
obstetrical risk f.
ovarian f.
perinatal risk f.
plasma thromboplastin
antecedent f.
platelet-activating f.
platelet-derived growth f.
prenatal risk f.
prognostic f.
prolactin inhibiting f. (PIF)
prolactin releasing f. (PRF)
Rh f.
rheumatoid f.
risk f.
Stuart f.
Stuart-Prower f.
testis-determining f. (TDF)
tissue f.
transfer f.
transforming growth f.
(TGF)
tubal f.
tumor angiogenesis f. (TAF)
tumor-limiting f.
tumor necrosis f. (TNF)
tumor necrosis f.-α (TNF-α)
uterine f.
f. V deficiency
f. VI deficiency
f. VII deficiency
f. VIII deficiency
f. VIII inhibitor
f. VII inhibitor
von Willebrand f. (vWF)
f. X deficiency
f. XI deficiency
f. XII deficiency
f. XIII deficiency
Fact Plus
Factrel
fadir sign
FAE
fetal alcohol effect
Fagan Test of Infant Intelligence
failed forceps delivery
failure
acute renal f.
bone marrow f.
cardiac f.
congestive heart f.

contraceptive f.
fertility f.
fimbrial f.
gonadal f.
heart f.
hypothalamic f.
implantation f.
kidney f.
multiple organ f.
ovarian f.
f. to progress
renal f.
reproductive f.
f. to thrive (FTT)
failure-to-thrive syndrome
falciform hymen
Falk-Shukuris operation
falling of the womb
fallopian
    f. pregnancy
    f. tube
    f. tube carcinoma
    f. tube mass
    f. tube metastasis
Fallot
    pentology of F.
    pink tetralogy of F.
    F. syndrome
    tetralogy of F. (TF, TOF)
    trilogy of F.
Falope
    F. ring
    F. ring applicator
false
    f. conjugate
    f. heteroovular twins
    f. knot of umbilical cord
    f. labor
    f. mole
    f. pains
    f. pregnancy
    f. twins
    f. waters
falx laceration
familial
    f. aortic ectasia
    f. aortic ectasia syndrome

f. atypical multiple mole
    melanoma syndrome
f. bipolar mood disorder
f. cardiac myxoma
    syndrome
f. cholesterolemia
f. diathesis
f. dysautonomia
f. erythroblastic anemia
f. erythrophagocytic
    lymphohistiocytosis (FEL)
f. exudative
    vitreoretinopathy
f. familial cardiac myxoma
f. hirsutism
f. hypercholesterolemia
f. hyperprolinemia
f. hypofibrinogenemia
f. infertility
f. juvenile nephrophthisis
    (FJN)
f. lipodystrophy
f. lipoid adrenal hyperplasia
f. Mediterranean fever
f. multiple endocrine
    adenomatosis
f. osteochondrodystrophy
f. tendency
f. trait
f. visceral neuropathy
family
    F. Adaptability and
    Cohesion Scale-III
    (FACES-III)
    F. Apgar Questionnaire
    f. dysfunction
    dysfunctional f.
    F. Environment Scale (FES)
    f. history
    f. planning
Fanconi
    F. anemia
    F. syndrome
Fanconi-Albertini Zellweger
    syndrome
Fanconi-Petrassi syndrome
fan douche

NOTES

Fansidar
faradism
Farber
    F. disease
    F. test
Farre white line
Farris test
FAS
    fetal alcohol syndrome
fascia
    Camper f.
    Colles f.
    Cooper f.
    cremasteric f.
    endopelvic f.
    obturator f.
    perirectal f.
    Scarpa f.
    subserous f.
fascial
    f. necrosis
    f. sling procedure
    f. strip
fasciculation
fasciitis
    diffuse f.
    eosinophilic f.
    necrotizing f.
fascioscapulohumeral
Fastin
fasting blood sugar
fast neutron
fat
    f. density
    f. depot
    dietary f.
    f. flap
    f. metabolism
    f. necrosis
    unsaturated f.
fate mapping
fatty
    f. acid-coenzyme A
    f. halo
    f. infiltration
    f. liver of pregnancy
faun tail nevus
Fazio-Londe atrophy
5-FC
    5-fluorocytosine
FD
    forceps delivery

Fe
    iron
        Loestrin Fe
        Norlestrin Fe
        Slow Fe
fear
    pregnancy f.
feature
    epidemiological f.
    grotesque f.'s
    mongoloid f.'s
febrile
    f. convulsion
    f. seizure
fecal
    f. diversion colostomy
    f. impaction
    f. streptococci
fecalith
    appendiceal f.
feces
FECO$_2$
    fraction in expired gas of carbon
    dioxide
fecund
fecundability
fecundate
fecundation
fecundity
fed
    breast f.
    nipple f.
Federation
    F. of Gynecology and
        Obstetrics classification
    F. International de
        Gynecologie et Obstetrique
        (FIGO)
    F. of International
        Gynecology and Obstetrics
        (FIGO)
Federici sign
feed
    bottle f.
feeder
    Brecht f.
feeding
    ad lib f.
    Alimentum f.
    breast f.
    enteral f.
    enteric f.
    Finkelstein f.

gastric enteral f.
gavage f.
nasoduodenal f.
nipple f.
f. regimen
syringe f.
transpyloric enteral f.
Feer disease
feet
rockerbottom f.
FEL
familial erythrophagocytic
lymphohistiocytosis
Felty syndrome
female
f. condom
f. eunuchoidism
f. fertility efficiency
f. fertility inefficiency
f. pseudohermaphroditism
Femcaps
feminization
f. syndrome
testicular f.
feminizing
f. adrenal tumor
f. testes syndrome
Feminone
Femogen Forte
Femogex
femoral
f. artery
f. artery catheter
f. artery catheterization
f. circumflex artery
f. hernia
f. lymph node
f. nerve
f. neuropathy
Femstat
F. Prefill
femur
f. length (FL)
FEN
fluids, electrolytes, nutrition
fenamate
fencing reflex

fenestrata
placenta f.
fenestration
laparoscopic f.
fenfluramine
fenoterol
fentanyl
f. citrate
f. lollipop
Fenton vaginoplasty
Fe₃O₄
magnetite
Feosol
Ferguson reflex
Fer-In-Sol
F.-I.-S. supplement
F.-I.-S. vitamins
fern
f. leaf pattern
f. leaf tongue
f. test
ferning
f. technique
fern-leaf crystallization
fern-positive Nitrazine
Ferralet
ferric sulfate
Ferriman-Gallwey
F.-G. hirsutism score
F.-G. hirsutism scoring
system
Ferris Smith-Sewall retractor
ferritin
Ferrold-Hisaw unit
ferrous
f. fumarate
f. gluconate
f. sulfate ($FeSO_4$)
fertile
f. period
f. phase
fertility
f. cycle
f. failure
f. rate
subsequent f.
fertilizable life span

NOTES

151

fertilization
> f. age
> ex vivo f.
> in vitro f. (IVF)
> in vivo f.

fertilized ovum

FES
> Family Environment Scale

FeSO$_4$
> ferrous sulfate

fetal
> f. abdominal circumference
> f. abnormality
> f. acid-base balance
> f. acidemia
> f. acidosis
> f. acoustic stimulation test
> f. activity
> f. activity test
> f. adrenal gland
> f. age
> f. alcohol effect (FAE)
> f. alcohol syndrome (FAS)
> f. anatomy
> f. anomaly
> f. anoxia
> f. aorta
> f. arrhythmia
> f. asphyxia
> f. aspiration syndrome
> f. attitude
> f. biometry
> f. biparietal diameter
> f. blood
> f. blood flow
> f. blood gases
> f. blood glucose
> f. blood oxygen-carrying capacity
> f. blood pH
> f. blood sampling
> f. blood study
> f. blood value
> f. blood volume
> f. body movement
> f. bradycardia
> f. brain
> f. brain death
> f. brain disruption sequence
> f. breathing
> f. cardiac activity
> f. cardiac function
> f. cardiac motion
> f. cartilage
> f. cell
> f. cellular growth
> f. circulation
> f. condition
> f. congenital hyperplasia
> f. cortisol infusion
> f. cotyledon
> f. cranial artery
> f. crowding
> f. death
> f. death rate
> f. demise
> f. descent
> f. development
> f. diagnosis
> f. disappearance
> f. distress
> f. distress syndrome
> F. Dopplex
> F. Dopplex monitor
> f. dose limit
> f. drug therapy
> f. duplication
> f. dystocia
> f. electrocardiography
> f. engraftment
> f. exsanguination
> f. face syndrome
> f. factor
> f. fracture
> f. gigantism
> f. growth
> f. growth measurement
> f. growth parameters
> f. growth restriction (FGR)
> f. growth retardation
> f. habitus
> f. head
> f. head:abdominal circumference ratio
> f. head position
> f. heart
> f. heart action
> f. heart disease
> f. heart rate (FHR)
> f. heart rate deceleration
> f. heart rate monitor
> f. heart rate monitoring
> f. heart rate pattern
> f. heart rate reactivity
> f. heart rate variability
> f. heart sounds

f. hemoglobin (HbF)
f. hemorrhage
f. hiccup
f. hormone
f. hydantoin syndrome (FHS)
f. hydrops
f. hypoxia
f. imaging
f. infection
f. intracranial anatomy
f. jeopardy
f. karyotype
f. LDL level
f. lie
f. limb
f. liver
f. lung liquid
f. lung maturation
f. lung maturity (FLM)
f. maceration
f. macrosomia
f. malformation
f. malpresentation
f. maturity
f. membrane
f. metabolism
f. monitor
f. monitoring
f. morbidity
f. mortality
f. movement
f. nuchal translucency thickness
f. nutrition
f. oculocerebrorenal syndrome of Lowe
f. outcome
f. outline
f. ovarian cyst
f. oxygenation
f. phenytoin syndrome
f. physiologist
f. pole
f. position
f. postural abnormality
f. posture

f. reduction
f. rejection
f. resorption
f. retention
f. risk
f. scalp blood sampling
f. scalp electrode
f. scalp oxygenation
f. serum
f. sexual differentiation
f. skeletal dysplasia
f. skin sampling
f. skull depression
f. small parts
f. somatic activity
f. souffle
f. station
f. steroid concentration
f. surgery
f. surveillance
f. swallowing
f. thoracic abnormality
f. tissue implant
f. tissue transplant
f. toxoplasmosis
f. transfusion
f. trauma
f. trimethadione syndrome
f. ultrasound
f. urination
f. uropathy
f. varicella syndrome (FVS)
f. vascular anomaly
f. viability
f. warfarin syndrome
f. wastage
f. weight
f. well-being

Fetalert fetal heart rate monitor
fetalis
chondromalacia f.
erythroblastosis f.
hydrops f.
ichthyosis f.
maternal hydrops f.
maternal parvovirus f.

NOTES

fetalis *(continued)*
    opisthotonos f.
    rachitis f.
fetalism
fetal-maternal
    f.-m. communication
    f.-m. exchange
    f.-m. hemorrhage
    f.-m. medicine
fetal-neonatal transition
fetal-pelvic index
fetal-placental
    f.-p. steroidogenesis
    f.-p. unit
FetalPulse Plus monitor
Fetasonde fetal monitor
fetation
feticide
fetoamniotic
    f. shunt
fetofetal
    f. transfusion
    f. transfusion syndrome
fetography
fetology
fetomaternal
    f. hemorrhage
    f. transfusion
fetometry
    ultrasonic f.
    ultrasound f.
feto-neonatal estrogen-binding protein
fetopathy
    diabetic f.
fetopelvic disproportion
fetoplacental
    f. access
    f. anasarca
    f. circulation
    f. function
    f. transfusion
fetoprotein
α-fetoprotein *(var. of* alpha-fetoprotein*)*
fetoscope
fetoscopy
fetotoxic
fetouterine cell
fetu
    fetus in f.
fetus, pl. **fetuses**
    acardiac f.

f. acardius
amorphous f.
f. amorphus
asynclitic position of f.
calcified f.
coexistent f.
f. compressus
f. in fetu
f. growth elevation
growth-retarded f.
habitus of f.
harlequin f.
HLA-compatible f.
ichthyosis f.
impacted f.
macerated f.
mummified f.
nonstressed f.
nonviable f.
paper-doll f.
papyraceous f.
f. papyraceus
parasitic f.
presentation of f.
previable f.
retroperitoneal f.
f. sanguinolentis
singleton f.
sireniform f.
stressed f.
stunted f.
triploid f.
viable f.
fetus-to-fetus transplant
Feulgen stain
FEV
    forced expiratory volume
fever
    absorption f.
    acute rheumatic f. (ARF)
    artificial f.
    aseptic f.
    cat-scratch f.
    childbed f.
    Colorado tick f.
    dehydration f.
    drug f.
    Ebola hemorrhagic f.
    ephemeral f.
    eruptive f.
    familial Mediterranean f.
    Haverhill f.
    hay f.

hemorrhagic f.
inanition f.
intermittent f.
milk f.
paratyphoid f.
parturient f.
periodic f.
puerperal f.
Q f., Queensland f.
quotidian f.
rat-bite f.
relapsing f.
rheumatic f.
Rocky Mountain spotted f.
scarlet f.
South African tick f.
spotted f.
tactile f.
tick f.
typhoid f.
typhus f.
undulant f.
unexplained f.
f. of unknown etiology
  (FUE)
f. of unknown origin (FUO)
Valley f.
West Nile f.
yellow f.
Fèvre-Languepin syndrome
FFP
  fresh frozen plasma
FGFa
  acidic fibroblast growth factor
FGR
  fetal growth restriction
FG syndrome
FHR
  fetal heart rate
FHS
  fetal hydantoin syndrome
FIA
  fluorescent immunoassay
fiber
  Dacron f.
  dietary f.
  Purkinje f.'s

FiberCon
Fibiger-Debré-Von Gierke
  syndrome
fibrillation
  atrial f.
fibrillin
fibrin
  f. degradation product
  f. sheath
  f. stabilizing factor
Fibrindex test
fibrinogen
  f. abnormality
  f. deficiency
  plasma f.
fibrinogen-fibrin conversion
  syndrome
fibrinoid
fibrinolysis
fibrinolytic
  f. agent
  f. and clotting system
fibrinous polyp
fibroadenolipoma
  degenerated f.
fibroadenoma
  giant f.
  intracanalicular f.
  pericanalicular f.
fibroblast
  f. growth factor
  human embryo f. (HEF)
  f. pneumocyte factor
fibrocystic
  f. breast
  f. breast change
  f. disease
fibroelastosis
  endocardial f. (EFE)
fibroid
  intramural f.
  uterine f.
fibroidectomy
fibroma
  histiocytic f.
  f. molle gravidarum

NOTES

155

fibroma *(continued)*
    ovarian f.
    vulvar f.
fibromatosis
    gingival f.
    pelvic f.
fibromectomy
fibromuscular cervical stroma
fibromyalgia
    childhood f.
fibromyoma, pl. fibromyomata
    uterine f.
fibronectin
    oncofetal f.
fibroplasia
    retrolental f.
fibrosa
    osteitis f.
fibrosarcoma
fibrosing
    f. adenomatosis
    f. adenosis
fibrosis
    cystic f. (CF)
    focal f.
    hepatic f.
    horseshoe f.
    postradiation periureteral f.
    pulmonary f.
fibrosum
    molluscum f.
fibrotic ophthalmoplegia
fibrous
    f. connective tissue
    f. dysplasia of jaw
fibroxanthoma
Fick
    F. method
    F. principle
fiddle-string adhesion
field
    visual f.
fifth
    f. disease
    f. venereal disease
FIGLU
    formiminoglutamic acid
FIGO
    Federation International de
        Gynecologie et Obstetrique
    Federation of International
        Gynecology and Obstetrics

International Federation of
    Gynecology and Obstetrics
    FIGO nomenclature
    FIGO staging
figure
    mitotic f.
filament
    myosin f.
Filatov-Dukes disease
Filibon
fillet
Filshie
    F. clip
    F. clip applicator
    F. clip minilaparotomy
        applicator
filter
    vena caval f.
filtered specimen trap
filtration
    glass-wool f.
    glomerular f.
    rate of fluid f. (Qf)
fimbria, pl. fimbriae
    flowering-out of f.
    mushrooming of f.
    f. ovarica
fimbrial
    f. evacuation
    f. failure
    f. obstruction
fimbriated end of fallopian tube
fimbriectomy
fimbriocele
fimbrioplasty
    Bruhat laser f.
finasteride
finding
    clinical f.
    endovaginal f.
    histopathological f.
    laboratory f.
    pathologic f.
    sonographic f.
    ultrasonic endovaginal f.
Findley folding pessary
fine-needle
    f.-n. aspiration (FNA)
    f.-n. aspiration biopsy
finger
    f. cot
    f. grasp
    Madonna f.

seal f.
spider f.
webbed f.
fingerbreadth
fingerprinting
DNA f.
fingerstick
fingertip dilated
Finkelstein feeding
first
f. arch syndrome
f. degree prolapse
f. parallel pelvic plane
F. Response
F. Response ovulation
predictor
f. stage of labor
f. trimester
FISH
fluorescence in situ
hybridization
Fisher
F. exact test
F. and Paykel RD1000
resuscitator
Fisher-Yates test
fish-mouth cervix
fish skin
FISS
Flint Infant Security Scale
fissure
Ammon f.
f. in ano
palpebral f.
fistula, pl. **fistulae, fistulas**
arteriovenous f.
branchial f.
bronchobiliary f.
cervicovaginal f.
colovaginal f.
enterovaginal f.
gastrointestinal f.
genitourinary f.
H-type f.
intestinal f.
lacteal f.
mammary f.

metroperitoneal f.
perineovaginal f.
postradiation f.
rectolabial f.
rectovaginal f.
rectovestibular f.
rectovulvar f.
systemic arteriovenous f.
tracheoesophageal f.
umbilical f.
urachal f.
ureter f.
ureterovaginal f.
urethrovaginal f.
urinary f.
urogenital f.
uteroperitoneal f.
vesicouterine f.
vesicovaginal f.
vesicovaginorectal f.
vitelline f.
Fitz-Hugh and Curtis syndrome
five-hour glucose tolerance test
fixation
complement f.
Nichols sacrospinous f.
fixator
Ilizarov external f.
FJN
familial juvenile nephrophthisis
FL
femur length
flaccid
f. extremity
flag sign
Flagyl
flail
f. foot
f. value
flammeus
nevus f.
flank pain
flap
bladder f.
Boari f.
bulbocavernosus fat f.
butterfly f.

NOTES

flap *(continued)*
    Byers f.
    endorectal f.
    fat f.
    Martius bulbocavernosus
      fat f.
    McCraw gracilis
      myocutaneous f.
    myocutaneous f.
    Pontén fasciocutaneous f.
    Warren f.
flaring
    f. of ala nasi
    alar f.
    f. and grunting
    grunting and f.
    nasal f.
flash
    hot f.
flat
    f. pelvis
    f. wart
flatfoot
flatus vaginalis
flecainide acetate
Fleet enema
Fleming
    F. afterloading tandem
    F. ovoid
fleshy mole
Fletcher-Suit
    F.-S. afterloading tandem
    F.-S. applicator
flexion
flexure
    splenic f.
Fliess treatment
Flint Infant Security Scale (FISS)
FLM
    fetal lung maturity
flood
flooding
floor
    pelvic f.
floppy infant syndrome
flora
    microbial f.
    vaginal f.
Florical
Florida pouch
florid complexion
flow
    blood f. ($\dot{Q}$)

    cardiac f.
    cerebral blood f.
    cutaneous blood f.
    Doppler f.
    fetal blood f.
    menstrual f.
    myocardial blood f.
    pulmonary blood f. (PBF)
    f. rate
    renal plasma f.
    retrograde menstrual f.
    umbilical blood f.
    urine f.
    uterine blood f.
    uteroplacental blood f.
    f. velocity waveform
    volume f.
flowering-out of fimbria
FlowGel
    F. barrier material
flowmeter
    laser-Doppler f.
Flowtron DVT prophylaxis unit
flow-volume loop
Floxin
floxuridine in hepatic metastasis
Fluanxol
fluconazole
flucytosine
flufenamic acid
Fluhmann test
fluid
    amniotic f. (AF)
    Bamberger f.
    body f.
    cerebrospinal f. (CSF)
    f.'s, electrolytes, nutrition
      (FEN)
    extracellular f.
    follicular f.
    human oviduct f. (HOF)
    meconium-stained
      amniotic f. (MSAF)
    f. overload
    peritoneal f.
    f. replacement
    serosanguineous f.
    sperm-counting f.
    f. therapy
    transcapillary f.
    f. wave
fluke
flumecinol

fluocinolone acetonide
Fluogen
fluorescein-conjugated monoclonal
    antibody test
fluorescein-labeled milk
fluorescein treponema antibody test
fluorescence-activated cell sorter
    (FACS)
fluorescence in situ hybridization
    (FISH)
fluorescent
    f. immunoassay (FIA)
    f. polarization
    f. treponema antibody
      (FTA)
    f. treponemal antibody
      absorption (FTA-ABS)
    f. treponemal antibody-
      absorption test
fluoridation
fluoride
    slow-release sodium f.
    sodium f.
fluorinated corticosteroid
fluorine
5-fluorocytosine (5-FC)
fluorodeoxyuridine (FUDR)
9-fluorohydrocortisone
fluorophosphate
    diisopropyl f.
Fluoroplex
fluoroscopy
fluorouracil
5-fluorouracil (5-FU)
    intraperitoneal 5-f.
Fluothane
fluoxetine HCl
fluoxymesterone
flupenthixol
fluphenazine
flurazepam
flurbiprofen
flush
    breast f.
    hot f.
    f. method
    orgasmic f.

flutamide
fluted drain
flutter
    atrial f.
Fluzone
fly
    Spanish f.
flying-T pelvis
FNA
    fine-needle aspiration
FNA-21
    F. needle
    F. syringe
foam
    Because vaginal f.
    contraceptive f.
    intravaginal f.
    Sklar f.
    f. stability index
    f. stability test
focal
    f. change
    f. dermal hypoplasia
      syndrome
    f. epilepsy
    f. fibrosis
    f. lobular carcinoma
    f. neurological deficit
    f. spot size
focally dilated duct
focus, pl. foci
    endometriotic f.
Foerster sign
folate
fold
    aryepiglottic f.
    Duncan f.'s
    epicanthal f.
    genitocrural f.
    head and tail f.
    f. of Hoboken
    Juvara f.
    Pawlik f.
    rectouterine f.
    rugal f.
    skin f.

NOTES

fold *(continued)*
    splanchnic f.
    urogenital f.
Foldan
folding frequency
Foley catheter
folic
    f. acid
    f. acid antagonist
    f. acid deficiency
folinic acid
follicle
    antral f.
    f. aspiration tube
    atretic f.
    dominant f.
    graafian f.
    luteinized unruptured f.
    f. maturation stimulation
    nabothian f.
    preantral f.
    preovulatory f.
    primary f.
    primordial f.
    f. regulatory protein (FRP)
    f. steroidogenesis
follicle-stimulating
    f.-s. hormone (FSH)
    f.-s. hormone antagonist
    f.-s. hormone binding
      inhibitor
    f.-s. hormone inhibition
    f.-s. hormone inhibitor
    f.-s. hormone secretion
follicular
    f. attrition
    f. cyst
    f. development arrest
    f. factor
    f. fluid
    f. function
    f. hematoma
    f. maturation
    f. phase
    f. phase gonadotropin
      secretion
    f. urethritis
    f. vulvitis
follicularis
    keratosis f.
folliculitis
folliculogenesis
folliculostatin

Folling disease
follistatin
follitropin
followup, follow-up
    f. care
    Carnation F.'s
    long-term f.
follow up
Follutein
Folvite
fontanel, fontanelle
    anterolateral f.
    Casser f.
    casserian f.
    Gerdy f.
    mastoid f.
    posterior f.
    posterolateral f.
    sagittal f.
    scaphoid f.
    f. sign
    sphenoid f.
    sunken f.
Fontan procedure
fonticulus, pl. **fonticuli**
foot
    athlete's f.
    club f.
    flail f.
    Freidreich f.
    Morand f.
    f. presentation
    reel f.
    rockerbottom f.
    spatula f.
foot-drop
footling
    f. breech presentation
    f. presentation
footprinting
foramen, pl. **foramina**
    f. of Monro
    f. ovale
    pleuroperitoneal f.
    f. primum
    f. secundum
Forane
Forbes-Albright syndrome
Forbes disease
force
    compression f.
    expulsive f.
    physician-applied f.

forcé
    eccouchement f.
forced
    f. expiratory volume (FEV)
    f. grasping reflex
forceps
    Adson f.
    alligator f.
    Allis f.
    Allis-Abramson breast
      biopsy f.
    Apple Medical bipolar f.
    atraumatic f.
    axis-traction f.
    Barton f.
    Baumberger f.
    BiCoag f.
    Bierer ovum f.
    Billroth tumor f.
    Bill traction handle f.
    bipolar laparoscopic f.
    Bozeman uterine dressing f.
    Brown-Adson tissue f.
    cephalic f.
    Chamberlen f.
    Clarke ligator scissor f.
    cold biopsy f.
    Corey ovum f.
    Corson myoma f.
    Crile f.
    DeBakey tissue f.
    DeLee f.
    f. delivery (FD)
    DeWeese axis traction f.
    Dewey obstetrical f.
    dressing f.
    Elliot f.
    ENDO-ASSIST endoscopic f.
    Eppendorfer biopsy f.
    Evershears bipolar
      laparoscopic f.
    Gellhorn f.
    Haig-Fergusson f.
    Halsted mosquito f.
    Hawk-Dennen f.
    Heaney f.
    Heaney-Ballentine f.

    Heaney-Hyst f.
    Hirst placental f.
    Hodge f.
    hot biopsy f.
    Hunt bipolar f.
    Kevorkian-Younge biopsy f.
    Kjelland f.
    Kjelland-Barton f.
    Kjelland-Luikart f.
    Kleppinger bipolar f.
    Lahey f.
    Laufe polyp f.
    Levret f.
    low f.
    Luikart f.
    f. maneuver
    McGill f.
    McLane f.
    Naegele f.
    nonfenestrated f.
    obstetrical f.
    Ochsner f.
    Palmer ovarian biopsy f.
    Péan f.
    pelvic f.
    Perez-Castro f.
    Phaneuf uterine artery f.
    Piper f.
    Pistofidis cervical biopsy f.
    Polaris reusable f.
    punch biopsy f.
    Quinones-Neubüser uterine-
      grasping f.
    Quinones uterine-grasping f.
    Randall stone f.
    Reiner-Knight f.
    Rochester-Ochsner f.
    Rochester-Péan f.
    Roger f.
    f. rotation
    Russian tissue f.
    Saenger ovum f.
    Schroeder tenaculum f.
    Schroeder vulsellum f.
    Schubert uterine biopsy f.
    Seitzinger tripolar cutting f.
    Shearer f.

NOTES

forceps *(continued)*
    Shute f.
    Simpson f.
    Singley f.
    Sopher ovum f.
    sponge f.
    sponge-holding f.
    Tarnier axis-traction f.
    Thomas-Gaylor biopsy f.
    Tischler cervical biopsy f.
    Tischler-Morgan uterine
     biopsy f.
    tissue f.
    trial f.
    Tucker-McLane f.
    Tucker-McLane-Luikhart f.
    uterine tenaculum f.
    Willett f.
    Winter placental f.
    Yeoman f.
Fordyce
    F. disease
    F. granule
    F. spot
forebag
foregut malformation
foreign
    f. body
    f. body salpingitis
forekidney
foremilk
foreplay
foreskin
forewaters
fork
    replication f.
form
    Doppler flow-velocity
     wave f.
formaldehyde
formation
    blood vessel f.
    bone f.
    chiasma f.
    echo f.
    somite f.
formative yolk
forme fruste
formiminoglutamic acid (FIGLU)
formula
    Advance f.
    20-calorie f.
    24-calorie f.

dextro f.
Enfamil Next Step
  toddler f.
Enfamil Premature 20 F.
evaporated milk f.
fortified f.
full-strength f.
glucose f.
goat's milk f.
Good Nature f.
Good Start HA f.
half-strength f.
Hardy-Weinberg f.
high-calorie f.
high-fructose f.
high-glucose f.
hypercaloric f.
Infalyte f.
Isomil f.
I-Soyalac f.
Lactofree f.
lactose-free f.
Lonalac f.
Lytren f.
Mall f.
MCT oil f.
Mead-Johnson f.
menstrual f.
Neocate f.
Nursoy f.
Nutramigen f.
Osmolite f.
Pedialyte f.
PediaSure f.
PEF-24 f.
PM-60/40 f.
Polycose f.
Portagen f.
Pregestimil f.
Premature f.
Premature Special Care f.
ProSobee f.
Pulmocare f.
quarter-strength f.
Rehydralyte f.
Rice-Lyte f.
Sabbagha f.
Similac f.
Similac Special Care f.
Sim SC-20 f.
Sim SC-24 f.
S-M-A f.
sodium-free f.

Soyalac f.
Spearman-Brown
  prediction f.
Special Care f.
SSC-20 f.
SSC-24 f.
sucrose-free f.
Sustacal f.
Sustagen f.
three-quarter strength f.
fornix, pl. **fornices**
  posterior f.
**Forsius-Eriksson type ocular
  albinism**
Forssman antigen
Fortaz
Fortel ovulation test
fortified formula
fortifier
  Enfamil human milk f.
  human milk f.
fosinopril
fossa
  f. navicularis
Fothergill-Donald operation
Fothergill-Hunter operation
Fothergill operation
founder chromosome
four-cell embryo
four-chamber view
fourchette
four-day syndrome
four-flap Z-plasty
four-hour rule
**Fourier transform infrared
  microspectroscopy**
Fournier teeth
fourth
  Bartholomew rule of f.'s
  f. parallel pelvic plane
  f. venereal disease
Fowler position
Fowler-Stephens orchiopexy
Fox-Fordyce disease
fraction
  f. of alveolar carbon
    dioxide ($FACO_2$)

f. in expired gas of carbon
  dioxide ($FECO_2$)
plasma f.
S phase f.
fractional dilation and curettage
fractionated radiation therapy
fractionation
fracture
  birth f.
  Colles f.
  fetal f.
  hip f.
  intrauterine f.
  maternal f.
  osteoporotic f.
  pelvic f.
  skull f.
  spinal compression f.
  vertebral compression f.
fractured chromosomes
fragile
  f. X
  f. X carrier
  f. X chromosome
  f. X syndrome
fragment
  f. antigen binding
  Okazaki f.
  placental f.
Franceschetti-Jadassohn syndrome
Franceschetti-Klein syndrome
Franceschetti syndrome
Francois syndrome
**Frangenheim-Goebel-Stoeckel
  operation**
frank
  f. breech presentation
  F. nonsurgical perineal
    autodilation
  F. procedure
  F. technique
  F. technique of dilation
Frankenhäuser
  F. ganglion
  F. plexus
Franklin Diagnostics
Franklin-Dukes test

NOTES

Frank-Starling
    F.-S. principle
    F.-S. relation
frappage therapy
Fraser syndrome
fraternal twins
FRAXE-associated mental
  retardation
FRC
  functional residual capacity
FreAmine
Fredet-Ramstedt
    F.-R. operation
    F.-R. procedure
free
    F. & Active
    f. androgen index
    f. beta
    f. beta test
    f. estradiol
    f. fatty acid
    f. hydroxyl radical
    f. testosterone
    f. testosterone index
    f. thyroxine index
Freeman-Sheldon syndrome
freezing process
Frei
    F. antibody
    F. test
Freiberg
    F. disease
    F. infraction
Freidman splint
Freidreich foot
French
    F. Gesco catheter
    F. lock
French-American-British (FAB)
frenectomy
frenoplasty
frenotomy
frenulum, pl. **frenula**
frenum
frequency
    folding f.
    Nyquist f.
    pulse f.
    urinary f.
fresh frozen plasma (FFP)
freudian
Freud theory

Freund
    F. adjuvant
    F. operation
Freyer suprapubic drain
Friberg microsurgical agglutination
  test
Friedman
    F. curve
    F. rabbit test
Friedman-Lapham test
Friedreich ataxia
Friedrich
    F. criteria
    F. criteria for dyspareunia
Friend syndrome
frigid
frigidity
Fritsch
    F. douche
    F. syndrome
Fritsch-Asherman syndrome
frogleg
    f. position
    f. view
froglegged
Fröhlich syndrome
frondlike
frontal
    f. bossing
    f. horns
    f. suture
frontoanterior
    left f. position (LFA)
    f. position
    right f. position (RFA)
frontometaphyseal dysplasia
frontoposterior
    left f. position (LFP)
    f. position
    right f. position (RFP)
frontotransverse
    left f. position (LFT)
    f. position
    right f. position (RFT)
frostbite
frozen
    f. egg
    f. embryo
    f. ovum
    f. pelvis
    f. plasma
    f. red cells
    f. section

f. semen
f. sperm
f. zygote
FRP
follicle regulatory protein
fructokinase
fructose
f. galactokinase deficiency
f. intolerance
fructosuria
frusemide
fruste
forme f.
Fryne syndrome
FSH
follicle-stimulating hormone
FTA
fluorescent treponema antibody
FTA test
FTA-ABS
fluorescent treponemal antibody
absorption
(FTB)
Mono-Test (FTB)
FTBD
full term, born dead
FTT
failure to thrive
5-FU
5-fluorouracil
fucosidosis
FUDR
fluorodeoxyuridine
FUE
fever of unknown etiology
fugax
amaurosis f.
fugue state
Fujinon flexible hysteroscope
fulguration
full-breech presentation
Fuller shield
full-strength formula
full term, born dead (FTBD)
full-term pregnancy

full-thickness skin graft
fulminans
purpura f.
fulminant
f. hepatitis
Fulvicin
fumarate
ferrous f.
function
adrenocortical f.
bladder f.
bowel f.
cardiac f.
cardiorespiratory f.
corpus luteum f.
fetal cardiac f.
fetoplacental f.
follicular f.
hypothalamic-pituitary f.
kidney f.
leukocyte f.
luteal f.
myocardial f.
oromotor f.
ovarian f.
pituitary gland f.
pituitary-ovarian f.
pulmonary f.
renal f.
renal tubular f.
reproductive f.
sexual f.
thyroid f.
urethral f.
ventricular f.
functional
f. dysmenorrhea
f. murmur
f. ovarian cyst
f. prepubertal castrate
syndrome
f. residual capacity (FRC)
fundal height
fundectomy

NOTES

fundoplication
    Nissen f.
    Toupet f.
fundus, pl. fundi
    optic f.
fundusectomy
fungal
    f. infection
fungating mass
fungi (*pl. of* fungus)
Fungizone
Fungoid Tincture
fungus, pl. fungi
    f. ball
    umbilical f.
funic
    f. presentation
    f. reduction
    f. souffle
funicular souffle
funiculus, pl. funiculi
    f. umbilicalis
funipuncture
funis
funnel
    accessory müllerian f.
    f. chest

funnel-shaped pelvis
Funston syndrome
FUO
    fever of unknown origin
Furadantin
Furalan
furan
furazolidone
furosemide
Furoxone
furuncle
furunculosis
fusanic acid
fusion
    f. of eyelids
    f. implantation
    labial f.
    müllerian duct f.
    robertsonian f.
Fusobacterium
    F. gonidiaformans
    F. mortiferum
    F. necrophorum
    F. nucleatum
FVS
    fetal varicella syndrome

G
   gravida
      G band
      G protein
G$_0$
   gap$_0$
G$_1$
   gap$_1$
G$_2$
   gap$_2$
GA
   gestational age
Gabastou hydraulic method
GAG
   glycosaminoglycan
gag reflex
Gailliard syndrome
gain
   weight g.
gait
   broad-based g.
   toe-in g.
galactacrasia
galactagogue
galactic
galactobolic
galactocele
galactography
galactokinesis
galactopoiesis
galactorrhea
galactorrhea-amenorrhea syndrome
galactose
galactosemia
galactosis
galactotherapy
Galbiati bilateral fetal
  ischiopubiotomy
galea
Galeazzi sign
Gallant reflex
gallbladder
   g. disease
Galli-Mainini test
gallinatum
   pectus g.
gallstone
   g. pancreatitis
galoche chin
Galtonian-Fisher genetics

galtonian trait
Galton law of regression
Gamble-Darrow syndrome
gametangium
gamete
   aging g.
   g. intrafallopian transfer
   (GIFT)
   g. manipulation
gametic chromosome
gametogenesis
   ovarian g.
Gamimune N
gamma
   g. globulin
   g. glutamyl transferase
   (GGT)
   g. interferon
   g. ray
gamma-benzene hexachloride
Gamma BHC
gamma-chain disorder
Gammagard
   G. S/D
gamma-loop disorder
Gamper bowing reflex
gampsodactyly
Gamulin Rh
gangliocytoma
ganglion, pl. ganglia
   basal g.
   Frankenhäuser g.
   g. trigger theory
ganglioneuroma
ganglioneuromatosis
ganglionic blocker
ganglioside storage disease
gangliosidosis
   generalized g.
   juvenile g.
gangrene
   gas g.
   pulmonary g.
   spontaneous g. of newborn
gangrenosa
   varicella g.
Gantanol
   Azo G.
Gantrisin
   Azo G.

GAP
 gonadotropin releasing hormone-
 associated peptide
gap_0 (G_0)
gap_1 (G_1)
gap_2 (G_2)
gap
 anion g.
 g. junction
Garamycin
Gardnerella
 G. vaginalis
 G. vaginalis
 chorioamnionitis
 G. vaginitis
Gardner syndrome
gargantuan mastitis
gargoylism
Gariel pessary
Gartner
 G. cyst
 G. duct
gartnerian
 g. cyst
 g. duct
gas, pl. gases
 g. anesthetic
 arterial blood g. (ABG)
 blood gases
 capillary blood g. (CBG)
 cord blood g. (CBG)
 g. embolus
 fetal blood gases
 g. gangrene
 inspired g. (I)
 intervillous blood g.
 sweep g.
 g. transfer
 venous blood g. (VBG)
 volume of expired g. (VE)
GASA
 growth-adjusted sonographic age
Gas-Pak jar
Gasser syndrome
gastric
 g. bubble
 g. bypass
 g. dysrhythmia
 g. emptying
 g. emptying time
 g. enteral feeding
 g. fluid aspiration
 g. lavage

 g. reduction surgery
 g. volvulus
gastritis
gastroacephalus
gastroamorphus
gastrocolic reflex
gastrodidymus
gastroenteritis
 eosinophilic g.
gastroesophageal
 g. incompetence
 g. reflux (GER)
Gastrografin
gastrointestinal
 g. disorder
 g. fistula
 g. infection
 g. malignancy
 g. obstruction
 g. series
 g. tract
 g. tuberculosis
gastromelus
gastropagus
gastroplasty
gastroschisis
 Silastic silo reduction of g.
gastrostomy
gastrothoracopagus
gastrula
gate control theory
Gaucher disease
Gauss sign
gauze
 g. dissection
 g. wick
gavage
 g. feeding
GAX collagen
GCI
 gestational carbohydrate
 intolerance
G-CSF
 granulocyte colony-stimulating
 factor
GDM
 gestational diabetes mellitus
Gee disease
Gee-Herter disease
Gee-Herter-Heubner
 G.-H.-H. disease
 G.-H.-H. syndrome
Gehrung pessary

gel

Accoustix conductivity g.
Aquagel lubricating g.
Aquasonic 100 ultrasound
transmission g.
Cerviprost g.
Comfort personal
lubricant g.
dinoprostone cervical g.
1D sodium dodecyl
sulfate g.
Electro-Gel conductivity g.
electrophoresis g.
Itch-X g.
MetroGel-Vaginal g.
metronidazole vaginal g.
Monsel g.
Prepidil G.
PRO/Gel ultrasound
transmission g.
prostaglandin E_2 g.
Scan ultrasound g.
gelastic seizure
gelatin agglutination test
gelatinous
g. skin
g. varix
geleophysic dwarfism
Gelfoam
Gellhorn
G. forceps
G. pessary
Gelpi-Lowrie retractor
Gelpi-Lowry hysterectomy
Gelpi perineal retractor
gel-transfer
gemellary pregnancy
gemellipara
geminus, pl. gemini
gemmule
Hoboken g.'s
Gemonil
Genapax
Gencalc 600
gender
g. assignment
g. determination

g. dysphoria syndrome
g. reversal
g. role

gene

g. action
adhalin g.
allelic g.
g. amplification
autosomal g.
cell interaction g.
chimeric g.
g. cloning
c-*myc* g.
codominant g.
complementary g.'s
g. complex
cumulative g.
g. deletion
derepressed g.
dominant g.
g. duplication
dystrophin g.
H g.
histocompatibility g.
holandric g.'s
homeobox-2 g.
homeotic g.'s
housekeeping g.
immune response g.
immune suppressor g.
immunoglobulin g.
Ir g.
Is g.
jumping g.
leaky g.
lethal g.
g. library
g. location
g. locus
major g.
g. map
g. mapping
marker g.
MOMP g.
mutant g.
g. mutation
nonstructural g.

NOTES

gene *(continued)*
    od g.
    operator g.
    partner g.'s
    penetrant g.
    pleiotropic g.
    g. pool
    g. probe
    recessive g.
    reciprocal g.'s
    regulator g.
    repressed g.
    repressor g.
    g. sequencing
    sex-conditioned g.
    sex-influenced g.
    sex-limited g.
    sex-linked g.
    silent g.
    g. splicing
    structural g.
    sublethal g.
    supplementary g.'s
    suppressor g.
    syntenic g.'s
    tdy g.
    g. therapy
    g. transcription
    wild-type g.
    X-linked g.
    Y-linked g.
    Z-linked g.
Genentech
    G. biosynthetic human
      growth hormone
    G. growth chart
general anesthesia
generalisata
    osteitis condensans g.
generalized
    g. gangliosidosis
    g. linear interactive
      modeling (GLIM)
generational
generator
    Valleylab Force IC
      electrosurgical g.
genesial cycle
genetic
    g. abnormality
    g. amniocentesis
    g. anomaly
    g. burden

    g. code
    g. counseling
    g. defect
    g. diagnosis
    g. disease
    g. disorder
    g. drift
    g. engineering
    g. equilibrium
    g. linkage
    g. locus
    g. marker
    g. material
    g. model
    g. screening
    g. sex
    g. susceptibility
    g. switch
    g. test
geneticist
genetics
    behavioral g.
    classical g.
    epidemiological g.
    Galtonian-Fisher g.
    modern g.
    multilocal g.
    prenatal g.
    reproductive g.
    reverse g.
genetotrophic
    g. disease
genetous
genital
    g. ambiguity
    g. cord
    g. corpuscle
    g. crisis of newborn
    g. development
    g. differentiation
    g. duct
    g. elephantiasis
    g. herpes
    g. infection
    g. lesion
    g. mycoplasma
    g. ridge
    g. tract
    g. tract embryology
    g. tract malignancy
    g. tract trauma
    g. tract tumor
    g. tubercle

g. ulcer
g. ulcer syndrome
g. wart
genitalia
ambiguous g.
external g.
indifferent g.
internal g.
lymphatic drainage of g.
genitalis
herpes g.
genitocrural fold
genitofemoral nerve
**Genitor mini-intrauterine
insemination cannula**
genitourinary
g. abnormality
g. defect
g. fistula
genoblast
genocopy
genome
g. DNA
Genoptic
G. S.O.P.
Genora
G. 0.5/35
G. 1/35
G. 1/50
genotype
genotypic
Gen-Probe test
Gentacidin
Gent-AK
gentamicin
g. sulfate
gentian violet
Gentrasul
genu
g. recurvatum
g. valgum
genucubital position
Genupak tampon
genupectoral position
genus
Bordetella g.
Geocillin

geographic tongue
Geopen
geophagia
Gepfert procedure
GER
gastroesophageal reflux
Gerace reflex
Gerdy fontanel
Geref
Gerimed
germ
g. cell
g. cell ovarian neoplasm
g. cell teratoma
g. cell testicular tumor
g. cell tumor
g. layer
g. line
g. ridge
German
G. lock
G. measles
germinal
g. epithelium
g. epithelium of Waldeyer
g. membrane
g. pole
g. vesicle
g. vesicle breakdown
(GVBD)
germinoma
Gerstmann syndrome
**GE RT 3200 Advantage II
ultrasound**
Gesco
G. cannula
G. catheter
Gesell
G. Developmental Scale
G. test
G. test with Knobloch
modification
gestagen
gestagenic
gestation
anembryonic g.
multiple g.

NOTES

gestation *(continued)*
    prolonged g.
    term g.
    tubal g.
    twin g.
    unruptured tubal g.
gestational
    g. abnormality
    g. age (GA)
    g. age assessment
    g. age estimation
    g. carbohydrate intolerance (GCI)
    g. diabetes
    g. diabetes mellitus (GDM)
    g. edema
    g. hypertension
    g. lupus
    g. proteinuria
    g. psychosis
    g. ring
    g. sac
    g. sac mean diameter
    g. surrogate
    g. trophoblastic disease (GTD)
    g. trophoblastic neoplasia (GTN)
    g. trophoblastic tumor
gestator
Gesterol
gestodene
Gestogen
gestosis, pl. gestoses
Gestrinone
GF
    growth factor
GFR
    glomerular filtration rate
GGT
    gamma glutamyl transferase
GH
    growth hormone
Ghon
    G. complex
    G. tubercle
GH-RH
    growth hormone-releasing hormone
GHST
    growth hormone stimulation test
Gianotti-Crosti syndrome

giant
    g. baby
    g. cell hepatitis
    g. cell pneumonia
    g. chromosome
    g. fibroadenoma
Gianturco spring embolus
giardiasis
gibbous deformity
gibbus
Gibco BRL sperm preparation media
GI cocktail
Giemsa
    G. banding
    G. stain
Gierke disease
GIFT
    gamete intrafallopian transfer
    cervical GIFT
    intrauterine GIFT
    vaginal GIFT
gigantism
    cerebral g.
    eunuchoid g.
    exomphalos, macroglossia, and g. (EMG)
    fetal g.
    hyperpituitary g.
    pituitary g.
gigantoblast
gigantomastia
giggle incontinence
Gigli
    G. operation
    G. saw
Gilbert disease
Gilbert-Dreyfus syndrome
Gilbert-Lereboullet syndrome
gill
    g. arch skeleton
    G. respirator
Gilles de la Tourette syndrome
Gilliam
    G. operation
    G. round ligament
Gilliam-Doleris
    G.-D. operation
    G.-D. uterine suspension
Gimbernat reflex ligament
gingival fibromatosis
gingivitis
    herpetic g.

gingivostomatitis
  herpetic g.
Giordano operation
girdle
  Hitzig g.
gitalin
Gittes
  G. operation
  G. procedure
  G. technique
gland
  adrenal g.
  apocrine g.
  Bartholin g.
  bulbourethral g.
  Cowper g.
  Duverney g.
  eccrine g.
  endocrine g.
  external genitalia/Bartholin,
    urethral, and Skene g.'s
    (EG/BUS)
  fetal adrenal g.
  Littre g.
  mammary g.
  Mery g.
  Montgomery g.'s
  nabothian g.
  parathyroid g.
  paraurethral g.
  parotid g.
  periurethral g.
  Philip g.
  pineal g.
  pituitary g.
  salivary g.
  Skene g.
  sublingual g.
  submaxillary g.
  thymus g.
  thyroid g.
  urethral g.
  uterine g.
  vestibular g.
glandular
  g. cells
  g. hyperplasia

  g. mastitis
  g. tissue
glans
Glanzmann
  G. disease
  G. syndrome
  G. thrombasthenia
Glanzmann-Riniker syndrome
glass factor
glass-wool filtration
glassy cell carcinoma
glaucoma
  congenital g.
  primary congenital g.
Glaucon
Glazunov tumor
Gleeson FloVAC Hi-Flo
  laparoscopic suction/irrigation
  system
gleet
  vent g.
gleety discharge
Glen Anderson
  ureteroneocystostomy
Glenard disease
Glenn operation
GLIM
  generalized linear interactive
  modeling
glioma
  optic g.
  pontine g.
gliosis
  g. uteri
glipizide
global aphasia
globe cell anemia
globin
  α-g.
  β-g.
globoid cell leukodystrophy
globulin
  anti-D gamma g.
  anti-D immune g.
  antithymocyte g.
  corticosteroid-binding g.
  (CBG)

NOTES

globulin *(continued)*
    gamma g.
    hepatitis B immune g.
     (HBIG, HBIg)
    hepatitis immune g.
    human g.
    hyperimmune serum g.
    immune g.
    immune serum g. (ISG)
    pregnancy-associated g.
    rabies immune g.
    Rho immune g.
    sex hormone-binding g.
     (SHBG)
    testosterone-estrogen-
     binding g.
    tetanus immune g.
    thyroid-binding g. (TBG)
    thyroxine-binding g.
    varicella-zoster immune g.
     (VZIG)
    zoster immune g. (ZIG)
globus hystericus
glomerular
    g. capillary endotheliosis
    g. change
    g. filtration
    g. filtration rate (GFR)
    g. insufficiency
    g. proteinuria
    g. sclerosis
glomeruli (*pl. of* glomerulus)
glomerulonephritis
    membranous g.
glomerulopathy
glomerulosclerosis
glomerulotubular
glomerulus, pl. **glomeruli**
glossitis
glossopalatine ankylosis syndrome
glossoptosis
glove
    Biogel g.
    Micro-Touch Platex
     medical g.
gloving
    double g.
glubionate
    calcium g.
glucagon
Glucamide
glucocorticoid
    g. excess

glucocorticosteroid therapy
glucoglycinuria
Glucola
    G. screen
Glucolet Endcaps
glucometer
    Accu-Chek II g.
    G. Elite diabetes care
     system
    G. II
gluconate
    calcium g.
    ferrous g.
    potassium g.
gluconeogenesis
glucose
    blood g.
    g. challenge test
    fetal blood g.
    g. formula
    hypertonic g.
    g. intolerance
    g. meter
    g. tolerance
    g. tolerance test (GTT)
    urinary g.
glucose-galactose intolerance
glucose-6-phosphate
    g.-p. dehydrogenase (G6PD)
    g.-p. dehydrogenase
     deficiency
glucosiduronate
Glucostix
glucosuria
Glucotrol
glucuronate pregnanediol
glucuronide
    3α-androstanediol g.
    5α-androstane-3α,17β-diol g.
     (3α-diol-G)
    androsterone g.
    virilizing 3α-
     androstanediol g.
Glukor
glutamate
    arginine g.
    g. cycle
glutamyl transpeptidase (GTP)
glutaraldehyde
glutaric acidemia
glutathionemia
gluteal lymph node
gluten-free diet

glyburide
glycemia
glycemic control
glycerin
    g., lanolin and peanut oil
    g. suppository
glycerol
    iodinated g.
glycerophospholipid
glyceryl
    g. guaiacolate
    g. trinitrate (GTN)
glycinuria
glycocalyx
glycogen
glycogenesis
glycogenolysis
    von Gierke g.
glycogenosis
    type 7 g.
glycogen-storage disease
    g.-s. d. type 1
glycohemoglobin
glycoprotein
    heterodimeric integral
      membrane g.
glycopyrrolate
glycorrhachia
glycosaminoglycan (GAG)
glycoside
    cardiac g.
glycosuria
glycosylated hemoglobin (HbA1C)
    g. h. A
Glyrol
gm
    gram
GM-CSF
    granulocyte-macrophage colony-
      stimulating factor
gnathocephalus
GnRH
    gonadotropin-releasing hormone
    G. agonist
GnRH-facilitated
    G.-f. FSH release
    G.-f. LH release

Goa antigen
goat's milk formula
Goebell-Frangenheim-Stoeckel
    technique
Goebell procedure
Goebell-Stoeckel-Frangenheim
    procedure
Goffe colporrhaphy
GOG
    Gynecologic Oncology Group
goiter
    g. development
    simple colloid g.
gold
    g.-198 (^{198}Au)
    radioactive g.
    g. salt
    g. seeds
    g. sodium thiomalate
    g. therapy
Goldenhar syndrome
Golden sign
Goldstein
    G. disease
    G. sign
Golgi bodies
Goltz-Gorlin syndrome
Goltz syndrome
GoLYTELY
Gomco
    G. bell
    G. circumcision clamp
    G. technique
gonad
    indifferent g.'s
    maternal g.
    streak g.'s
    undifferentiated g.
gonadal
    g. agenesis
    g. agenesis syndrome
    g. aplasia
    g. axis
    g. dysgenesis
    g. failure
    g. mosaicism
    g. ridge

NOTES

gonadal *(continued)*
    g. sex
    g. steroid suppression
    g. streak
    g. stroma
    g. stromal ovarian tumor
gonadarche
gonadectomy
gonadoblastoma
    ovarian g.
gonadocrinin
gonadoliberin
gonadorelin
    g. acetate
gonadostat
gonadotrope
gonadotrophin *(var. of*
  gonadotropin)
**gonadotrophin-releasing hormone-
like protein**
**gonadotrophin-resistant ovary
syndrome**
gonadotropic deficiency
gonadotropin, gonadotrophin
    chorionic g. (CG)
    exogenous g.
    human chorionic g. (hCG,
      HCG)
    human menopausal g.
      (HMG)
    g. level
    pituitary g.
    pulsatile human
      menopausal g.
    g. pulsatile release
    g. regulation
    g. release
    g. releasing hormone-
      associated peptide (GAP)
    g. secretion
    g. secretion inhibitor
    urinary chorionic g. (UCG)
**gonadotropin-induced ovarian
hyperstimulation**
gonadotropin-releasing
    g.-r. hormone (GnRH)
    g.-r. hormone agonist
    g.-r. hormone analogue
    g.-r. hormone antagonist
    g.-r. hormone-like peptide
    g.-r. peptide
gonadotropin-resistant testis
gonane

Gonic
gonidiaformans
    Fusobacterium g.
gonoblennorrhea
gonococcal
    g. conjunctivitis
    g. infection
    g. ophthalmia
gonococcus
Gono Kwik test
gonorrhea
    g. culture
    disseminated g.
gonorrheal
    g. cervicitis
    g. ophthalmia
    g. salpingitis
gonorrhoeae
    Neisseria g.
Gonozyme test
Gonzales blood group
Good
    G. Nature formula
    G. Start HA formula
Goodall-Power operation
Goodell
    G. dilator
    G. sign
Goodman syndrome
Goodpasture syndrome
gooseneck deformity
Gordan-Overstreet syndrome
Gore-Tex surgical membrane
Gorlin-Psaume syndrome
goserelin
    g. acetate
    g. acetate implant
gossypol
Gott-Balfour blade
Gott-Harrington blade
Gott malleable retractor
Gott-Seeram blade
Gougerot-Carteaud syndrome
Goulet retractor
gouty diathesis
Gower-1
    hemoglobin G.
Gower-2
    hemoglobin G.
Gowers sign
gown
    Barrier g.

G6PD
glucose-6-phosphate
dehydrogenase
GPMAL
gravida, para, multiple births,
abortions, live births
G-protein-coupled receptor
graafian
g. follicle
g. vesicle
gracilis
g. flap technique
g. muscle
grade
placental g.
Gradenigo syndrome
gradient
A-a g.
g. recalled acquisition in a
steady state (GRASS)
grading
histopathological g.
placental g.
tumor g.
Graefenberg ring
Grafco breast pump
graft
allogeneic fetal g.
bilateral myocutaneous g.
full-thickness skin g.
heterologous g.
isogeneic g.
polytetrafluoroethylene g.
split-thickness g.
graft-versus-host
g.-v.-h. disease (GVHD)
g.-v.-h. reaction
Graham-Rosenblith scale
Graham Steell murmur
gram (gm)
oxy-CR g.
Gram-negative, gram-negative
G.-n. bacilli
G.-n. bacteria
G.-n. cocci
G.-n. organism

G.-n. pneumonia
G.-n. rods
Gram-positive, gram-positive
G.-p. bacilli
G.-p. bacteria
G.-p. cocci
G.-p. organism
G.-p. rods
Gram stain
Gram-Weigert stain
grand
g. climacteric
g. mal
g. mal epilepsy
g. multipara
g. multiparity
g. pregnancy
grandmother theory
Granger sign
Grant-Ward operation
granular
g. cell myoblastoma
g. lung
g. urethritis
granulation tissue
granule
argyrophilic g.
Birbeck g.
cortical g.
Fordyce g.
sulfur g.
granulocyte colony-stimulating
factor (G-CSF)
granulocyte-macrophage colony-
stimulating factor (GM-CSF)
granulocytic leukemia
granuloma, pl. granulomata
g. annulare
g. gravidarum
g. inguinale
Langhans giant cell g.
pyogenic g.
telangiectatic g.
granulomatosis
Wegener g.
granulomatous
g. calcification

NOTES

granulomatous *(continued)*
    g. colitis
    g. infection
    g. mastitis
    g. salpingitis
granulosa
    g. cell
    g. cell tumor
    g. lutein cell
granulosa-stromal cell tumor
grape mole
graphesthesia
grasp
    finger g.
    pincer g.
    g. reflex
grasper
    Polaris reusable g.
GRASS
    gradient recalled acquisition in a
    steady state
        GRASS MRI
        GRASS MRI technique
grating sound
Graves
    G. bivalve speculum
    G. disease
gravid
    g. uterus
gravida (G)
gravida, para, multiple births,
    abortions, live births (GPMAL)
gravidarum
    chorea g.
    epulis g.
    hydrops g.
    hyperemesis g.
gravidic
    g. retinitis
    g. retinopathy
gravidism
graviditas
    g. examnialis
    g. exochorialis
gravidity
Gravindex test
gravis
    icterus g.
    myasthenia g.
    neonatal myasthenia g.
Gravlee jet washer
Gravol

gray
    g. baby syndrome
    g. syndrome
gray-scale ultrasonography
great
    g. arteries
    g. vessels
Greenfield disease
Green uterine curette
Gregersen U-elevator
Greig syndrome
Greulich and Pyle bone age
grid
gridiron incision
Grifulvin V
grimace
Grimelius stain
Grisactin
Griscelli syndrome
griseofulvin
Grisolle sign
Grisovin
Gris-PEG
groin
    g. dissection
    g. hernia
grommet
groove
    Harrison g.
    neural g.
    primitive g.
    g. sign
grotesque features
ground-glass appearance
group
    g. A streptococcus
    blood g.
    g. B streptococcus
    Cartwright blood g.
    Children's Cancer Study G.
      (CCSG)
    determinant g.
    g. D streptococcus
    Gonzales blood g.
    Gynecologic Oncology G.
      (GOG)
    Kidd blood g.
    Lewis blood g.
    Lutheran blood g.
    Pediatric Oncology G.
      (POG)
    private blood g.
    Rh blood g.

streptococcal g.
support g.
grouping
blood g.
growth
bacterial g.
g. discordancy
epiphyseal g.
g. factor (GF)
fetal g.
fetal cellular g.
g. hormone (GH)
g. hormone release
g. hormone-releasing
hormone (GH-RH)
g. hormone-secreting
adenoma
g. hormone stimulation test
(GHST)
longitudinal g.
nonestrogen-regulated g.
placental g.
g. problem
pubertal g.
g. retardation
retarded fetal g.
skeletal g.
growth-adjusted sonographic age
(GASA)
growth-discordant twins
growth-like factor
growth-retarded fetus
Gruber syndrome
Grünfelder reflex
grunting
flaring and g.
g. and flaring
g. respirations
G-spot
GTD
gestational trophoblastic disease
GTN
gestational trophoblastic
neoplasia
glyceryl trinitrate
GTP
glutamyl transpeptidase

guanosine triphosphate
guanosine 5'-triphosphate
GTT
glucose tolerance test
guaiac
g. test
guaiacolate
glyceryl g.
guaifenesin
guanabenz
guanadrel
guanethidine
guanfacine
guanine
guanosine
g. triphosphate (GTP)
g. 5'-triphosphate (GTP)
gubernaculum
guidance
ultrasound g.
Guillain-Barré-Landry syndrome
gulf
Lecat g.
gumma
gun
Bard Biopty g.
Cobe g.
coring biopsy g.
Günther disease
Guthrie
G. card
G. muscle
G. test
gut suture
guttata
g. parapsoriasis
g. psoriasis
gutter
pelvic g.
GVBD
germinal vesicle breakdown
GVHD
graft-versus-host disease
gymnast's wrist
GYN
gynecologic

NOTES

GYN *(continued)*
    gynecologist
    gynecology
gynandroblastoma
gynatresia
gynecic
gynecogenic
gynecography
gynecoid
    g. obesity
    g. pelvis
gynecologic, gynecological (GYN)
    g. cancer
    g. cancer patient
    g. history
    g. oncology
    G. Oncology Group (GOG)
gynecologist (GYN)
    American College of
      Obstetricians and G.'s
      (ACOG)
gynecology (GYN)

    adolescent g.
    Council on Resident
      Education in Obstetrics
      and G. (CREOG)
    International Federation
      Obstetrics and G.
    pediatric g.
gynecomastia
Gyne-Lotrimin
Gyne-Sulf
gyniatrics
gyniatry
gynogenetic
Gynogen L.A.
Gynol II contraceptive jelly
gynopathy
gynoplasty, gynoplastics
GynoSampler endometrial aspirator
Gynos perineometer
gyrata
    cutis verticis g.

Haase rule
HABA
  hydroxybenzeneazobenzoic acid
  HABA binding test
habit
  bladder h.'s
  bowel h.'s
  eating h.'s
  sexual h.'s
  sleeping h.'s
habitual
  h. aborter
  h. abortion
habituation
habitus
  body h.
  Buddha-like h.
  fetal h.
  h. of fetus
HAC
  hexamethylmelamine with
  doxorubicin and
  cyclophosphamide
Hacker hypospadias
Hadlock equation
Haemophilus
  H. ducreyi
  H. influenzae
  H. influenzae type B (HIB)
  H. pertussis
  H. pertussis vaccine (HPV)
  H. vaginalis
  H. vaginitis
Hageman factor
Hahn sign
Haig-Fergusson forceps
Haight baby retractor
Hailey-Hailey disease
hair
  h. growth phase
  lanugo h.
  h. loss
  h. monster
  pubic h.
  sexual h.
  terminal h.
  vellus h.

HAIR-AN
  hyperandrogenism, insulin
  resistance, acanthosis nigricans
  HAIR-AN syndrome
hairball
hairpin vessel
hairy tongue
Hajdu-Cheney syndrome
Hakim-Adams syndrome
Hakim syndrome
Halban
  H. culdoplasty
  H. syndrome
Halbrecht syndrome
Haldol
half-life
half-strength formula
half-value layer (HVL)
Halle
  H. infant nasal speculum
  H. point
Hallermann-Streiff-François
  syndrome
Hallermann-Streiff syndrome
Hallervorden-Spatz
  H.-S. disease
  H.-S. syndrome
Hallopeau-Siemens syndrome
Hall-Pallister syndrome
Hall-Riggs syndrome
hallux valgus
halo
  fatty h.
  h. nevus
  h. sign
  h. sign of hydrops
halogen acne
haloperidol
Halotestin
halothane
Halsted
  H. mastectomy
  H. mosquito forceps
  H. operation
halstedian concept of tumor spread
hamartoma
  mesenchymal h.
Hamilton method
Hamman-Rich syndrome

hammer
Quisling h.
h. toe
hammock
Mersilene gauze h.
Hamou
H. colpomicrohysteroscope
H. contact
microhysteroscope
H. hysteroscope
H. Microcolpohysteroflator
H. Micro-Hysteroflator
H. technique
hamster
h. egg penetration assay
h. ovum
hand
ape h.
h. and head presentation
lobster-claw h.
mitten h.
vaginal h.
h. ventilation
hand-foot-mouth syndrome
hand-foot syndrome
hand-foot-uterus syndrome
Hand-Schüller-Christian
H.-S.-C. disease
H.-S.-C. syndrome
Hanely-McDermitt pelvimeter
hanging-drop test
Hanhart syndrome
Hanks dilator
Hansen disease
H₂-antagonist
histamine H.-a.
haploid
h. cell
h. set
h. sperm
haploinsufficiency
haplotype
maternal HLA h.
happy puppet syndrome
hapten
haptoglobin
HARD
hydrocephalus, agyria, retinal
dysplasia
HARD syndrome
Hardy-Weinberg
H.-W. equilibrium

H.-W. formula
H.-W. law
harelip
harlequin
h. color change
h. fetus
h. ichthyosis
h. reaction
h. sign
Harmonic scalpel
harness
Pavlik h.
Wheaton Pavlik h.
Harpenden
H. calipers
H. stadiometer
Harrington retractor
Harris
H. growth arrest line
H. uterine injector (HUI)
**Harris-Kronner uterine
manipulator/injector (HUMI)**
Harrison
H. groove
H. method
Hartmann solution
Hartman sign
Hartnup disease
Hart syndrome
Hashimoto thyroiditis
hashish
Hasson cannula
hat
measuring h.
Hata phenomenon
hatching
assisted zonal h. (AZH)
HATT
hemagglutination treponemal
test
Haultain operation
Hautain uterine inversion
Haverhill fever
Hawk-Dennen forceps
Hawthorne effect
hay fever
Hay-Wells syndrome
hazy lung
HB
Recombivax H.
HbA1C
glycosylated hemoglobin

HBAg
hepatitis B antigen
HbF
fetal hemoglobin
HBIG, HBIg
hepatitis B immune globulin
HbP
primitive (fetal) hemoglobin
HbS
hemoglobin S
sickle cell hemoglobin
HBsAg
hepatitis B surface antigen
HbsC
sickle cell hemoglobin C
HbSS
homozygosity for hemoglobin S
HbS-Thal
sickle thalassemia
HC
head circumference
β-HCG
human chorionic gonadotropin
beta-subunit
hCG, HCG
human chorionic gonadotropin
Clearview hCG
OvuDate hCG
Pro-Step hCG
Tandem Icon II hCG
Test Pack hCG
HCl
hydrochloride
Cleocin HCl
fluoxetine HCl
oxytetracline HCl
phenazopyridine HCl
sertraline HCl
Hct
hematocrit
pretransfusion Hct
HCTZ
hydrochlorothiazide
HDL
high-density lipoprotein
HDL-cholesterol

HDN
hemolytic disease of the
newborn
head
breech h.
h. circumference (HC)
h. circumference/abdominal
circumference ratio
h. compression
dolichocephalic h.
engaged h.
fetal h.
hourglass h.
molding of h.
h. presentation
H. reflex
h. and tail fold
transillumination of h.
h. ultrasound
headache
migraine h.
preeclampsia h.
spinal h.
vascular h.
head:body ratio
headlight
Keeler fiberoptic h.
Healthdyne
H. apnea monitor
H. oximeter
H. ventilator
Heaney
H. clamp
H. curette
H. forceps
H. needle holder
H. operation
H. technique
Heaney-Ballentine forceps
Heaney-Hyst
H.-H. forceps
H.-H. retractor
heart
h. block
crisscross h.
cushion defect of h.
h. disease

NOTES

183

heart *(continued)*
   h. failure
   fetal h.
   h. rate
   h. rate monitoring
   h. sounds
   h. valve replacement
heartburn
heart-hand syndrome
heart-shaped
   h.-s. pelvis
   h.-s. uterus
heat
   h. loss
   prickly h.
   h. transfer mechanism
heavy chain
heavy-ion
   h.-i. irradiation
   h.-i. mammography
hebetic
HEC
   human endothelial cell
Hecht pneumonia
heelstick
heel-to-ear maneuver
HEF
   human embryo fibroblast
Hegar
   H. dilator
   H. sign
height
   fundal h.
   midparental h.
   h. table
Heineke-Mikulicz pyloroplasty
Heinz
   H. bodies
   H. body anemia
HeLa
   Henrietta Lack
   HeLa cells
helcomenia
helix, pl. helices
   alpha h.
   double h.
   H. endocervical curette
   H. uterine biopsy curette
   Watson-Crick h.
Hellendall sign
Heller-Belsey operation
Heller-Döhle disease
Heller-Nissen operation

Heller test
Hellin law
Hellin-Zeleny law
HELLP
   hemolysis, elevated liver
   enzymes, and low platelet
   count
   HELLP syndrome
Helmex
helminth
helminthic disease
helper
   h. factor
   h. T cell
Hemabate
hemagglutinating inhibition
  antibody (HIA)
hemagglutination
   h. inhibition (HI, HI titer)
   h. treponemal test (HATT)
hemagglutinin
hemagogue
hemangioblastoma
hemangioectasia hypertrophicans
hemangioma
   cavernous h.
   epidural h.
   macular h.
   port-wine h.
   strawberry h.
   vulvar h.
hemangioma-thrombocytopenia
  syndrome
hemangiomatosis
hemarthrosis
hematemesis
Hematest
   H. positive
   H. test
hematocele
   pelvic h.
   pudendal h.
hematocephalus
hematochezia
hematocolpometra
hematocolpos
hematocrit (Hct)
   mean menstrual cycle h.
   spun h.
hematologic
   h. disorder
   h. neoplasia
hematological change

hematology
hematoma
    axillary h.
    h. drainage
    extradural h.
    follicular h.
    interstitial and loculated h.
    intrauterine h.
    puerperal h.
    subdural h.
    sublingual h.
    submental h.
    uterine h.
    vaginal h.
    vulvar h.
hematometra
hematometrocolpos
hematomphalocele
hematopoiesis
    extramedullary h.
hematopoietic
    h. disorder
    h. stem cell (HSC)
    h. system stimulator
hematosalpinx
hematotrachelos
hematuria
heme
    h. metabolism disorder
    h. positive
hemelytrometra
hemiacardius
hemiacephalus
hemiagnathia
hemianencephaly
hemiatrophy
hemibody irradiation
hemicardia
hemicephalia
hemicervix
hemicolectomy
hemicrania
hemi-Fontan procedure
hemimelia
    dysplasia epiphysealis h.
hemimelus
hemipagus

hemiparesis
hemiplegia
hemiuterus
hemivertebra
hemivulvectomy
hemizona assay
hemoblastic leukemia
Hemoccult test
hemochorial
    h. placenta
hemochorioendothelial placentation
hemochromatosis
hemoconcentration
HemoCue
    H. blood glucose analyzer
    H. blood glucose system
    H. Blood-Glucose tester
    H. blood hemoglobin
      analyzer
    H. blood hemoglobin
      system
    H. Blood-Hemoglobin tester
    H. glucose test
    H. hemoglobin photometer
    H. hemoglobin test
    H. microcurette
hemocytometer
    Neubauer h.
hemodialysis
hemodynamic monitoring
hemodynamics
hemofilter
hemofiltration
    continuous arteriovenous h.
    (CAVH)
hemoglobin
    h. A
    h. A_{Ic} determination
    h. Bart, Bart h.
    h. C disease
    h. E
    h. F
    fetal h. (HbF)
    glycosylated h. (HbA1C)
    h. Gower-1
    h. Gower-2
    h. H

NOTES

hemoglobin *(continued)*
    h. H disease
    h. level
    h. M disease
    mean corpuscular h. (MCH)
    h. Portland
    primitive (fetal) h. (HbP)
    h. S (HbS)
    serum free h.
    sickle cell h. (HbS)
hemoglobinemia
hemoglobinopathy
hemoglobin-oxygen dissociation
hemoglobinuria
    paroxysmal nocturnal h.
hemolysin
hemolysis
    microangiopathic h.
hemolysis, elevated liver enzymes, and low platelet count (HELLP)
hemolytic
    ABO h. disease of the newborn
    h. anemia
    h. disease of the newborn (HDN)
    h.-uremic syndrome
β-hemolytic streptococcus
hemolyzed specimen
hemometra
hemopathy
    maternal h.
hemoperitoneum
hemophilia
    h. A
    h. B
hemophiliac
hemopneumothorax
hemoptysis
hemorrhage
    accidental h.
    antepartum h.
    concealed h.
    epidural h.
    external h.
    fetal h.
    fetal-maternal h.
    fetomaternal h.
    intracranial h. (ICH)
    intrapartum h.
    intraventricular h. (Grade I, II, III, IV) (IVH)

    periventricular-intraventricular h.
    placental h.
    postpartum h.
    scleral h.
    sternocleidomastoid h.
    subarachnoid h.
    subchorionic h.
    subdural h.
    subependymal h. (SEH)
    transplacental h.
    unavoidable h.
hemorrhagic
    h. cystitis
    h. disease
    h. disease of the newborn
    h. endovasculitis
    h. fever
    h. scurvy
    h. shock
    h. telangiectasia
hemorrhagica
    purpura h.
hemorrhoid
hemorrhoidal
    h. artery
    h. nerve
hemosalpinx
hemosiderosis
    pulmonary h.
hemostasis
hemostat
    Crile h.
    curved h.
    Endo-Avitene microfibrillar collagen h.
hemostatic staple line
Henderson-Hasselbalch equation
Henle
    loop of H.
Henoch disease
Henoch-Schönlein purpura
Henrietta Lack (HeLa)
Henschke colpostat
Hepalean
heparin
    calcium h.
    h. challenge test
    h. lock (hep-lock)
    low-dose h.
    minidose h.
    prophylactic h.
    h. sodium

heparinization
hepatic
  h. disorder
  h. fibrosis
  h. focal nodular hyperplasia
  h. infantilism
  h. metastasis
  h. necrosis
  h. neoplasm
  h. porphyria
  h. pregnancy
  h. rupture
hepatitis
  h. A
  h. A virus
  h. B
  h. B antigen (HBAg)
  h. B immune globulin
  (HBIG, HBIg)
  h. B surface antigen
  (HBsAg)
  h. B vaccine
  h. B virus
  h. C
  chronic h.
  h. D, delta h.
  fulminant h.
  giant cell h.
  h. immune globulin
  h. immunization
  infectious h.
  maternal h.
  neonatal h.
  non-A, non-B h.
  h. screening
  serum h.
hepatobiliary
hepatoblastoma
hepatocellular
  h. carcinoma
  h. damage
hepatoerythropoietic porphyria
hepatolenticular
  h. degeneration
hepatoma
hepatomegaly
hepatorenal

hepatosplenomegaly
Hep-B-Gammagee
hep-lock
  heparin lock
Heprofile ELISA test
Heptavax-B
HER-2/neu proto-oncogene
Heraeus LaserSonics InfraGuide
herald bleed
herbicide
Herbst registry
Hercules
  infant H.
hereditaria
  adynamia episodica h.
  alopecia h.
  anemia hypochromica
  siderochrestica h.
  atrophia bulborum h.
  porphyria cutanea tarda h.
hereditary
  h. benign intraepithelial
  dyskeratosis syndrome
  h. bone dysplasia
  h. clubbing
  h. deforming
  chondrodystrophy
  h. disease
  h. dysplastic nevus
  syndrome
  h. ectodermal polydysplasia
  h. edema
  h. nonspherocytic anemia
  h. orotic aciduria
  h. spherocytosis
  h. syphilis
  h. trait
heredity
  autosomal h.
  sex-linked h.
  X-linked h.
heredoataxia
heredobiologic
heredoconstitutional disease
heredodegeneration
heredodegenerative disease
heredodiathesis

NOTES

heredofamilial
heredoimmunity
heredolues
heredopathia atactica
heredosyphilis
Hering-Breuer reflex
heritability
heritable
Hermansky-Pudlak syndrome
hermaphrodite
hermaphroditism
    true h.
    XX h.
hermaphroditismus
hernia
    abdominal h.
    Bochdalek h.
    broad ligament h.
    diaphragmatic h.
    epigastric h.
    femoral h.
    groin h.
    hiatal h.
    incarcerated h.
    incisional h.
    inguinal h.
    labial h.
    Morgagni h.
    paraduodenal h.
    peritoneal h.
    pleuroperitoneal h.
    reducible h.
    retrocecal h.
    retrosternal h.
    Richter h.
    sliding h.
    spigelian h.
    strangulated h.
    transmesenteric h.
    umbilical h.
    h. uteri inguinalis
    h. uterine inguinale
    ventral h.
herpangina
Herp-Check test
herpes
    acute neonatal h.
    genital h.
    h. genitalis
    h. gestationis
    intrauterine h.

    h. labialis
    neonatal h.
    h. simplex
    h. simplex virus (HSV)
    h. simplex virus type II
    (HSV II)
    h. zoster
    h. zoster virus (HZV)
Herpesvirus
    H. hominis
    H. suis
    H. varicellae
herpesvirus
    h. type 1 (HSV-1)
    h. type 2 (HSV-2)
herpetic
    h. gingivitis
    h. gingivostomatitis
    h. stomatitis
herpeticum
    eczema h.
herpetiformis
    dermatitis h.
Herplex Liquifilm
Herrick anemia
Hers disease
Herter infantilism
Hertig-Rock ovum
hertz (Hz)
Hesselbach triangle
hetacillin
heteradelphus
heteralius
heterocephalus
heterochromia
heterodimer
heterodimeric integral membrane
    glycoprotein
heterodymus
heterogamete
heterograft
heterologous
    h. graft
    h. insemination
    h. surfactant
    h. twins
    h. uterine sarcoma
heteromorphous
heteroovular
    h. twins
heteropagus

heterophil
   h. antigen
heterophilic
heteroploid
heteroprosopus
heterosexual
   h. precocious puberty
heterosomal aberration
heterotaxia syndrome
heterotopia
   neuronal h.
heterotopic
   h. pregnancy
heterotropic
   h. chromosome
heterotypic
heterotypical chromosome
heterozygosity
heterozygote
   obligate h.
heterozygous
   h. carrier
Heuser membrane
Hexa-Betalin
Hexa-CAF
   hexamethylmelamine,
   cyclophosphamide,
   doxorubicin, and 5-fluorouracil
hexachloride
   gamma-benzene h.
hexachlorocyclohexane
hexadactyly
Hexadrol
Hexalen
hexamethonium chloride
hexamethylmelamine
hexamethylmelamine,
   cyclophosphamide, doxorubicin,
   and 5-fluorouracil (Hexa-CAF)
hexamethylmelamine with
   doxorubicin and
   cyclophosphamide (HAC)
hexamine
hexaploidy
hexenmilch
hexestrol
hexocyclium methylsulfate

hexoprenaline sulfate
hexosaminidase
   h. A deficiency
Heyman capsules
Heyman-Herndon clubfoot
   procedure
Heyns abdominal decompression
   apparatus
HFJ
   high-frequency jet
   HFJ ventilation
HFJV
   high-frequency jet ventilation
   HFJV ventilator
HFO
   high-frequency oscillatory
   HFO ventilation
HFOV
   high-frequency oscillatory
   ventilation
   HFOV ventilator
HFPP
   high-frequency positive pressure
   HFPP ventilation
HFPPV
   high-frequency positive pressure
   ventilation
   HFPPV ventilator
H gene
HG factor
hGH
   human growth hormone
HGSIL
   high-grade squamous
   intraepithelial lesion
H-H neonatal shunt
HI
   hemagglutination inhibition
   HI titer
HIA
   hemagglutinating inhibition
   antibody
5-HIAA
   5-hydroxyindoleacetic acid
21-HIAA
   21-hydroxyindoleacetic acid
hiatal hernia

NOTES

hiatus
    urogenital h.
HIB
    Haemophilus influenzae type B
    HIB polysaccharide vaccine
hiccup, hiccough
    fetal h.
Hicks version
hidradenitis suppurativa
hidradenoma
    papillary h.
hidrotic ectodermal dysplasia
HIE
    hypoxic-ischemic
      encephalopathy
high
    h. altitude perinatal
      mortality
    h. fetal order
    h. forceps delivery
    h. intrauterine insemination
    h. molecular weight dextran
high-calorie
    h.-c. diet
    h.-c. formula
high-contrast Bucky imaging
high-density lipoprotein (HDL)
high-dose chemotherapy
high-fiber diet
high-frequency
    h.-f. jet (HFJ)
    h.-f. jet ventilation (HFJV)
    h.-f. oscillatory (HFO)
    h.-f. oscillatory ventilation
      (HFOV)
    h.-f. positive pressure
      (HFPP)
    h.-f. positive pressure
      ventilation (HFPPV)
    h.-f. ventilator
high-fructose formula
high-glucose formula
high-grade
    h.-g. cervical dysplasia
    h.-g. squamous
      intraepithelial lesion
      (HGSIL)
high-pitched cry
high-resolution ultrasound
high-risk
    h.-r. infant
    h.-r. mother
    h.-r. obstetrician

    h.-r. patient
    h.-r. pregnancy
    h.-r. pregnancy assessment
Hi-Gonavis test
Higoumenakia sign
hilar
    h. cell hyperplasia
    h. cell pathology
    h. cell tumor
Hillis-Müller maneuver
hindbrain
hindgut
hindwater
Hinton test
hip
    h. bone density
    h. click
    congenital dislocated h.
      (CDH)
    h. deformity
    h. fracture
Hiprex
Hirschberg test
Hirschsprung disease
Hirst placental forceps
hirsute woman
hirsutism
    constitutional h.
    familial h.
    hormonal h.
    idiopathic h.
    male-pattern h.
    postmenopausal h.
His
    bundle of H.
    H. rule
histaminase
histamine
    h. H_2-antagonist
Histantil
Histatan
Histerone
histidinemia
histidinuria
histiocyte
histiocytic fibroma
histiocytoma
histiocytosis
    Langerhans cell h.
    malignant h.
    sinus h.
    h. X

histocompatibility
   h. antigen
   h. gene
   h. locus antigen
Histofreezer cryosurgical system
histogenesis
histoimmunological origin
histoincompatibility
   maternal-fetal h.
histologic
   h. architecture
   h. diagnosis
histology
   endometrial h.
histomorphometry
histone
   h. H1 kinase
histopathological
   h. diagnosis
   h. finding
   h. grading
   h. study
histopathology
histoplasmosis
   pulmonary h.
history
   family h.
   gynecologic h.
   menstrual h.
   obstetric h.
   occupational h.
   reproductive h.
   sexual h.
   urologic h.
histrelin
Histussin NC
Hitachi EUB-405 imaging system
hitchhiker thumb
Hitzig girdle
HIV
   human immunodeficiency virus
   HIV classification
   HIV test
HIVAGEN test
HLA
   human leukocyte antigen

HLA-A3
HLA-B
HLA-B14,DR1
HLA-D
HLA-DR
HLA-compatible fetus
HLHS
   hypoplastic left heart syndrome
   HLHS syndrome
HLI
   human leukocyte interferon
HMD
   hyaline membrane disease
hMG, HMG
HN
   Two-Cal H.
hobnail cell
Hoboken
   fold of H.
   H. gemmules
   H. nodule
Hodge
   H. forceps
   H. maneuver
   H. pessary
Hodgkin
   H. disease
   H. lymphoma
Hoehne sign
HOF
   human oviduct fluid
Hofbauer cell
Hogben test
Hogness box
holandric
   h. genes
   h. inheritance
hole
   Murphy h.
Holinger
   H. infant bougie
   H. infant bronchoscope
   H. infant esophageal
   speculum
   H. infant esophagoscope
   H. infant laryngoscope

NOTES

Hollister collecting device
holmium:yttrium-aluminum-garnet
  (Ho:YAG)
holoacardius
holoblastic
  h. ovum
hologastroschisis
Hologic
  H. 1000 QDR densitometer
  H. 1000 QDR dual-energy
    absorptiometer
hologynic inheritance
holoprosencephaly
  h. anomalad
holorachischisis
holosystolic murmur
Holter monitor
Holt-Oram
  H.-O. atriodigital dysplasia
  H.-O. syndrome
Homans sign
homatropine
HOME
  Home Observation for the
  Measurement of the
  Environment
home
  h. birth
  H. Observation for the
    Measurement of the
    Environment (HOME)
  h. oxygen
  h. pregnancy test
  h. uterine monitoring
    (HUM)
homeobox-2 gene
homeostasis
  carbohydrate h.
homeostatic lag
homeotic genes
hominis
  Herpesvirus h.
  poliovirus h.
homochronous inheritance
homocystinemia
homocystinuria
homogamete
homogeneity
  tissue h.
homograft
homolog
homologous
  h. chromosomes

h. disease
h. insemination
h. uterine sarcoma
homology
homophilic
homosexuality
homotropic inheritance
homotypic
homozygosity for hemoglobin S
  (HbSS)
homozygote
homozygous
honeymoon cystitis
hood
  clitoral h.
  h. mist
  h. O_2
  h. oxygen
  Oxy-Hood oxygen h.
  H. procedure
  Rock-Mulligan h.
  vaginal h.
hook
  Mayo h.
  Miya h.
  tenaculum h.
Hooker-Farbes test
hookworm
Hope resuscitation bag
hordeolum
horizon
  Streeter h.
horizontal transmission of virus
hormonal
  h. abnormality
  h. antineoplastic therapy
  h. contraception
  h. effect
  h. hirsutism
  h. implant
  h. level
  h. pregnancy test tablets
  h. treatment
hormone
  adrenocortical h.
  adrenocorticotropic h.
    (ACTH)
  anterior pituitary-like h.
  antidiuretic h. (ADH)
  anti-müllerian h. (AMH)
  h. assay
  bioactive h.
  calcitropic h.

cancer and steroid h.
  (CASH)
chorionic gonadotropic h.
chorionic growth h.
circulating h.
h. complex receptor
corticotropin-releasing h.
  (CRH)
endogenous h.
exogenous h.
fetal h.
follicle-stimulating h. (FSH)
Genentech biosynthetic
  human growth h.
gonadotropin-releasing h.
  (GnRH)
growth h. (GH)
growth h.-releasing hormone
  (GH-RH)
human chorionic
  adrenocorticotropic h.
human growth h. (hGH)
human urinary follicle-
  stimulating h. (hu-FSH)
Humatrope growth h.
hypothalamic luteinizing
  hormone-releasing h.
inappropriate antidiuretic h.
  (IADH)
LATS h.
luteinizing h. (LH)
luteinizing hormone-
  releasing h. (LH-RH)
lutein-stimulating h. (LSH)
melanocyte-stimulating h.
ovarian h.
parathyroid h.
pituitary h.
placental h.
pregnancy h.
Protropin growth h.
purified h.
h. receptor
recombinant human
  growth h.
h. replacement therapy
  (HRT)

sex h.
somatrem growth h.
somatropin growth h.
steroid h.
syndrome of inappropriate
  antidiuretic h. (SIADH)
h. therapy
thyroid h.
thyroid-stimulating h. (TSH)
thyrotropic h.
thyrotropin-releasing h.
  (TRH)
tropic h.
urinary-derived human
  follicle-stimulating h. (u-
  hFSH)
**hormone-receptor complex
  internalization**
**hormone-stimulated endometrial
  change**
hormonogenesis
hormonotherapy
horn
  frontal h.'s
  noncommunicating
    uterine h.
  rudimentary uterine h.
  uterine h., h. of uterus
horseshoe
  h. fibrosis
  h. placenta
host
  h. defense mechanism
  h. response mechanism
hot
  h. biopsy
  h. biopsy forceps
  h. cross bun skull
  h. flash
  h. flush
hot-knife conization
Hottentot apron
hour
  cubic centimeters per h.
    (cc/hr)

NOTES

193

hourglass
  h. head
  h. uterus
24-hour urinary free cortisol
housekeeping gene
Howell-Jolly bodies
Ho:YAG
  holmium:yttrium-aluminum-
    garnet
    Ho:YAG laser
HP
  Profasi HP
H.P.
  Mission Prenatal H.P.
HPA
  hypothalamic-pituitary-adrenal
  HPA axis
hPL, HPL
  human placental lactogen
HPV
  Haemophilus pertussis vaccine
  human papillomavirus
  human papilloma virus
H-ras p21 protein
HRHS
  hypoplastic right heart syndrome
HRT
  hormone replacement therapy
HS
  hysterosalpingography
HSC
  hematopoietic stem cell
    HSC Scale
3βHSD
  3β-hydroxysteroid
    dehydrogenase
HSG
  hysterosalpingography
    HSG tray
HSI
  human seminal (plasma)
  inhibitor
HSV
  herpes simplex virus
HSV-1
  herpesvirus type 1
HSV-2
  herpesvirus type 2
HSV II
  herpes simplex virus type II
HTLV
  human T-cell leukemia virus
    HTLV-I

human T-cell leukemia
  virus type I
HTLV-II
  human T-cell leukemia
  virus type II
HTLV-III
  human T-cell leukemia
  virus type III
H-type fistula
Hudson T Up-Draft II disposable
  nebulizer
Huffman
  H. infant vaginal speculum
  H. infant vaginoscope
Huffman-Huber
  H.-H. infant urethrotome
  H.-H. infant vaginoscope
hu-FSH
  human urinary follicle-
  stimulating hormone
Huguier circle
Huhner test
HUI
  Harris uterine injector
  HUI Mini-Flex
Hulka-Clemens clip
Hulka clip
HUM
  home uterine monitoring
human
  h. chorionic
    adrenocorticotropic
    hormone
  h. chorionic gonadotropin
    (hCG, HCG)
  h. chorionic gonadotropin
    beta-subunit (β-HCG)
  h. chorionic gonadotropin
    level
  h. embryo fibroblast (HEF)
  h. endothelial cell (HEC)
  H. Genome Project
  h. globulin
  h. growth hormone (hGH)
  h. immunodeficiency virus
    (HIV)
  h. immunodeficiency virus
    test
  Insulatard NPH h.
  h. leukocyte antigen (HLA)
  h. leukocyte interferon
    (HLI)
  h. lymphocyte antigen

h. lymphocyte antigen-locus D
h. lymphocyte antigen-locus DR
h. menopausal gonadotropin (HMG)
h. milk fortifier
h. oviduct fluid (HOF)
h. ovum fertilization test
h. papillomavirus (HPV)
h. papilloma virus (HPV)
h. placental lactogen (hPL, HPL)
h. seminal (plasma) inhibitor (HSI)
H. Surf surfactant
h. T-cell leukemia virus (HTLV)
h. T-cell leukemia virus type I (HTLV-I)
h. T-cell leukemia virus type II (HTLV-II)
h. T-cell leukemia virus type III (HTLV-III)
h. urinary follicle-stimulating hormone (hu-FSH)
Velosulin H.
Humatin
Humatrope
H. growth hormone
HUMI
Harris-Kronner uterine manipulator/injector
humidification ventilator
humidifier
Ohio h.
humoral
h. antibody
h. factor
h. immunity
Humorsol
hump
buffalo h.
dowager's h.
dromedary h.
Humulin 50/50
Humulin 70/30

Humulin L
Humulin N
Humulin R
Humulin U Ultralente
Hünermann disease
Hunner interstitial cystitis
Hunt bipolar forceps
hunterian chancre
Hunter syndrome
Huntington
H. chorea
H. disease
H. Reproduction Center
Hunt-Reich cannula
Hurler-Scheie syndrome
Hurler syndrome
hurry
intestinal h.
Hurtig dilator
husband
artificial insemination by h. (AIH)
Hutchinson
H. sign
H. syndrome
H. triad
Hutchinson-Gilford syndrome
Hutinel disease
Hutterite
Huxley respirator
HVF ventilator
HVL
half-value layer
hyaline
h. cast
h. membrane
h. membrane disease (HMD)
h. membrane syndrome
h. myoma degeneration
hyaluronidase
H-Y antigen
Hybolin
H. Decanoate
H. Improved
hybridization
DNA h.

NOTES

hybridization *(continued)*
    dot-blot h.
    fluorescence in situ h.
    (FISH)
    papillomavirus h.
    in situ h.
    in situ nucleic acid h.
hybridoma technique
Hybritech
hyclate
    doxycycline h.
Hycodan
hydatid
    h. cyst
    h. cyst of Morgagni
    h. disease
    h. mole
    h. polyp
    h. pregnancy
hydatidiform mole
hydraemica
    plethora h.
hydralazine
hydramnion, hydramnios
hydranencephaly
Hydrate
hydrate
    chloral h.
hydration
    maternal h.
Hydrazide
Hydrea
hydrencephalocele
hydrencephalomeningocele
hydriodic acid
hydroa
    h. aestivale
    h. gestationis
    h. puerorum
    h. vacciniforme
hydrocele
    h. feminae
    Maunoir h.
    h. muliebris
    Nuck h.
hydrocelectomy
hydrocephalic
hydrocephalocele
hydrocephaloid
    h. disease
hydrocephalus
    normal pressure h. (NPH)

hydrocephalus, agyria, retinal
    dysplasia (HARD)
hydrocephaly
Hydro-chlor
hydrochloride (HCl)
    arginine h.
    butriptyline h.
    chlorcyclizine h.
    ciprofloxacin h.
    cyclopentolate h.
    cycrimine h.
    cyproheptadine h.
    dihydromorphinone h.
    dobutamine h.
    dopamine h.
    doxapram h.
    doxorubicin h.
    esmolol h.
    ethopropazine h.
    isoprenaline h.
    mechlorethamine h.
    mitoxantrone h.
    naftifine h.
    naloxone h.
    paroxetine h.
    phenazopyridine h.
    propranolol h.
    quinacrine h.
    ritodrine h.
    sertraline h.
    sulfamethox-
      azole/phenazopyridine h.
    sulfisox-
      azole/phenazopyridine h.
    tetracycline h.
    tolazoline h.
    trimethobenzamide h.
    tritodrine h.
    vancomycin h.
hydrochlorothiazide (HCTZ)
hydrocodone
hydrocolpocele, hydrocolpos
hydrocortisone
hydrodissection
HydroDIURIL
hydroepiandrosterone
hydroflotation
hydroflumethiazide
hydrogen
    h. peroxide
    h. peroxide-producing
    lactobacillus

hydrolysate
    casein h.
hydrolysis-resistant
hydromeningocele
hydrometra
hydrometrocolpos
hydromicrocephaly
hydromorphone
Hydromox
hydromphalus
hydromyelocele
hydromyelomeningocele
hydronephrosis
hydroparasalpinx
hydropertubation
hydrophobia
hydrophthalmos
hydrops
    h. amnii
    fetal h., h. fetalis
    h. folliculi
    h. gravidarum
    immune fetal h.
    maternal h.
    nonimmune fetal h.
    h. ovarii
    h. tubae profluens
hydrorrhea
    h. gravidae, h. gravidarum
hydrosalpinx
    intermittent h.
hydrothorax
hydrotubation
hydroureter
hydrovarium
hydroxide
    magnesium h.
    potassium h. (KOH)
11β-hydroxyandrosterone
hydroxybenzeneazobenzoic acid (HABA)
17-hydroxycorticosteroid
11-hydroxyetiocholanolone
21-hydroxyindoleacetic acid (21- HIAA)
5-hydroxyindoleacetic acid (5- HIAA)

hydroxyindole-*o*-methyltransferase
hydroxylase
    phenylalanine h.
17-hydroxylase
    17-h. deficiency
    17-h. deficiency syndrome
17α-hydroxylase
21-hydroxylase
    21-h. deficiency syndrome
    21-h. gene deletion
hydroxylation
hydroxylysine
3-hydroxy-3-methylglutaryl coenzyme A
hydroxyphenyluria
17-hydroxypregnenolone
17α-hydroxypregnenolone
hydroxyprogesterone
    h. caproate
17-hydroxyprogesterone (17-OHP)
    17-h. caproate
17α-hydroxyprogesterone
    17α-h. caproate
hydroxyprogesterone and estradiol valerate
hydroxyproline
hydroxyprolinemia
15-hydroxyprostaglandin dehydrogenase
hydroxysteroid
    3β-h. dehydrogenase (3βHSD)
    18-h. dehydrogenase
hydroxyurea
1,25-hydroxyvitamin D
25-hydroxyvitamin-D$_3$
hydroxyzine
hyfrecation
hyfrecator
Hy-Gene seminal fluid collection kit
Hy-Gestrone
hygiene
    perineal h.
hygroma
    cystic h.
Hygroton

NOTES

Hylorel
Hylutin
hymen
    h. bifenestratus, h. biforis
    cribriform h.
    denticulate h.
    falciform h.
    imperforate h.
    infundibuliform h.
    redundant h.
    h. sculptatus
    septate h.
    h. subseptus
    vertical h.
    virginal h.
hymenal
    h. band
    h. membrane
    h. ring
    h. tag
hymenectomy
hymenitis
hymenorrhaphy
hymenotomy
hyobranchial cleft
hyoscine
    h. methylbromide
hypamnion, hypamnios
Hypaque
    H. Meglumine
Hyperab
hyperacidity
hyperactive bowel sounds
hyperactivity
hyperadrenalism
hyperalaninemia
hyperaldosteronism
hyperalimentation
    central h.
    Intralipid h.
    intravenous h. (IVH)
    Pedtrace-4 h.
    peripheral h.
    TrophAmine h.
hyperalphalipoproteinemia
hyperammonemia, hyperammoniemia
    cerebroatrophic h.
hyperandrogenemia
hyperandrogenism
    adrenal h.
    cryptic h.
    h., insulin resistance,

    acanthosis nigricans
    (HAIR-AN)
    h., insulin resistance,
    acanthosis nigricans
    syndrome (HAIR-AN
    syndrome)
    ovarian h.
    h. reversal
hyperandrogenism,
hyperargininemia
hyperbaric
    h. chamber
    h. oxygen
    h. oxygen therapy
    h. oxygen treatment
hyperbilirubinemia
hyperbilirubinemic
hypercalcemia
    idiopathic h.
hypercalcemic crisis
hypercalciuria
hypercaloric formula
hypercapnia
hypercarbia
hyperchloremic renal acidosis
hypercholesterolemia
    familial h.
hyperchromic acidosis
hypercoagulability
hypercortisolism
hypercyesis, hypercyesia
hyperdactyly
hyperdibasicaminoaciduria
hyperdiploid
hyperdynamia
    h. uteri
hyperechogenic
hyperechoic
    h. bowel
    h. endometrium
hyperelastica
    cutis h.
hyperemesis
    h. gravidarum
    h. lactentium
hyperencephalus
hyperexpansion
hyperfolliculoidism
hypergalactosis
hypergenitalism
hyperglycemia
    ketotic h.
    nonketotic h.

hyperglycinemia
    nonketotic h.
hypergonadism
hypergonadotropic
    h. amenorrhea
    h. eunuchoidism
    h. hypogonadism
hypergynecosmia
hyperhaploidy
HyperHep
hyperimmune serum globulin
hyperimmunoglobulin E
hyperinsulinemia
hyperinsulinism
hyperinvolution
hyperkalemia
hyperkeratosis
    epidermolytic h.
hyperlactation
hyperlacticacidemia
hyperlaxity
    joint h.
hyperlipidemia
hyperlipoproteinemia
hyperlucency
hyperlucent lung syndrome
hyperluteinization
hyperlysinemia
hypermagnesemia
hypermastia
hypermenorrhea
hypernatremia
    h. dehydration
hyperopia
hyperornithinemia
hyperosmolar coma
hyperosmotic agent
hyperostosis
    infantile cortical h.
hyperovarianism
hyperoxia
hyperparathyroidism
    maternal h.
hyperphenylalaninemia
hyperphosphatemia
hyperpigmentation
hyperpigmented lesion

hyperpituitary gigantism
hyperplasia
    adenomatous h.
    adenomatous endometrial h.
    adrenal h.
    adult-onset congenital
      adrenal h.
    congenital adrenal h. (CAH)
    cystic h.
    cystic h. of the breast
    cystic glandular h.
    ductal h.
    endometrial h. (EH)
    epithelial h.
    familial lipoid adrenal h.
    fetal congenital h.
    glandular h.
    hepatic focal nodular h.
    hilar cell h.
    late-onset h.
    Leydig cell h.
    lipoid adrenal h.
    lymphoid h.
    microglandular cervical h.
    polypoid h.
    sebaceous h.
    Swiss cheese h.
    vulvar squamous h.
hyperplastic
    h. polyp
hyperploidy
hyperprolactinemia
    tumorous h.
hyperprolactinemia-associated luteal
  phase
hyperprolactinemic amenorrhea
hyperprolinemia
    familial h.
hyperpyrexia
hyperreactio luteinalis
hyperreflexia
hyperreflexic
hyperrelaxinemia
hypersecretion
hypersegmentation
hypersensitivity
    delayed h.

NOTES

hypersensitization
hypersplenism
Hyperstat
hyperstimulation
    gonadotropin-induced
      ovarian h.
    ovarian h.
hypertelorism
    Bixler h.
    ocular h.
hypertelorism-hypospadias syndrome
hypertension
    chronic h.
    gestational h.
    intracranial h.
    malignant h.
    maternal h.
    portal h.
    postpartum h.
    pregnancy-induced h. (PIH)
    pulmonary h.
hypertensive encephalopathy
Hyper-Tet
hyperthecosis
    h. ovarii
    stromal h.
hyperthermia
hyperthyroid
hyperthyroidism
hypertonia
hypertonic
    h. glucose
    h. saline
    h. uterine dysfunction
hypertransaminasemia
hypertrichosis
hypertrophic
    h. cirrhosis
    h. stenosis
hypertrophicans
    hemangioectasia h.
hypertrophy
    clitoral h.
    left ventricular h. (LVH)
    massive breast h.
    myocardial h.
    ovarian h.
    septal h.
    virginal breast h.
hyperuricemia
hyperuricosuria
hypervalinemia
hyperventilation

hyperviscosity
    h. syndrome
hypervitaminosis
hypha, pl. hyphae
hyphema
hypnotic effect
hypoactive bowel sounds
hypoadrenalism
hypoalbuminemia
hypoallergenic
hypocalcemia
    neonatal h.
hypocapnia
hypochloremia
hypochondriasis
hypochondroplasia
    h. syndrome
hypocycloidal tomography
hypodactyly
hypodermoclysis
hypodiploid
hypoechogenic
hypoechoic density
hypoestrogenic woman
hypofertility
hypofibrinogenemia
    congenital h.
    familial h.
hypofolliculogenesis
hypogalactia
hypogalactous
hypogammaglobulinemia
    acquired h.
    congenital h.
    physiologic h.
    transient h.
    X-linked h.
hypogastric
    h. artery
    h. artery ligation
    h. lymph node
    h. pain
    h. plexus
hypogastropagus
hypogastroschisis
hypogenitalism
hypoglossia-hypodactyly syndrome
hypoglycemia
    neonatal h.
hypoglycemic
    oral h.
hypognathus
    cyclops h.

hypogonadal woman
hypogonadism
  eugonadotropic h.
  hypergonadotropic h.
  hypogonadotropic h.
hypogonadotropic
  h. amenorrhea
  h. eunuchoidism
  h. hypogonadism
hypohaploidy
hypokalemia
hypomagnesemia
hypomastia, hypomazia
hypomelanosis
  h. of Ito
hypomenorrhea
hyponatremia
hyponatremic
hypoosmotic swelling test
hypoovarianism, hypovarianism
hypoparathyroidism
hypopharynx
hypophosphatasia
hypophosphatemia
hypophosphatemic rickets
hypophysectomy
hypophysial, hypophyseal
  h. amenorrhea
  h. dwarfism
  h. infantilism
hypophysitis
  lymphocytic h.
hypopituitarism
hypoplasia
  biliary h.
  congenital adrenal h.
  lipoid adrenal gland h.
  müllerian h.
  pulmonary h.
  transient erythroid h.
hypoplastic
  h. anemia
  h. congenital anemia
    syndrome
  h. left heart syndrome
    (HLHS)
  h. lung

  h. penis
  h. right heart syndrome
    (HRHS)
hypopotassemia
hypoproteinemia
hypoprothrombinemia
hyposegmentation
hyposensitization
hypospadias
  balanic h., balanitic h.
  Hacker h.
hyposplenism
hypostatic pneumonia
hypotelorism
  ocular h.
hypotension
  maternal h.
  orthostatic h.
hypothalamic
  h. amenorrhea
  h. disease
  h. dysfunction
  h. failure
  h. luteinizing hormone-
    releasing hormone
hypothalamic-hypophyseal-ovarian-
  endometrial axis
hypothalamic-hypophyseal portal
  circulation
hypothalamic-pituitary
  h.-p. axis
  h.-p. axis dysfunction
  h.-p. disorder
  h.-p. function
hypothalamic-pituitary-adrenal
  (HPA)
hypothalamic-pituitary-gonadal axis
hypothalamus
hypothermia
  chronic scrotal h.
hypothesis, pl. hypotheses
  alternative h.
  bayesian h.
  critical weight h.
  estrogen window etiologic h.
  Korenman estrogen
    window h.

NOTES

hypothesis *(continued)*
    Lyon h.
    Neyman-Pearson
      statistical h.
    Wramsby h.
hypothyroid
    h. dwarfism
hypothyroidism
    athyrotic h.
    congenital h.
    subclinical h.
    transient congenital h.
hypotonia
    Oppenheim congenital h.
hypotonic
    h. bladder
    h. myometrium
    h. uterine dysfunction
hypotony
    ocular h.
hypotrichosis
hypouricemia
hypovarianism *(var. of*
  hypoovarianism)
hypoventilation
hypovitaminosis
hypovolemia
hypovolemic
    h. shock
hypoxemia
hypoxemic
hypoxia
    fetal h.
hypoxic cell sensitizer
hypoxic-ischemic
    h.-i. encephalopathy (HIE)
    h.-i. injury
HypRho-D
    H.-D. Mini Dose
Hyprogest
Hyproval
hypsarhythmia, hypsarrhythmia
hypsicephaly
Hyrexin
Hyskon
hysteralgia
hysteratresia
hysterectomized
hysterectomy
    abdominal h.
    abdominovaginal h.
    Bell-Buettner h.
    Bonney abdominal h.

    cesarean h.
    classic abdominal Semm h.
      (CASH)
    Dellepiane h.
    Döderlein method of
      vaginal h.
    Doyen vaginal h.
    Eden-Lawson h.
    extrafascial h.
    Gelpi-Lowry h.
    laparoscopic h.
    laparoscopic-assisted
      vaginal h. (LAVH)
    laparoscopic Döderlein h.
    Mayo h.
    Meigs-Werthein h.
    modified radical h.
    Munro and Parker
      classification for
      laparoscopic h.
    obstetrical h.
    paravaginal h.
    pelviscopic intrafascial h.
    Porro h.
    radical h.
    Reis-Wertheim vaginal h.
    Rutledge classification of
      extended h.
    supracervical h.
    total abdominal h. (TAH)
    vaginal h.
    Ward-Mayo vaginal h.
hysteresis
hystereurysis
hysteria
hysterical
    h. mother
    h. paralysis
    h. seizure
hystericus
    globus h.
hysterocele
hysterocleisis
hysterocolposcope
hysterocystopexy
hysterodynia
hysterogram
hysterograph
hysterography
hysterolith
hysterolysis
hysterometer
hysteromyoma

hysteromyomectomy
hysteromyotomy
hystero-oophorectomy
hysteropathy
hysteropexy
    abdominal h.
    Alexander-Adams h.
hysterophore
hysteroplasty
hysterorrhaphy
hysterorrhexis
hysterosalpingectomy
hysterosalpingography (HS, HSG)
hysterosalpingo-oophorectomy
hysterosalpingosonography
hysterosalpingostomy
hysteroscope
    Baggish h.
    Baloser h.
    Circon-ACMI h.
    diagnostic h.
    Fujinon flexible h.
    Hamou h.
    Liesegang LM-FLEX 7
     flexible h.
    Olympus h.
    Scopemaster contact h.
    Valle h.

hysteroscopic
    h. insufflator
    h. surgery
hysteroscopy
    laparoscopic-assisted
     vaginal h. (LAVH)
hysterospasm
hysterothermometry
hysterotomy
    abdominal h.
    vaginal h.
hysterotonin
hysterotrachelectomy
hysterotracheloplasty
hysterotrachelorrhaphy
hysterotrachelotomy
hysterotubography
hystersalpingography catheter
Hysto-vac drain
hystrix
    ichthyosis h.
Hytakerol
Hytuss
Hz
    hertz
HZV
    herpes zoster virus

NOTES

I
    inspired gas
^{131}**I**
    iodine-131
^{125}**I**
    iodine-125
IADH
    inappropriate antidiuretic
      hormone
      IADH syndrome
IAHS
    infection-associated
      hemophagocytic syndrome
iatrogenic
    i. dissemination
    i. effect
    i. event
    i. fetal distress
    i. menopause
    i. precocious puberty
    i. ureteral injury
IBC
    iron-binding capacity
IBR
    Infant Behavior Record
ibuprofen
iCa
    ionized calcium
I-cell disease
ICH
    intracranial hemorrhage
ichthyosis
    congenital i.
    i. fetalis
    i. fetus
    harlequin i.
    i. hystrix
    lamellar i.
    i. linearis circumflexa
    i. spinosa
    i. uteri
    i. vulgaris
    X-linked i.
Icon
    I. serum pregnancy test
    I. strep B test
    I. urine pregnancy test
ICRF 159
ICSI
    intracytoplasmic sperm injection

icteric
icterus
    i. gravis
    i. gravis neonatorum
    Liouville i.
    i. neonatorum
    physiologic i.
    i. precox
IDA
    iron deficiency anemia
IDDM
    insulin-dependent diabetes
      mellitus
identical twins
identity matrix
idiocy
    amaurotic familial i.
    Aztec i.
    Kalmuk i.
    xerodermic i.
idiopathic
    i. cholestasis of pregnancy
    i. hirsutism
    i. hypercalcemia
    i. hypertrophic subaortic
      stenosis
    i. infantile hypercalcemia
      syndrome
    i. infertility
    i. polyserositis
    i. precocious puberty
    i. respiratory distress
      syndrome (IRDS)
    i. short stature
    i. steatorrhea
    i. thrombocytopenic purpura
      (ITP)
idiot
    mongolian i.
IDM
    infant of diabetic mother
idoxuridine
IDS
    intrinsic sphincter deficiency
I/E
    inspiratory/expiratory
      I/E ratio
IFI
    intrafollicular insemination

IFN
    interferon
ifosfamide
Ig
    immunoglobulin
IgA
    immunoglobulin A
      IgA deficiency
      IgA HIV antibody test
      secretory IgA
IgE
    immunoglobulin E
      IgE deficiency
IGF
    insulin-like growth factor
IGF-1
IgF
    immunoglobulin F
IgG
    immunoglobulin G
IgM
    immunoglobulin M
      IgM antibody
      IgM deficiency
IGT
    impaired glucose tolerance
IL
    interleukin
      IL-1
        interleukin-1
      IL-2
        interleukin-2
ileal
    i. atresia
    i. conduit
    i. diversion
    i. perforation
ileitis
    terminal i.
ileocolic
    i. artery
    i. intussusception
ileocystoplasty
    Camey i.
ileoentectropy
ileoileal intussusception
ileostomy
    continent i.
Iletin
ileum
    duplication of i.
ileus
    adynamic i.

    duodenal i.
    meconium i.
    paralytic i.
    i. subparta
Ilfeldt splint
iliac
    i. artery
    i. node
    i. vein
iliococcygeal muscle
ilioneoureterocystotomy
iliopagus
iliopectinate line
iliopectineal line
iliothoracopagus
ilioxiphopagus
Ilizarov
    I. external fixator
    I. procedure
ill-defined mass
illegitimacy
illegitimate
illicit
    i. drug use
    i. sex
illness
    psychiatric i.
    systemic i.
Illumina
    I. Pro Series CO2 surgical
      laser system
    I. Pro series laparoscopic
      laser
illuminator
    Dyonic DyoBride 300 i.
Ilosone
Ilotycin
IM
    intramuscular
image recording system
imaging
    continuous-wave
      ultrasound i.
    diagnostic i.
    echoplanar magnetic
      resonance i.
    endovaginal i.
    fetal i.
    high-contrast Bucky i.
    magnetic resonance i. (MRI)
    M-mode i.
    Rho i.

imbalance
electrolyte i.
Imerslund-Graesback syndrome
Imerslund syndrome
**IMEXLAB vascular diagnostic
system**
IMEX Pocket-Dop OB Doppler
imidazole
imidazopyridine
iminoglycinuria
imipemide
imipenem-cilastaten sodium
imipramine
Imitrex
Imlach ring
immature
i. infant
i. ovarian teratoma
imminent abortion
immobilization
Treponema pallidum i.
(TPI)
immobilizer
Olympic Neostraint i.
immotile cilia
immune
i. clearance
i. deficiency
i. factor
i. fetal hydrops
i. globulin
i. monitoring technique
i. process
i. response
i. response gene
rubella i.
i. separation technique
i. serum globulin (ISG)
i. suppressor gene
i. surveillance
i. system
i. system anatomy
i. thrombocytopenia
i. thrombocytopenic purpura
(ITP)
immunity
Burnet acquired i.

cell-mediated i. (CMI)
cellular i.
humoral i.
passive i.
previous maternal i.
immunization
blood group i.
hepatitis i.
prophylactic i.
Rh i.
immunoassay
chemiluminescent i. (CIA)
Chlamydiazyme i.
enzyme i. (EIA)
fluorescent i. (FIA)
nonradioactive i.
nonreactive i.
radioactive i.
solid-phase enzyme i.
immunobead test
immunochemistry
immunochemotherapy
immunocompetent cell
immunocytochemical
immunodeficiency
combined i.
i. syndrome
immunodiagnosis
immunoelectrophoresis
immunofluorescence
immunofluorescent antibody test
immunogen
immunogenetics
immunoglobulin (Ig)
i. A (IgA)
antenatal anti-D i.
anti-D i.
i. deficiency
i. E (IgE)
i. F (IgF)
i. G (IgG)
i. gene
intravenous i.
intravenous anti-D i.
i. M (IgM)
Rh i.
$Rh_o(D)$ i.

NOTES

immunoglobulin *(continued)*
    surface i.
    thyroid-stimulating i.
immunohistochemical
    i. change
    i. stromal leukocyte
    characterization
immunologic
    i. assay
    i. change
    i. enhancement
    i. paralysis
    i. pregnancy test
    i. suppression
    i. surveillance
    i. tolerance
    i. unresponsiveness
immunology
    maternal i.
    placental i.
    transplantation i.
    tumor i.
immunoprophylaxis
immunoprotein
immunoradiometric assay (IRMA)
immunoreaction
immunoreactivity
immunoresistance
immunosuppression
immunosuppressive
    i. therapy
immunotherapy
    adoptive i.
    nonspecific i.
    specific i.
    systemic-active nonspecific i.
    tumor i.
Imodium
Imogam
Imovax
impacted
    i. fetus
    i. twins
impaction
    fecal i.
impaired
    i. glucose tolerance (IGT)
    i. secretion
impairment
    inherited androgen uptake i.
    opioidergic control i.
impedance
    acoustic i.

    i. plethysmography
    i. pneumography
    transcephalic i.
imperfecta
    osteogenesis i. (OI)
imperforate
    i. anus
    i. hymen
    i. urethra
impervious
    i. sheet
    i. stockinette
impetigo
    bullous i.
    i. contagiosa
    i. herpetiformis
    i. neonatorum
implant
    cesium i.
    collapsed subpectoral i.
    Contigen glutaraldehyde
    cross-linked collagen i.
    endometrial i.
    fetal tissue i.
    goserelin acetate i.
    hormonal i.
    iridium i.
    levonorgestrel i.
    metastatic i.
    Norplant i.
    Organon percutaneous E2 i.
    peritoneal i.
    radioactive i.
    radium i.
    saline i.
    silicone i.
    subdermal i.
    subdermal levonorgestrel i.
    (SLI)
    subpectoral i.
    transperineal i.
    transvaginal i.
implantation
    blastocyst i.
    cortical i.
    displacement i.
    i. failure
    fusion i.
    intrusive i.
    i. phase
    placental i.
    radioactive seed i.

i. theory
tubouterine i.
impotence
impotent
impregnate
Impril
Improved
Clearblue I.
Hybolin I.
Imuran
IMV
intermittent mandatory
ventilation
intermittent mechanical
ventilation
IMx Estradial Assay
^{111}In
indium-111
in
i. situ hybridization
i. situ nucleic acid
hybridization
toeing i.
i. utero exposure
i. vitro
i. vitro fertilization (IVF)
i. vitro fertilization-embryo
transfer (IVF-ET)
i. vivo
i. vivo fertilization
inactivated poliovirus vaccine (IPV)
inactivation pattern
inactive endometrium
inadequacy
luteal phase i.
inadequate luteal phase
inanition fever
inappropriate
i. antidiuretic hormone
(IADH)
i. lactation
Inapsine
inborn error of metabolism
inbreeding
coefficient of i.

incarcerated
i. hernia
i. placenta
incarceration
incessant ovulation
incest
incestuous
incipient abortion
incision
boutonierre i.
buttonhole i.
cervical i.
Cherney i.
classical transverse i.
i. closure
colpotomy i.
elliptical uterine i.
gridiron i.
Kehr i.
laparotomy i.
lazy-S i.
low-segment transverse i.
Maylard i.
midline i.
paramedian i.
periumbilical i.
Pfannenstiel i.
Rockey-Davis i.
Sanger i.
Schuchardt i.
Sellheim i.
smiling i.
supraumbilical i.
transverse i.
uterine i.
incisional hernia
inclination
pelvic i.
inclusion cyst
incompatibility
ABO i.
Rh i.
incompatible blood group antigen
incompetence
cervical i. (CI)
gastroesophageal i.
palatopharyngeal i.

NOTES

incompetent cervix
incomplete
    i. abortion
    i. breech presentation
    i. conjoined twins
    i. foot presentation
    i. knee presentation
    i. precocious puberty
    i. puberty
incompletus
    coitus i.
incontinence
    anal i.
    exercise-induced i.
    giggle i.
    key-in-lock i.
    i. of milk
    overflow i.
    paradoxical i.
    passive i.
    stress urinary i. (SUI)
    true i.
    urge i.
    urinary i.
    urinary exertional i.
    urinary stress i.
incontinentia
    i. pigmenti
    i. pigmenti achromiens
increase
    plasma prorenin i.
increta
    placenta i.
incubation
incubator
    double-walled i.
    Ohmeda Care-Plus i.
incudiform uterus
indapamide
independence
    causal i.
    stochastic i.
Inderal
    I. LA
index, pl. indices, indexes
    amniotic fluid i. (AFI)
    anterior cerebral artery
      pulsatility i. (ACAPI)
    body mass i. (BMI)
    Broders i.
    i. case
    deoxyribonucleic acid i.
    fetal-pelvic i.

    foam stability i.
    free androgen i.
    free testosterone i.
    free thyroxine i.
    karyopyknotic i.
    Mengert i.
    mental development i.
      (MDI)
    oxygenation i. (OI)
    Pearl i.
    pelvic i.
    pelvic support i. (PSI)
    placental i.
    ponderal i.
    Pourcelot i.
    psychomotor development i.
      (PDI)
    pulsatility i. (PI)
    Quetelet i.
    resistance i. (RI)
    short-increment sensitivity i.
      (SISI)
    Silverman-Anderson i.
    Stuart i.
    testosterone i.
    thyroid i.
    total testosterone i.
    urinary diagnostic i. (UDI)
    Wintrobe i.
Index-I
    State-Trait-Anxiety I.-I.
      (STAI-I)
Indiana pouch
India rubber skin
indicator
    prognostic i.
indices (*pl. of* index)
Indiclor test
indifferent
    i. genitalia
    i. gonadal stage
    i. gonads
indigenous neoplasm
indigo
    i. carmine
    i. carmine dye
indigotin
indirect placentography
indium-111 (^{111}In)
Indocid
Indocin
    I. I.V.
    I. SR

indolamine
indomethacin
induced
    i. abortion
    i. labor
    i. remission
induction
    labor augmentation i.
    menstrual cycle i.
    ovulation i.
    Pitocin i.
    Spemann i.
    superovulation i.
indusium, pl. **indusia**
inefficiency
    female fertility i.
inencephaly
inertia
    primary uterine i.
    secondary uterine i.
    true uterine i.
    uterine i.
inevitable abortion
Infalyte
    I. formula
infancy
    acropustulosis of i.
    spongy degeneration of i.
    transient
      hypogammaglobulinemia
      of i. (THI)
infant
    I. Behavior Record (IBR)
    i. death
    i. of diabetic mother (IDM)
    drug-depressed i.
    i. Hercules
    high-risk i.
    immature i.
    jittery i.
    large-for-dates i.
    liveborn i.
    low-birth-weight i. (LBWI)
    mature i.
    i. morbidity
    i. mortality
    i. mortality rate

    Neurodevelopmental
      Assessment Procedure for
      Preterm I.'s (NAPI)
    postmature i.
    postterm i.
    premature i. (PI)
    preterm i.
    i. respiratory distress
      syndrome
    Rh-positive i.
    small-for-gestational-age i.
    I. Star high-frequency
      ventilator
    i. Star ventilator
    stillborn i.
    term i.
    very-low-birth-weight i.
    vigorous i.
    well-oxygenated i.
infantile
    i. arteriosclerosis
    i. breath-holding response
    i. cataract
    i. celiac disease
    i. colic
    i. cortical hyperostosis
    i. diplegia
    i. dwarfism
    i. eczema
    i. myoclonic seizure
    i. myxedema
    i. neuroaxonal dystrophy
    i. polycystic kidney disease
      (IPKD)
    i. polyneuritis
    i. purulent conjunctivitis
    i. respiratory distress
      syndrome
    i. scurvy
    i. spasm
    i. spastic paraplegia
    i. spinal muscular atrophy
infantilis
    dystaxia cerebralis i.
    poliodystrophia cerebri
      progressiva i.

NOTES

infantilism
Brissaud i.
cachectic i.
celiac i.
dysthyroidal i.
hepatic i.
Herter i.
hypophysial i.
Levi-Lorain i.
Lorain i.
myxedematous i.
regressive i.
sexual i.
infantis
Bifidobacterium i.
infantum
anemia pseudoleukemica i.
cholera i.
dermatitis excoriativa i.
dermatitis exfoliativa i.
dermatitis gangrenosa i.
lichen i.
roseola i.
tabes i.
infarct
bilirubin i.
placental i.
uric acid i.
white i.
infarction
cerebral i.
myocardial i.
pulmonary i.
renal i.
Infasurf
infected abortion
infection
adnexal i.
asymptomatic i.
bacterial i.
benign papillomavirus i.
cervical i.
cervicovaginal i.
chlamydial i.
chorioamnionic i.
coxsackievirus i.
cytomegalovirus i.
disseminated i.
disseminated gonococcal i.
fetal i.
fungal i.
gastrointestinal i.
genital i.

gonococcal i.
granulomatous i.
intraabdominal i.
intraamniotic i.
intrauterine i.
IUD-related i.
latent herpes simplex
virus i.
lower genital tract i.
maternal i.
neisserial i.
neonatal i.
nosocomial i.
papillomavirus i.
paronychial i.
pelvic i.
pharyngeal gonococcal i.
postpartum i.
puerperal i.
recurrent i.
respiratory tract i.
retroperitoneal i.
streptococcal i.
surgical i.
symptomatic i.
Trichomonas i.
upper genital tract i.
upper respiratory i. (URI)
urinary tract i. (UTI)
uterine i.
vaginal i.
varicella i.
varicella-zoster virus i.
vertically-acquired i.
viral i.
vulvar i.
vulvovaginal premenarchal i.
wound i.
yeast i.
infection-associated hemophagocytic syndrome (IAHS)
infectiosum
erythema i.
infectious
i. colitis
i. disease
i. esophagitis
i. hepatitis
i. mononucleosis
infective endocarditis
infecundity
inferior
inferior i.

i. mesenteric artery
i. straight
i. vena cava
infertile
  i. patient
  i. woman
infertility
  i. agent
  anovulatory i.
  asymptomatic i.
  endometriosis-associated i.
  i. evaluation
  i. factor
  familial i.
  idiopathic i.
  inherited i.
  i. investigation
  male i.
  male factor i.
  i. management
  primary i.
  secondary i.
  i. treatment
  unexplained i.
infiltrate
  patchy i.
  streaky i.
infiltrating
  i. carcinoma
  i. small-cell lobular
    carcinoma
infiltration
  fatty i.
inflammation
  pelvic i.
inflammatory
  i. bowel disease
  i. carcinoma
influenza
  i. A
  i. B
  i. C
  i. vaccine
  i. virus
influenzae
  Haemophilus i.

informed
  i. consent
  i. consent disclosure rules
informosome
infraction
  Freiberg i.
InfraGuide
  I. delivery system
  Heraeus LaserSonics I.
inframammary
Infrasurf surfactant
infundibular
  i. stalk
  i. stenosis
infundibuliform hymen
infundibulopelvic ligament
infundibulum
infusion
  colloid i.
  continuous subcutaneous
    insulin i.
  fetal cortisol i.
  intraarterial i.
  intralymphatic i.
  intravenous i.
  vasopressin i.
Ingelman-Sundberg gracilis muscle procedure
ingestion
  alcohol i.
inguinal
  i. canal
  i. hernia
  i. lymphadenectomy
  i. lymph node
  i. lymph node metastasis
inguinale
  lymphogranuloma i.
inguinal-femoral node dissection
inguinalis
  hernia uteri i.
INH
  isoniazid
inhalation
  i. anesthesia
  smoke i.

NOTES

inhaler
    metered dose i. (MDI)
inheritance
    amphigonous i.
    autosomal dominant i.
    autosomal recessive i.
    biparental i.
    codominant i.
    complemental i.
    cytoplasmic i.
    dominant i.
    extrachromosomal i.
    holandric i.
    hologynic i.
    homochronous i.
    homotropic i.
    mendelian i.
    monofactorial i.
    multifactorial i.
    polygenic i.
    quantitative i.
    quasicontinuous i.
    recessive i.
    sex-linked i.
    unit i.
    X-linked dominant i.
    X-linked recessive i.
inherited
    i. androgen uptake
      impairment
    i. disorder
    i. infertility
inhibin
    i. concentration
inhibited sexual desire
inhibition
    follicle-stimulating
      hormone i.
    hemagglutination i. (HI, HI
      titer)
    labor i.
    luteinization i.
    pituitary gonadotropin i.
    premature uterine
      contraction i.
    prostaglandin synthesis i.
    steroid secretion i.
inhibitor
    alpha-1 protease i. (alpha-1
      PI)
    cell growth i.
    cholinesterase i.
    corticotropin-releasing i.

dihydrofolate reductase i.
    factor VII i.
    factor VIII i.
    follicle-stimulating
      hormone i.
    follicle-stimulating hormone
      binding i.
    gonadotropin secretion i.
    human seminal (plasma) i.
      (HSI)
    luteinization i.
    luteinizing hormone
      receptor-binding i.
    monoamine oxidase i.
    oocyte maturation i. (OMI)
    ovum-capture i.
    plasminogen activator i.
      type I, II
    prostaglandin synthetase i.
      (PGSI)
    protease i. (PI)
    serotonin reuptake i.
iniodymus
iniopagus
iniops
initial apnea
initiation
    labor i.
    lactation i.
    puberty i.
injectable
    i. bromocriptine
    i. contraceptive
injection
    adrenaline i.
    continuous subcutaneous
      insulin i.
    intracytoplasmic sperm i.
      (ICSI)
    local methotrexate i.
    paracervical i.
    silicone i.
    Teflon periurethral i.
injector
    Harris uterine i. (HUI)
    Mini-Flex flexible Harris
      uterine i.
injury
    accidental fetal i.
    birth i.
    brachial plexus i.
    congenital i.
    hypoxic-ischemic i.

iatrogenic ureteral i.
intraoperative
   gastrointestinal i.
irradiation i.
lumbosacral plexus i.
mechanical birth i.
muscular i.
nerve i.
neurological i.
obstetrical traction i.
pelvic nerve i.
pulmonary i.
spinal i.
spinal cord i.
thermal i.
traumatic i.
urological i.
vaginal i.
vascular i.
inlet
   conjugate diameter of
      pelvic i.
   pelvic i.
inner cell mass
innominate bone
Innova
   I. electrotherapy system
   I. feminine incontinence
      treatment system
   I. pelvic floor stimulator
Innovar
Inocor
inoculata
   varicella i.
inositol
   i. 1,4,5-triphosphate
   i. trisphosphate
inotropic
insemination
   artificial i. (AI)
   artificial intravaginal i.
   cervical i.
   cup i.
   direct intraperitoneal i.
   i. dish
   heterologous i.
   high intrauterine i.

homologous i.
intrafollicular i. (IFI)
intratubal i. (ITI)
intrauterine i. (IUI)
Makler i.
subzonal i. (SUZI)
i. swim-up technique
therapeutic i.
washed intrauterine i.
insensible fluid loss
insensitive ovary syndrome
insertion
   i. of chromosome
   marginal i.
   velamentous i.
insertional mutagenesis
InSight prenatal test
insipidus
   diabetes i.
insomnia
inspiration time (I-time)
inspiratory/expiratory (I/E)
inspiratory stridor
inspired gas (I)
inspissated
   i. bile syndrome
   i. milk syndrome
INSS
   International Staging System
instability
   detrusor i.
instillation
instrument
   EndoMax advanced
      laparoscopic i.
   Kevorkian-Younge cervical
      biopsy i.
   LDS i.
   myoma fixation i.
   Newport medical i.
   Polaris reusable i.
instrumentation
   DeLee i.
insufficiency
   ACTH i.
   adrenal i.
   adrenocortical i.

NOTES

insufficiency *(continued)*
    aortic i.
    aortic valve i.
    corpus luteum i.
    glomerular i.
    mitral i.
    mitral valve i.
    placental i.
    renal i.
    respiratory i.
    tricuspid i.
    uterine i.
    uteroplacental i.
insufflation
    i. needle
    peritoneal i.
    tubal i.
insufflator
    hysteroscopic i.
    Kidde tubal i.
    laparoscopic i.
    Neal i.
    Semm Pelvi-Pneu i.
Insulatard NPH human
insulin
    beef i.
    maternal i.
    neutral protamine
      Hagedorn i. (NPH
      insulin)
    Novolin i.
    NPH I.
    pork i.
    i. pump
    Regular I.
    Regular Purified Pork I.
    i. resistance
    i. shock
    i. tolerance test
    Ultralente i.
insulinase
insulin-dependent
    i.-d. diabetes mellitus
      (IDDM)
    i.-d. diabetic
insulinemia
insulin-like growth factor (IGF)
    i.-l. g. f. I
insulopenia
Insul-Sheath vaginal speculum
    sheath
intact membrane
intake and output (I&O)

Intal
integrin
    beta-1 i.
    beta-2 i.
integrin-binding
Intelligence
    Fagan Test of Infant I.
Intelligence-Revised
    Wechsler Preschool and
      Primary Scale of I.-R.
      (WPPSI-R)
intensity/duration (I/T)
interaction
    actin-myosin i.
    androgen i.
    sperm-oocyte i.
    stromal-epithelial i.
Interceed
    I. absorbable adhesion
      barrier
    I. barrier material
Intercept
intercostal retractions
intercourse
    sexual i.
intercross
interdigitation
interference
    acoustical i.
interferon (IFN)
    i. alfa-n3
    alpha i.
    alpha-recombinant i.
    beta i.
    gamma i.
    human leukocyte i. (HLI)
    leukocyte i.
    lymphoblastoid i.
Intergroup Rhabdomyosarcoma
    Study (IRS)
interleukin (IL)
    i.-1 (IL-1)
    i.-1β
    i.-2 (IL-2)
intermedia
    a-thalassemia i.
    thalassemia i.
intermenstrual
    i. bleeding
    i. pain
intermittent
    i. cyclical etidronate
      disodium

i. fever
i. hydrosalpinx
i. mandatory ventilation
(IMV)
i. mechanical ventilation
(IMV)
i. pneumatic compression
i. porphyria
i. positive pressure
breathing (IPPB)
i. positive pressure
ventilation (IPPV)
i. sterilization

interna
endometriosis i.

internal
i. conjugate
i. diameter
i. endometriosis
i. generative organ
i. genitalia
i. os
i. radiation therapy
i. rotation
i. version

internalization
hormone-receptor complex i.
receptor i.

international
I. Association for the Study
of Pain
i. classification of cancer of
cervix
I. Federation of Gynecology
and Obstetrics (FIGO)
I. Federation of Gynecology
and Obstetrics
classification
I. Federation Obstetrics and
Gynecology
I. Reference Preparation
(IRP)
I. Society for Gynecologic
Pathology (ISGP)
I. Society for the Study of
Vulvar Diseases (ISSVD)
I. Staging System (INSS)

I. Union Against Cancer
(UICC)

interobserver variation
interphase
interplant
interpretation
mirror image i.
i. variability

interrupted suture
interruption
vena caval i.

intersex
i. problem

intersexuality
interstitial
i. cell
i. deletion
i. irradiation
i. keratitis
i. and loculated hematoma
i. mastitis
i. nephritis
i. plasma cell pneumonia
i. pregnancy
i. therapy

intertriginous candidosis
intertrigo
intertuberous diameter
interval
Q-T i.

intervention
court-ordered obstetrical i.
legal i.

interventional procedure
intervillous
i. blood
i. blood gas
i. spaces

intestinal
i. bypass procedure
i. conduit
i. fistula
i. hurry
i. mesentery
i. obstruction
i. parasite

NOTES

217

intestinal *(continued)*
    i. peristalsis
    i. tract
intestinalis
    pneumatosis cystoides i.
intoeing
intolerance
    carbohydrate i.
    fructose i.
    gestational carbohydrate i.
     (GCI)
    glucose i.
    glucose-galactose i.
    lactose i.
intoxication
    intrarenal androgenic i.
    water i.
intraabdominal
    i. infection
    i. pressure
    i. surgery
intraamniotic infection
intraarterial infusion
Intrabutazone
intracanalicular fibroadenoma
intracavitary
    i. brachytherapy
    i. radium
intracellular mediator
intracervical tent
intracranial
    i. anatomy
    i. aneurysm
    i. dural vascular anomaly
    i. hemorrhage (ICH)
    i. hypertension
    i. tumor
intracystic papillary carcinoma
intracytoplasmic sperm injection
    (ICSI)
IntraDop probe
intraductal
    i. carcinoma
    i. papillary carcinoma
    i. papilloma
intradural spinal angioma
intraepithelial
    i. cervical dysplasia
    i. disease progression
    i. endometrial cancer
    i. lesion
    i. neoplasia

intrafallopian transfer
intrafollicular insemination (IFI)
intrahepatic cholestasis of
    pregnancy
intraligamentary pregnancy
intraligamentous myoma
Intralipid
    I. hyperalimentation
intralobular connective tissue
intralocal additivity
intraluminal upper airway
    obstruction
intralymphatic infusion
intramammary
    i. lymph node
intramural
    i. fibroid
    i. myoma
    i. pregnancy
    i. upper airway obstruction
intramuscular (IM)
intranatal
intranuclear virion
intraoperative
    i. complication
    i. gastrointestinal injury
    i. radiation
intrapartum
    i. asphyxiation
    i. cardiotocography
    i. hemorrhage
    i. monitor
    i. monitoring
    i. period
intrapelvic
intraperitoneal
    i. blood transfusion
    i. chemotherapy
    i. cisplatin
    i. cisplatin chemotherapy
    i. endometrial metastatic
     disease
    i. fetal transfusion
    i. 5-fluorouracil
    i. pregnancy
    i. radiation therapy
    i. therapy
intrapulmonary
    i. shunt
    i. shunt ratio (Qs/Qt)
intrarenal
    i. androgenic intoxication
    i. reflux

intrathoracic
    i. airway obstruction
    i. tuberculosis
intratubal insemination (ITI)
intrauterine
    i. adhesion
    i. amputation
    i. contraceptive device
      (IUCD)
    i. death
    i. device (IUD)
    i. diaphragm
    i. fetal monitoring
    i. fracture
    i. GIFT
    i. growth retardation
      (IUGR)
    i. hematoma
    i. herpes
    i. infection
    i. insemination (IUI)
    i. insemination cannula
    i. insemination cannula
      with mandrel
    i. intraperitoneal fetal
      transfusion
    i. parabiotic syndrome
    i. pneumonia
    i. pregnancy (IUP)
    i. pressure catheter (IUPC)
    i. pressure cycle
    i. pressure measurement
    i. resuscitation
    i. synechia
    i. transfusion
    i. volume
intravaginal
    i. condom
    i. contraceptive
    i. cream
    i. foam
    i. pouch
    i. sponge
intravascular transfusion
intravenous (I.V.)
    i. alimentation
    i. anti-D immunoglobulin

    i. drug
    i. glucose challenge
    i. hyperalimentation (IVH)
    i. immunoglobulin
    i. infusion
    i. leiomyomatosis
    i. line
    i. medication
    i. pyelogram (IVP)
    i. pyelography (IVP)
    i. urogram (IVU)
intraventricular
    i. hemorrhage (Grade I, II,
      III, IV) (IVH)
intravesical pressure
intrinsic
    i. dysmenorrhea
    i. pulsatility
    i. sphincter deficiency (IDS)
introital
introitus
    marital i.
    parous i.
    virginal i.
intromission
Intropin
intrusive implantation
intubation
    endotracheal i.
    tracheal i.
intussusception
    cecocolic i.
    colocolic i.
    ileocolic i.
    ileoileal i.
invaginata
    trichorrhexis i.
invagination
invasion
    early stromal i.
invasive
    i. cancer
    i. carcinoma
    i. cervical cancer
    i. hydatidiform mole
    i. mole
    i. neoplasia

NOTES

Inventory
    Children's Depression I.
      (CDI)
    Eyberg Child Behavior I.
      (ECBI)
    Minnesota Multiphasic
      Personality I. (MMPI)
    West Haven-Yale
      Multidimensional Pain I.
inverse square law
Inversine
inversion
    i. of chromosomes
    Hautain uterine i.
    paracentric i.
    pericentric i.
    i. of the uterus
inversus
    situs i.
inverted
    i. nipple
    i. pelvis
investigation
    infertility i.
involuntary sterilization
involution
    i. cyst
    i. of the uterus
involutional
    i. melancholia
    i. psychosis
involvement
    metastatic axillary i.
    neurologic i.
    nodal i.
    ocular i.
    pelvic i.
INVOS 3100 cerebral oximeter
I&O
    intake and output
Ioban
    I. drape
    I. 2 iodophor cesarean
      sheet
iocetamic acid
iodamide
iodide
    potassium i.
    sodium i.
    i. therapy
    i. trap defect
iodide-containing medication

iodinated glycerol
iodine
    i. douche
    i. 125-labeled fibrinogen
      scan
    i. stain
    i. supply
iodine-125 (^{125}I)
iodine-131 (^{131}I)
    antiferritin antibody linked
      to i.-131
iodipamide
iodomethyl-norcholesterol scanning
iodoquinol
iodothyronine
    i. level
iohexol
ion
    calcium i.
Ionamin
ionization
ionized calcium (iCa)
ionizing radiation
iopanoic acid
iothalamate sodium
Iowa trumpet
Ipecac
IPKD
    infantile polycystic kidney
      disease
ipodate sodium
IPPB
    intermittent positive pressure
      breathing
IPPV
    intermittent positive pressure
      ventilation
ipratropium bromide
iprindole
iproniazid
ipsilateral
IPV
    inactivated poliovirus vaccine
Ir
    iridium
^{192}Ir
    iridium-192
IRDS
    idiopathic respiratory distress
      syndrome
Ir gene
iridium (Ir)

i. implant
i. wire
iridium-192 (^{192}Ir)
iridocyclitis
iritis
    i. catamenialis
IRMA
    immunoradiometric assay
Iromin-G
iron (Fe)
    i. deficiency anemia (IDA)
    elemental i.
    I. interne retractor
    Pedicran with I.
    i. requirement
    serum i.
    Similac-24-LBW with whey
      and i.
    Similac 24 with i.
    i. turnover
iron-binding capacity (IBC)
Irospan
IRP
    International Reference
    Preparation
irradiation
    abdominal i.
    abdominopelvic i.
    cesium i.
    i. cystitis
    i. dermatitis
    external beam i.
    heavy-ion i.
    hemibody i.
    i. injury
    interstitial i.
    local i.
    paraaortic node i.
    pelvic i.
    surface i.
    whole-abdomen i.
    whole-body i.
    whole-pelvis i.
irregularity
    menstrual i.
Irrigant
    Neosporin G.U. I.

irrigation
irritable breast
IRS
    Intergroup Rhabdomyosarcoma
    Study
Irving tubal ligation
Isaac syndrome
ischemia
    myocardial i.
ischemic heart disease
ischiadelphus
ischiocavernosus muscle
ischiocavernous
ischiodidymus
ischiomelus
ischiopagus
ischiopubica
    osteochondritis i.
ischiopubic ramus
ischiopubiotomy
    Galbiati bilateral fetal i.
ischiothoracopagus
isethionate
    pentamidine i.
ISG
    immune serum globulin
Is gene
ISGP
    International Society for
    Gynecologic Pathology
Ishihara
    POU theory of I.
    I. theory
island
    Pander i.'s
islet
    i. cell adenoma
    i. cell tumor
    i.'s of Langerhans
Ismelin
isoamylase
isoantibody
isoantigen
Iso-Bid
isocarboxazid
isochemagglutinin

NOTES

isochromosome
    i. X
isodose curve
isoetharine
isofluorphate
isoflurane
isogeneic graft
isograft
isoimmune thrombocytopenia
isoimmunization
    D i.
    D-antigen i.
    Rh i.
Isojima test
isolated autosomal dominant
    syndrome
isolette
    bubble i.
    double-bubble i.
    double-walled bubble i.
Isolin
isologous neoplasm
isomer
isomerase
    triose phosphate i.
Isomil
    I. formula
isoniazid (INH)
Isopaque
Isophrin
isoprenaline hydrochloride
isopropamide iodide
isoproterenol
Isoptin
Isopto Carbachol
Isopto Carpine
Isopto Cetamide
Isopto Eserine
Isopto Frin
Isordil
isosexual idiopathic precocious
    puberty
isosorbide dinitrate
Isotamine
isothenuria
isotonic PBS
isotope
    i. cisternography
    radioactive i.
    i. scanning
Isotrate
isotretinoin
isovalericacidemia

isovaleric acidemia
iso-X chromosome
I-Soyalac formula
issue
    legal i.
    social i.
ISSVD
    International Society for the
    Study of Vulvar Diseases
isthmi (pl. of isthmus)
isthmica nodosa
isthmointerstitial anastomosis
isthmorrhaphy
isthmus, pl. isthmuses, isthmi
    cervical i.
Isuprel
I/T
    intensity/duration
    I/T ratio
itch-scratch cycle
Itch-X
    I.-X. gel
    I.-X. spray
ITI
    intratubal insemination
I-time
    inspiration time
Ito
    hypomelanosis of I.
    I. method
    nevus of I.
    I. nevus
ITP
    idiopathic thrombocytopenic
    purpura
    immune thrombocytopenic
    purpura
IUCD
    intrauterine contraceptive device
IUD
    intrauterine device
IUD-related infection
IUGR
    intrauterine growth retardation
IUI
    intrauterine insemination
        IUI disposable cannula
IUP
    intrauterine pregnancy
IUPC
    intrauterine pressure catheter
I.V.
    intravenous

Indocin I.V.
Metro I.V.
Monistat I.V.
Ivemark syndrome
IVF
  in vitro fertilization
IVF-ET
  in vitro fertilization-embryo
    transfer
IVH
  intravenous hyperalimentation

  intraventricular hemorrhage
    (Grade I, II, III, IV)
ivory bones
IVP
  intravenous pyelogram
IVP
  intravenous pyelogram
  intravenous pyelography
IVU
  intravenous urogram
Ivy bleeding time

NOTES

J
   joule
   J pulmonary receptors
Jabouley amputation
jackknife
   j. position
   j. seizure
Jackson
   J. membrane
   J. right-angle retractor
jacksonian epilepsy
Jackson-Pratt suction drain
Jacobsen-Brodwall syndrome
Jacobsen syndrome
Jacobs tenaculum
Jacob syndrome
Jacquemier sign
Jacquet
   J. dermatitis
   J. erythema
Jadassohn-Lewandowski syndrome
Jadassohn test
Jadassohn-Tieche nevus
Jaffe-Gottfried-Bradley syndrome
Jaffe-Lichtenstein syndrome
Jahnke syndrome
Jaksch
   J. anemia
   J. disease
   J. syndrome
jamais vu
Janacek reimplantation set
Janeway lesion
janiceps
   j. asymmetrus
   j. parasiticus
Janimine
Janosik embryo
Jansen syndrome
Jansky-Bielschowsky syndrome
Jansky classification
Janus report
jar
   Gas-Pak j.
Jarcho-Levin syndrome
Jarisch-Herxheimer reaction
Jarit
   J. disposable cannula
   J. disposable trocar
Jatene procedure

jaundice
   black j.
   breast milk j.
   catarrhal j.
   central j.
   cholestatic j.
   congenital hemolytic j.
   congenital nonhemolytic j.
   congenital obliterative j.
   neonatal cholestatic j.
   j. of newborn
   nuclear j.
   obstructive j.
   peripheral j.
   physiologic j.
   Schmorl j.
jaw
   bird-beak j.
   cleft j.
   fibrous dysplasia of j.
   j. myoclonus
   parrot j.
JDM
   juvenile diabetes mellitus
jejunoileal
   j. atresia
   j. bypass
jello sign
jelly
   Aci-Jel vaginal j.
   contraceptive j.
   Gynol II contraceptive j.
   K-Y lubricating j.
   Wharton j.
Jenamicin
Jenest-28
Jensen syndrome
jeopardy
   fetal j.
Jervell-Lange-Nielson syndrome
Jervis syndrome
jet
   high-frequency j. (HFJ)
Jeune
   J. disease
   J. syndrome
Jew
   Ashkenazi J.
Jewett classification
jitteriness

jittery
    j. baby
    j. infant
Job syndrome
Jocasta complex
JODM
    juvenile-onset diabetes mellitus
jogger's amenorrhea
Johanson-Blizzard syndrome
Johnson
    J. method
    J. syndrome
joint
    Clutton j.'s
    j. deformity
    j. hyperlaxity
    pelvic j.
    j. probability
    sacroiliac j.
Jones
    J. criteria
    J. and Jones wedge
       technique
Jorgenson scissors
Joseph
    J. disease
    J. syndrome
Josephs-Blackfan-Diamond
    syndrome
Joubert syndrome
joule (J)
Jr.
    Aerolate J.
    Caltrate, J.
    EpiPen J.
JRA
    juvenile rheumatoid arthritis
Juberg-Holt syndrome
jugular
    j. occlusion plethysmography
    j. venous pressure (JVP)
juice baby
Juliusberg
    J. pustulosis
    J. pustulosis vacciniformis
       acuta
jumping gene

junction
    gap j.
    squamocolumnar j.
    ureterovesical j. (UVJ)
junctional rhythm
Junius-Kuhnt syndrome
junky lung
justifiable abortion
Juvara fold
juvenile
    j. aldosteronism
    j. carcinoma
    j. diabetes
    j. diabetes mellitus (JDM)
    j. epithelial corneal
       dystrophy
    j. gangliosidosis
    j. osteomalacia
    j. papillomatosis
    j. pelvis
    j. pernicious anemia
    j. plantar dermatitis
    j. rheumatoid arthritis
       (JRA)
    j. spermatogonial depletion
    j. spinal muscular atrophy
    j. xanthogranuloma (JXG)
juvenile-onset
    j.-o. diabetes
    j.-o. diabetes mellitus
       (JODM)
juvenilis
    kyphoscoliosis dorsalis j.
    kyphosis dorsalis j.
    osteochondritis deformans j.
    osteodystrophia j.
    verruca plana j.
juxtaductal coarctation
juxtaglomerular
juxtamedullary
juxtaposition
Juzo-Hostess two-way stretch
    compression stockings
JVP
    jugular venous pressure
JXG
    juvenile xanthogranuloma

K
  potassium
    K cell
    K chain
Kabikinase
Kabuki make-up syndrome
Kagan staging system
Kahn
    K. cannula
    K. test
Kajava classification
KAL
kala-azar
Kalcinate
Kaliscinski ureteral procedure
kallikrein
Kallmann syndrome
Kalmuk idiocy
kanamycin
Kanana Banana
kangaroo
    K. Care
    k. pouch
kangarooing
Kanner syndrome
Kanter sign
Kantrex
Kantu sign
Kaochlor
kaolin clotting time
Kaon
    K.-Cl
Kapeller-Adler test
Kaplan-Meier
    K.-M. method
    K.-M. survival curve
Kaposi
    K. sarcoma
    K. varicelliform eruption
    K. varicelliform sarcoma
kappa chain
karaya
Karmen cannula
Karnofsky
    K. performance status
    K. performance status of
      chemotherapy
Karo syrup
Kartagener syndrome
karyogenesis

karyokinesis
karyopyknosis
karyopyknotic index
karyosome
karyothecakatadidymus
karyotype
    k. analysis
    fetal k.
    45,X k.
    XX k.
    46,XX k.
    XXX k.
    47,XXY k.
    XY k.
    46,XY k.
karyotyping
Kasabach-Merritt syndrome
Kasai
    K. peritoneal venous shunt
    K. procedure
Kashin-Beck disease
Kasnelson syndrome
Kasof
Kass criteria
Kato
Kaufman
    K. Assessment Battery for
      Children
    K. pneumonia
    K. syndrome
Kaufman-McKusick syndrome
Kawasaki disease (KD)
Kay Ciel
Kayexalate
Kaylixir
Kayser-Fleischer ring
kb
    kilobase
      kb pair
kc
    kilocycle
kcal
    kilocalorie
KD
    Kawasaki disease
KDC-Healthdyne nonfluorescent
  spotlight
KDF-2.3
    K. intrauterine catheter

KDF-2.3 *(continued)*
  K. intrauterine insemination
    cannula
Kearns-Sayre syndrome
keel chest
keeled breast
Keeler
  K. fiberoptic headlight
  K. loupe
to keep open (TKO)
keep vein open (KVO)
Keflex
Keflin
Keftab
Kefurox
Kefzol
Kegel exercises
Kehr
  K. incision
  K. technique
Keipert syndrome
Kell sensitization
Kelly
  K. clamp
  K. operation
  K. plication
  K. plication procedure
  K. retractor
Kelly-Gray curette
keloid
Kemadrin
Kendall McGaw Intelligent pump
Kennedy-Pacey operation
Kennedy procedure
Kenny-Caffey syndrome
Kenny-Linarelli-Caffey syndrome
Kent Infant Development Scale
  (KIDS)
Keofeed tube
keratin cyst
keratinization
keratitis
  interstitial k.
keratoconjunctivitis
  tuberculous k.
keratoconus
keratoderma
keratolysis neonatorum
keratoma hereditarium mutilans
keratopathy
  band k.
keratosis
  k. follicularis

  k. palmaris et plantaris
  k. pilaris
  seborrheic k.
Kergaradec sign
kerion
Kerlix gauze bandage
kernicterus
Kernig sign
Kerr cesarean section
Kesaree-Wooley syndrome
Kestrone
ketamine
ketoacidosis
  diabetic k. (DKA)
ketoconazole
3-ketodesogestrel
11-ketoetiocholanolone
17-ketogenic steroid
ketone bodies
ketonemia
ketonuria
ketoprofen
ketorolac tromethamine
ketosis
  starvation k.
ketosis-prone diabetes
ketosis-resistant diabetes
17-ketosteroid reductase deficiency
17-ketosteroids (17-KS)
ketotic
  k. hyperglycemia
Kety-Schmidt technique
kev
  kilo-electronvolt
Kevorkian
  K. curette
  K. punch biopsy
Kevorkian-Younge
  K.-Y. biopsy forceps
  K.-Y. cervical biopsy
    instrument
  K.-Y. curette
Keyes
  K. dermatologic punch
  K. punch biopsy
  K. vulvar punch
key-in-lock
  k.-i.-l. incontinence
  k.-i.-l. maneuver
kg
  kilogram
kHz
  kilohertz

Kibrick-Isojima infertility test
Kibrick test
kick count
Kidd blood group
Kidde
   K. cannula technique
   K. tubal insufflator
kidney
   k. biopsy
   cystic k.
   k. dialysis
   k. disease
   k. failure
   k. function
   k. morphology
   pelvic k.
   single k.
   solitary k.
   k. stone
   k. transplantation
kidney-derived growth factor
KIDS
   Kent Infant Development Scale
Kikuchi disease
Kilian pelvis
kill
   cell k.
   log cell k.
killed virus vaccine
killer
   k. cells
   natural k. cells (NK cells)
kilobase (kb)
   k. pair
kilocalorie (kcal)
kilocycle (kc)
kilo-electronvolt (kev)
kilogram (kg)
kilohertz (kHz)
Kimmelstiel-Wilson
   K.-W. disease (KW)
   K.-W. syndrome
kinase
   creatine k. (CK)
   histone H1 k.
   myosin light-chain k.

   pyruvate k. (PK)
   tyrosine k.
kind
   error of the first k.
   error of the second k.
kindred
   degree of k.
kinesiologic
kinetics
   cell k.
kinetocardiotocograph
kinin
kinked cord
kinky hair disease
kinky-hair syndrome
Kinsbourne syndrome
Kinyoun stain
KIO syndrome
Kirmisson respirator
kit
   Amplicor HIV-1 test k.
   Amplicor PCR k.
   Centocor CA 125
     radioimmunoassay k.
   Hy-Gene seminal fluid
     collection k.
   Male FactorPak seminal
     fluid collection k.
   Ortho diaphragm k.
   Otovent autoinflation k.
   OvuGen test k.
   OvuKIT Self-Test k.
   OvuQUICK Self-Test k.
   PregnaGen test k.
   rape evidence k.
   SAFE k.
   SureCell Chlamydia Test k.
   SureCell rapid test k.
   TAGO diagnostic k.
Kitchen postpartum gauze packer
Kitner dissector
Kitzinger method of childbirth
Kjelland-Barton forceps
Kjelland forceps
Kjelland-Luikart forceps
Klavikordal

NOTES

Klebsiella
    K. oxytoca
    K. pneumoniae
kleeblattschädel syndrome
Kleihauer-Betke
    K.-B. stain
    K.-B. test
Klein-Waardenburg syndrome
Kleppinger
    K. bipolar forceps
    K. envelope sign
Klinefelter syndrome
Kline test
Kling bandage
Klippel-Feil syndrome
Klippel-Trenaunay syndrome
Klippel-Trenaunay-Weber syndrome
Kloepfer syndrome
Klonopin
K-Lor
Klor-Con
Klorvess
Klotrix
Klotz syndrome
Kluge method
Klumpke
    K. palsy
    K. paralysis
Klumpke-Dejerine paralysis
Klüver-Bucy syndrome
K-Lyte
KM-1 breast pump
knee
    knock k.'s
    k. presentation
knee-chest position
knee-elbow position
Kniest
    K. dwarfism
    K. dysplasia
    K. syndrome
Knobloch-Gesell test
knock knees
knot
    Aberdeen k.
    clinch k.
    false k. of umbilical cord
    primitive k.
    syncytial k.
    true k.'s of umbilical cord
knuckle of tube
Kobayashi vacuum extractor
Köbner phenomenon

Koby syndrome
Kocher clamp
Kocher-Debré-Sémélaigne syndrome
kocherize
Koch postulates
Kock pouch
Kocks operation
Kodak
    K. hCG serum test
    K. SureCell Chlamydia Test
    K. SureCell hCG-Urine Test
    K. SureCell Herpes (HSV) Test
    K. SureCell LCH in-office pregnancy test
    K. SureCell Strep A test
Koerber-Salus-Elschnig syndrome
Kogan endocervical speculum
KoGENate
KOH
    potassium hydroxide
    KOH prep
    KOH stain
    KOH test
Kohdschnetter disease
Köhler bone disease
koilocyte
koilocytic atypia
koilocytosis
koilocytotic cell
koilonychia
Kolmer-Kline-Kahn test
Kolmer test
kolpos
Konakion
Kono procedure
Kontron electrode
Kopan needle
Koplik spot
Korenman estrogen window hypothesis
Koromex
Kosenow-Sinios syndrome
Kostmann
    K. infantile agranulocytosis
    K. neutropenia
    K. syndrome
Kovalevsky canal
Kozlowski disease
Krabbe
    K. disease
    K. leukodystrophy
Kramer disease

Kraske position
kraurosis vulvae
Krause
   K. disease
   K. syndrome
Kreiselman infant warmer
Krisovski sign
Kristeller
   K. maneuver
   K. method
Kroner tubal ligation
Krönig technique
Kronner
   K. Manipujector
   K. Manipujector uterine
     manipulator/injector
Krukenberg tumor
Kruskal-Wallis test
17-KS
   17-ketosteroids
K-Tab
Kučera equation
Kufs disease
Kugelberg-Welander disease
Kun colocolpopoiesis
Kupperman test
Kurzrok-Miller test

Kurzrok-Ratner test
Kussmaul respiration
Küstner
   K. law
   K. sign
Kveim
   K. antibody
   K. test
KVO
   keep vein open
KW
   Kimmelstiel-Wilson disease
kwashiorkor
   k. disease
Kwell
Kwellada
K-Y lubricating jelly
kynocephalus
Kyotest
kyphoscoliosis
   k. dorsalis juvenilis
kyphoscoliotic heart disease
kyphosis
   k. dorsalis juvenilis
   Scheuermann juvenile k.
kyphotic pelvis

NOTES

231

L

L
    liter
L-A
    Bicillin L.-A.
LA
    Inderal L.
    Zephrex L.
L.A.
    Gynogen L.
    Theoclear L.
LA:A
    left atrial to aortic ratio
labetalol
labia (*pl. of* labium)
    l. majora
    l. minora
labial
    l. agglutination
    l. fusion
    l. hernia
    l. reflex
labialis
    herpes l.
labioperineal pouch
labioscrotal
    l. swelling
labium, pl. labia
    l. majus pudendi
labor
    abnormal l.
    active l.
    active phase of l.
    arrest of l.
    l. augmentation
    l. augmentation induction
    l. and delivery (L&D)
    desultory l.
    dry l.
    false l.
    first stage of l.
    induced l.
    l. inhibition
    l. initiation
    latent phase of l.
    mimetic l.
    missed l.
    oxytocin stimulation of l.
    l. pains
    precipitate l.
    precipitous l.

    premature l.
    preterm l.
    prodromal l.
    prolonged l.
    second stage of l.
    spontaneous l.
    third stage of l.
    l. trial
    true l.
laboratory
    Abbott L.'s
    l. finding
    l. test
    Wampole L.'s
labor, delivery, and recovery (LDR)
Labotect catheter
labyrinthine
    l. placenta
    l. reflex
labyrinthitis
laceration
    aortic l.
    birth canal l.
    bladder l.
    cervical l.
    falx l.
    perineal l.
    tentorial l.
    vaginal l.
Lack
    Henrietta L. (HeLa)
lacmoid staining solution
lacrimal
β-lactamase-resistant antistaphylococcal antibiotic
lactate
    amrinone l.
    cyclizine l.
    l. dehydrogenase (LDH)
lactated
    l. Ringer
    l. Ringer solution
lactating
    l. adenoma
    l. breast
    l. woman
lactation
    l. amenorrhea
    inappropriate l.

lactation *(continued)*
    l. initiation
    l. letdown response
lactational
    l. mastitis
lactea
    crusta l.
lacteal
    l. cyst
    l. fistula
lactic
    l. acid dehydrogenase
    l. acidemia
    l. acidosis
lactiferous
    l. duct
lactifugal
lactifuge
lactigenous
lactigerous
Lactina breast pump
lactobacillus, pl. lactobacilli
    hydrogen peroxide-
        producing l.
Lactobacillus acidophilus
lactobezoar
lactocele
lactoflavin
Lactofree formula
lactogen
    human placental l. (hPL,
        HPL)
    placental l.
lactogenesis
lactogenic
lactorrhea
lactose
    l. intolerance
lactose-free formula
lactosuria
lactotropin
lactulose
    l. enema
lacuna, pl. lacunae
lacunar skull
LAD
    left atrial dimension
Ladd
    L. bands
    L. procedure
    L. syndrome
Ladin sign
Laerdal resuscitator

laetrile
Lafora body disease
lag
    anaphase l.
    homeostatic l.
lagophthalmos
Lahey forceps
LAIT
    latex agglutination inhibition test
LAK
    lymphokine-activated killer cell
lake
    subchorial l.
La Leche League
Lamaze method
lambda suture line
Lambert
    L. canals, canals of L.
lamellar
    l. desquamation of newborn
    l. exfoliation
    l. ichthyosis
lamina, pl. laminae
    basal l.
    l. propria
Laminaria
    L. digitata
laminaria
    l. cervical dilator
    Dilapan l.
    l. tent
lamination
laminin
L-amino acid
lamp
    Nightingale examining l.
    Wood l.
lampbrush chromosome
Landau
    L. reflex
    L. test
Landouzy-Dejerine
    facioscapulohumeral
        syndrome of L.-D.
    L.-D. muscular dystrophy
Landovski nucleoid
Landry-Guillain-Barré syndrome
Landry palsy
Langdon Down disease
Lange-Akeroyd syndrome
Langer
    L. dysplasia

L. mesomelic dwarfism
L. syndrome
Langer-Giedion syndrome
Langerhans
L. cell histiocytosis
L. cells
L. granule
L. islands
islets of L.
Langer-Petersen-Spranger syndrome
Langer-Saldino syndrome
Lange test
Langhans
L. cells
L. giant cell granuloma
L. stria
Laniazid
Lanophyllin
Lanoxin
lanuginous
lanugo
l. hair
Lanvis
lap
laparotomy
ex l.
exploratory laparotomy
laparohysterectomy
laparohystero-oophorectomy
laparohysteropexy
laparohysterosalpingo-oophorectomy
laparohysterotomy
laparomyomectomy
laparosalpingectomy
laparosalpingo-oophorectomy
laparosalpingotomy
laparoscope
Lent l.
Storz l.
Weerda l.
Wolf l.
laparoscopic
l. cautery
l. Döderlein hysterectomy
l. electrocautery
l. fenestration
l. hysterectomy

l. insufflator
l. management
l. multiple-punch resection
laparoscopic-assisted
l.-a. vaginal hysterectomy
(LAVH)
l.-a. vaginal hysteroscopy
(LAVH)
Laparoscopists
American Association of
Gynecologic L. (AAGL)
laparoscopy
laser l.
operative l.
pelvic l.
second-look l.
laparotomy (lap)
exploratory l. (ex lap, ex
lap)
l. incision
second-look l.
laparotrachelotomy
laparouterotomy
Lapides technique
Lapwall sponge
Largactil
large
l. endometrioma
l. for gestational age (LGA)
l. intestine neoplasm
l. loop excision of
transformation zone
(LLETZ)
large-for-dates
l.-f.-d. infant
l.-f.-d. uterus
Larmarck theory
Larodopa
Laron syndrome
Laron-type dwarfism
Larsen syndrome
larva
l. currens
l. migrans
laryngeal
l. cleft
l. papillomatosis

NOTES

235

laryngeal *(continued)*
    l. stridor
    l. web
laryngitis
laryngomalacia
laryngoscope
    Andrews infant l.
    Holinger infant l.
    pencil-handled l.
    Siker l.
laryngoscopy
laryngospasm
laryngotracheobronchitis
laryngotracheoesophageal
laryngotracheomalacia
larynx
Larzel anemia
laser
    l. ablation
    argon l.
    l. blanching
    carbon dioxide l.
    l. cervical conization
    CO_2 l.
    Culpolase l.
    l. ejecta
    Er:YAG l.
    Ho:YAG l.
    Illumina Pro series
      laparoscopic l.
    l. laparoscopy
    Merimack 1040 CO2 l.
    l. method
    Nd:YAG l.
    OPMILAS CO2 l.
    l. photocoagulation
    l. photovaporization
    l. reaction
    l. surgery
    Surgicenter 40 CO2 l.
    Surgilase 55W l.
    l. therapy
    l. treatment
    l. uterosacral nerve ablation
      (LUNA)
    YAG l.
    yttrium-aluminum-garnet l.
laser-Doppler flowmeter
lasered
Lash
    L. operation
    L. procedure
Lasix

last
    l. menstrual period (LMP)
    l. normal menstrual period
      (LNMP)
lata
    condylomata l.
    tensor fascia l. (TFL)
late
    l. apnea
    l. decelerations
    l. embryonic testicular
      regression syndrome
    l. pregnancy
    l. replicating chromosome
latent
    l. carrier
    l. diabetes
    l. herpes simplex virus
      infection
    l. phase
    l. phase of labor
late-onset hyperplasia
lateral
    l. oblique view
    l. recumbent position
    l. resolution
    l. wall retractor
lateralization
lateris
    nevus unius l.
lateromedial oblique view
lateroversion
latex
    l. agglutination
    l. agglutination inhibition
      test (LAIT)
    l. fixation test
Latrobe retractor
LATS
    long-acting thyroid stimulator
      L. hormone
LATS-protector
latum
    condyloma l.
    Diphyllobothrium l.
Latzko cesarean section
Latzko colpocleisis
Laufe polyp forceps
Launois-Cléret syndrome
Launois syndrome
Laurence-Moon-Bardet-Biedl
    syndrome
Laurence-Moon syndrome

LAV
    lymphadenopathy-associated
      virus
lavage
        bronchopulmonary l.
        gastric l.
        peritoneal l.
LAVH
    laparoscopic-assisted vaginal
      hysterectomy
    laparoscopic-assisted vaginal
      hysteroscopy
law
        Diday l.
        Hardy-Weinberg l.
        Hellin l.
        Hellin-Zeleny l.
        inverse square l.
        Küstner l.
        Leopold l.
        l. of mass action
        Mendel l.'s
        Poiseville l.
Läwen-Roth syndrome
laxa
        cutis l.
layer
        Bowman l.
        germ l.
        half-value l. (HVL)
        Nitabuch l.
        Rauber l.
Lazarus-Nelson technique
lazy leukocyte syndrome
lazy-S incision
LBW
    low birth weight
LBWI
    low-birth-weight infant
LC
    living children
LCA
    Leber congenital amaurosis
L-Caine
L&D
    labor and delivery

LDH
    lactate dehydrogenase
LDL
    low-density lipoprotein
LDL-cholesterol
l-dopa
    levo-dopamine
LDR
    labor, delivery, and recovery
        LDR room
LDS
    ligate-divide-staple
        LDS instrument
LE
    lupus erythematosus
lead
        l. blocks
        l. pipe urethra
        l. poisoning
leading ancestor
leaf of broad ligament
League
        La Leche L.
leakage
        placental l.
        silicone implant l.
leaky gene
Lear complex
Learning to Eat **manual**
Lea Shield
least squares estimator
Leber
        L. congenital amaurosis
        (LCA)
        L. disease
Leboyer
        L. method
        L. technique
lecanopagus
Lecat gulf
lecithin
        disaturated l.
lecithin/sphingomyelin (l/s)
        l./s. ratio
Lecompte maneuver
lectin

NOTES

Lectromed urinary investigation
  system
Ledbetter-Politano procedure
Ledercillin VK
Leder stain
LEEP
  loop electrosurgical excision
  procedure
    LEEP Redi-kit
Lee-White clotting time
LeFort
  L. operation
  L. partial colpocleisis
LeFort-Neugebauer operation
LeFort-Wehrbein-Duplay
  hypospadias repair
left
  l. atrial to aortic ratio
    (LA:A)
  l. atrial dimension (LAD)
  l. frontoanterior position
    (LFA)
  l. frontoposterior position
    (LFP)
  l. frontotransverse position
    (LFT)
  l. mentoanterior position
    (LMA)
  l. mentoposterior position
    (LMP)
  l. mentotransverse position
    (LMT)
  l. occipitoanterior position
    (LOA)
  l. occipitoposterior position
    (LOP)
  l. occipitotransverse position
    (LOT)
  l. to right (L-R)
  l. sacroanterior
  l. sacroanterior position
    (LSA)
  l. sacroposterior position
    (LSP)
  l. sacrotransverse position
    (LST)
  l. scapuloanterior position
    (LScA)
  l. scapuloposterior position
    (LScP)
  l. ventricle (LV)
  l. ventricular hypertrophy
    (LVH)

left-sidedness
  bilateral l.-s.
left-to-right shunt
leg
  baker l.
  bayonet l.
  l. cramp
  l. edema
  milk l.
  white l.
legal
  l. intervention
  l. issue
Legat point
leg-compression stockings
Legg-Calvé-Perthes disease
leggings
Legionnaire disease
Leigh
  L. disease
  encephalomyopathy of L.
  L. syndrome
Leiner disease
leiomyoma, pl. leiomyomata
  cervical l.
  endometrial metastasizing l.
  ovarian l.
  parasitic l.
  submucous l.
  leiomyomatata uteri
  uterine leiomyomata
  vascular l.
leiomyomatosis
  intravenous l.
  l. peritonealis disseminata
    (LPD)
leiomyosarcoma (LMS)
Leisegang colposcope
leishmaniasis
  cutaneous l.
  mucocutaneous l.
Leiter test
Lejeune syndrome
Lem-Blay circumcision clamp
lemon sign
lemon-squeezer obstetrical elevator
length
  crown-heel l. (CHL)
  crown-rump l. (CRL)
  femur l. (FL)
Lennox-Gastaut syndrome
Lennox syndrome

lens
>Barkan infant l.
>l. culinaris agglutinin

Lente Iletin I
Lente Iletin II
Lente L
lentigines
lentigo, pl. **lentigines**
lentis
>ectopia l.

lentivirus
Lent laparoscope
Lenz syndrome
leonine facies
LEOPARD syndrome
Leopold
>L. law
>L. maneuvers

LePad breast exam training pad
leperous salpingitis
Lepore thalassemia
leprechaun facies
leprechaunism
leprosum
>erythema nodosum l.

leprosy
leptomeningitis
leptospirosis
leptotene
>l. phase of meiosis
>l. stage

leptotrichosis
Leri
>L. pleonosteosis
>L. syndrome

Leri-Weill syndrome
Leroy
>L. syndrome

LeRoy ventricular catheter
lesbian
lesbianism
Leschke syndrome
Lesch-Nyhan syndrome
lesion
>anal squamous
>>intraepithelial l. (ASIL)
>axillary skin l.

barrel-shaped l.
benign l.
cervical l.
cutaneous l.
ductal-dependent l.
genital l.
high-grade squamous
>intraepithelial l. (HGSIL)
hyperpigmented l.
intraepithelial l.
Janeway l.
low-grade squamous
>intraepithelial l. (LGSIL)
lumbosacral plexus l.
lumbosacral root l.
lytic l.
metastatic l.
pigmented l.
plexus l.
precancerous l.
premalignant l.
radial sclerosing l.
satellite l.
sclerosing l.
SIL/ASCUS l.
skin l.
spiculated l.
squamous intraepithelial l.
>(SIL)
violaceous l.
vulvar pigmented l.
vulvovaginal l.

LET
>linear energy transfer

letdown
>milk l.
>l. reflex

lethal
>l. dwarfism
>l. equivalent
>l. gene
>l. multiple pterygium
>>syndrome

lethargic
lethargy
Letterer-Siwe disease

NOTES

leucine
    l. aminopeptidase
    l. tolerance test
leucocyte detection strip
leucovorin
leukanakmesis
leukapheresis
leukemia
    acute lymphocytic l.
    acute nonlymphocytic l.
    aplastic l.
    basophilic l.
    eosinophilic l.
    granulocytic l.
    hemoblastic l.
    leukopenic l.
    lymphocytic l.
    lymphosarcoma cell l.
    mast cell l.
    megakaryocytic l.
    micromyeloblastic l.
    myeloblastic l.
    myelogenous l.
Leukeran
leukocoria
leukocyte
    l. count
    l. function
    l. interferon
    l. transfusion
leukocytosis
leukocyturia
leukodystrophy
    cerebral l.
    globoid cell l.
    Krabbe l.
    metachromatic l.
    sudanophilic l.
leukoencephalopathy
leukokraurosis
leukomalacia
    periventricular l.
leukopenic leukemia
leukophlegmasia
    l. dolens
leukoplakia
    l. vulvae
leukoplakic vulvitis
leukorrhagia
leukorrhea
    menstrual l.
leukorrheal
Leukotrap red cell collector

leukotriene
leuprolide
    l. acetate
levallorphan tartrate
levamisole
levarterenol
Levate
levator
    l. ani
    l. ani muscle
    l. ani spasm
    l. sling
LeVeen shunt
level
    ACD l.
    alpha antitrypsin l.
    amniotic fluid l.
    arachidonic acid l.
    blood l.
    blood alcohol l. (BAL)
    cesium-137 l.
    cortisol l.
    developmental l.
    endothelin plasma l.
    estradiol l.
    estriol l.
    estrogen l.
    fetal LDL l.
    gonadotropin l.
    hemoglobin l.
    hormonal l.
    human chorionic
      gonadotropin l.
    iodothyronine l.
    maternal estriol l.
    maternal serum l.
    peak-and-trough l.'s
    peripheral hormone l.
    plasma l.
    postmenopausal l.
    progesterone l.
    progesterone myometrial l.
    prolactin l.
    relaxin serum l.
    serum l.
    somatomedin l.
    sweat chloride l.
    theophylline l.
    uterine lysosome l.
Levi-Lorain
    L.-L. dwarfism
    L.-L. infantilism
Levlen

levocardia
levodopa (L-dopa)
levo-dopamine (l-dopa)
Levo-Dromoran
Levoid
levonorgestrel
    ethinyl estradiol and l.
    l. and ethinyl estradiol
    l. implant
Levophed
levoposition
Levoprome
levorotatory alkaloid
levorphan
levorphanol tartrate
levoscoliosis
Levothroid
levothyroxine
    l. test
levotransposition (L-transposition)
levoversion
Levret
    L. forceps
    L. maneuver
Levsin
Levsinex
Lewandowsky
    nevus elasticus of L.
Lewis
    L. blood group
    L. recording cystometer
Leyden-Möbius muscular dystrophy
Leydig
    L. cell aplasia
    L. cell embryology
    L. cell hyperplasia
    L. cells
    L. cell tumor
LFA
    left frontoanterior position
LFP
    left frontoposterior position
LFT
    left frontotransverse position
LGA
    large for gestational age

LGSIL
    low-grade squamous
      intraepithelial lesion
LGV
    lymphogranuloma venereum
LH
    luteinizing hormone
      LH Color test
      LH surge
LH-RH
    luteinizing hormone-releasing
    hormone
libidinal change
libido
    decreased l.
library
    DNA l.
    gene l.
Librax
Librium
lice (*pl. of* louse)
Licentiate in Midwifery (L.M.)
lichen
    l. infantum
    l. nitidus
    l. planus
    l. ruber planus (LRP)
    l. sclerosus
    l. sclerosus et atrophicus
    (LS)
    l. scrofulosorum
    l. simplex
    l. spinulosus
    l. striatus
lichenification
lichenoides
    pityriasis l.
Liddle test
lidocaine
Lidoject
lie
    anterior l.
    fetal l.
    longitudinal l.
    oblique l.
    posterior l.

NOTES

lie *(continued)*
    transverse l.
    unstable l.
Liesegang LM-FLEX 7 flexible hysteroscope
life
    l. event
    l. expectancy
    l. stress
    l. table method
    l. table survival
    wrongful birth and l.
LifePak defibrillator
Li-Fraumeni cancer syndrome
Liga clip
liga-clipped
ligament
    Adams advancement of round l.'s
    broad l.
    Carcassone perineal l.
    cardinal l.
    cardinal-uterosacral l.
    Cooper suspensory l.'s
    Gilliam round l.
    Gimbernat reflex l.
    infundibulopelvic l.
    leaf of broad l.
    Mackenrodt l.'s
    ovarian l.
    Petit l.
    Poupart l.
    round l.
    transverse cervical l.
    l. of Treitz
    triangular l.
    umbilical l.
    uteroovarian l.
    uterosacral l.
    Waldeyer preurethral l.
ligamentopexis, ligamentopexy
ligamentum
    l. teres
    l. venosum
ligand-binding
ligand-receptor
ligase
    DNA l.
ligate-divide-staple (LDS)
ligation
    bleeding site l.
    hypogastric artery l.
    Irving tubal l.

    Kroner tubal l.
    modified Irving-type tubal l.
    Pomeroy tubal l.
    tubal l. (TL)
ligature
    chromic gut pelviscopic loop l.
    Deschamps l.
light
    bili l.'s
    l. chain
    double-bank bili l.'s
    Right Light examination l.
    Solar Beam medical examination l.
    Wood l.
lightening
lightning seizure
Lightwood-Albright syndrome
lignocaine
Liley
    L. curve
    L. three-zone chart
Lilliput neonatal oxygenator
limb
    l. bud
    fetal l.
    l. motion
    l. reduction
    short l.'s
    vertebral, anal, cardiac, tracheal, esophageal, renal, l. (VACTERL)
Limberg technique
limb-girdle
    l.-g. dystrophy
    l.-g. muscular dystrophy
limbic bands
limit
    confidence l.'s
    fetal dose l.
    radiation dose l.
limp infant syndrome
limulus amebocyte lysate assay
Lincocin
lincomycin
lindane
line
    art l.
      arterial line
    arterial l. (A-line, art line)
    Beau l.

black l.
canthomeatal l.
central l.
central venous l. (CVL)
central venous pressure l.
CVP l.
Farre white l.
germ l.
Harris growth arrest l.
hemostatic staple l.
iliopectinate l.
iliopectineal l.
intravenous l.
lambda suture l.
long l.
multiple resistant cell l.'s
neonatal l.
percutaneous l.
peripheral l.
peripheral arterial l.
radial arterial l.
sagittal suture l.
Shenton l.
Sydney l.
l. of Toldt
umbilical artery l.
V l.
venous l.
linea, pl. **lineae**
lineae albicantes
lineae atrophicae
l. nigra
l. terminalis
linear
l. accelerator
l. atelectasis
l. atrophy
l. energy transfer (LET)
l. salpingostomy
lingua, pl. **linguae**
l. nigra
short frenulum linguae
linkage
l. analysis
genetic l.
linoleic acid
Lioresal

liothyronine
liotrix
Liouville icterus
lip
cleft l. (CL)
nodular blueberry l.'s
l. phenomenon
l. reflex
lipase
lipid
l. cell
l. cell neoplasm
l. cell ovarian tumor
l. cell tumor
l. metabolism
l. metabolism disorder
lipid-associated sialic acid
lipidosis
lipochondrodystrophy
lipodystrophy
familial l.
lipogenic dyshepatia
lipogranulomatosis subcutanea
lipoid
l. adrenal gland hypoplasia
l. adrenal hyperplasia
l. ovarian neoplasm
l. ovarian tumor
l. pneumonia
l. proteinosis
lipolysis
lipoma, pl. **lipomata**
vulvar l.
lipomatosis
lipomyelomeningocele
liponecrosis microcystica calcificans
lipopolysaccharide (LPS)
l. endotoxin
lipoprotein
l. concentration
high-density l. (HDL)
low-density l. (LDL)
l. receptor-related protein
(LRP)
very low-density l. (VLDL)
lipoprotein-cholesterol metabolism

NOTES

Liposyn
    L. II
lipotropin
    β-l.
    μ-l.
Lippes loop
Lippes-type intrauterine device
Lipschütz ulcer
Liquaemin
liquefaction
    semen l.
liquid
    fetal lung l.
    Sklar Kleen l.
Liquiprin
liquor folliculi
Lisch nodule
lisinopril
Lisolipin
lissencephaly
Listeria
    L. meningitis
    L. monocytogenes
listeriosis
Lister scissors
liter (L)
    millequivalent per l.
    (mEq/L)
    l.'s per minute (L/min)
Lithane
lithiasis
lithium
Lithobid
lithokelyphopedion
Lithonate
lithopedion, lithopedium
Lithotabs
lithotomy
    marian l.
    l. position
    vaginal l.
Little disease
Littmann ECG electrode
Littre gland
Litzmann obliquity
Livadatis circular myotomy
livebirth, live birth
liveborn infant
live poliovirus vaccine
liver
    acute fatty l.
    cirrhosis of l.
    l. disease

    fetal l.
    l. function tests
    l. metastasis
    l. transplant
    l. transplantation
    l. tumor
live-virus vaccine
living children (LC)
LLETZ
    large loop excision of
    transformation zone
LLETZ-LEEP active loop electrode
Lloyd-Davies stirrups
L.M.
    Licentiate in Midwifery
LMA
    left mentoanterior position
L/min
    liters per minute
LMP
    last menstrual period
    left mentoposterior position
LMS
    leiomyosarcoma
LMT
    left mentotransverse position
LNMP
    last normal menstrual period
LOA
    left occipitoanterior position
lobar pneumonia
Lobstein
    L. disease
    L. syndrome
lobster-claw
    l.-c. deformity
    l.-c. hand
lobular
    l. carcinoma
    l. neoplasia
lobule
local
    l. anesthesia
    l. anesthetic
    l. excision
    l. irradiation
    l. methotrexate injection
    l. ovarian condition
localization
    epithelial autoantibody l.
    estrogen receptor l.
    needle l.
    placental l.

location
> gene l.

lochia
> l. alba
> l. cruenta
> l. purulenta
> l. rubra
> l. sanguinolenta
> l. serosa

lochial
lochiometra
lochiometritis
lochioperitonitis
lochiorrhagia
lochiorrhea
loci (*pl. of* locus)
lock
> English l.
> French l.
> German l.
> heparin l. (hep-lock)
> pivot l.
> sliding l.

locked twins
Locke solution
Locke-Wallace Marital Adjustment test
locus, pl. loci
> gene l.
> genetic l.
> operator l.

Loeb deciduoma
Loehlein diameter
Loestrin
> L. 1.5/30
> L. 1/20
> L. 21 1/20
> L. Fe

Lofene
Löffler syndrome
log cell kill
lollipop
> fentanyl l.

Lomanate
Lomotil
lomustine

Lonalac
> L. formula

long
> l. arm of chromosome
> l. line

long-acting
> l.-a. contraception
> l.-a. contraceptive
> l.-a. contraceptive steroid
> l.-a. thyroid stimulator (LATS)

long-axis view
longitudinal
> l. growth
> l. lie
> l. oval pelvis
> l. presentation
> l. scan

long-term
> l.-t. followup
> l.-t. sequelae
> l.-t. survival

Loniten
Lonox
loop
> cutting l.
> l. diathermy cervical conization
> l. electrode
> l. electrosurgical excision procedure (LEEP)
> flow-volume l.
> l. of Henle
> Lippes l.
> low-voltage diathermy l.
> Medevice surgical l.
> polysomnogram with flow-volume l.'s
> Schroeder tenaculum l.
> somatic nervous system feedback l.
> tenaculum hook l.
> vaginal speculum l.

Loosett maneuver
Lo/Ovral
LOP
> left occipitoposterior position

NOTES

lop ear
loperamide
lophosphamide
Lopressor
Loprox
Lorabid
loracarbef
Lorain infantilism
lorazepam
Lorcet
lordosis
loss
        blood l.
        bone l.
        early embryonic l.
        early pregnancy l.
        embryonic l.
        estrogen l.
        excessive blood l.
        hair l.
        heat l.
        insensible fluid l.
        menstrual blood l.
        normal blood l.
        postmenopausal bone l.
        pregnancy l.
        rapid bone l.
        recurrent pregnancy l.
        repetitive pregnancy l.
        l. of resistance technique
        sensory l.
        spinal bone l.
        surgical weight l.
        vertebral bone l.
        water l.
        weight l.
Lossen rule
Lostorfer bodies
LOT
    left occipitotransverse position
lotion
        Polysonic ultrasound l.
Lotrimin
        L. AF
Louis-Bar syndrome
loupe
        Keeler l.
        l. magnification
louse, pl. lice
        crab l.
Lovas training
Lovset maneuver

low
        l. birth weight (LBW)
        l. cervical cesarean section
        l. forceps
        l. forceps delivery
        l. molecular weight dextran
        l. rectal resection
        l. steroid content combined
            oral contraceptive
        l. transverse cesarean (LTC)
        l. transverse cesarean
            section
low-back pain
low-birth-weight infant (LBWI)
low-cholesterol diet
low-density lipoprotein (LDL)
low-dose
        l.-d. danazol
        l.-d. heparin
        l.-d. oral contraceptive
        l.-d. steroids
Lowe
        fetal oculocerebrorenal
            syndrome of L.
        L. oculocerebrorenal
            syndrome
lower
        l. abdominal pain
        l. abdominal tenderness
        l. genital tract infection
        l. limb ossification center
        l. uterine segment transverse
            (LUST)
        l. uterine segment transverse
            cesarean section (LUST C-
            section)
lower-segment scar
Lowe-Terry-Machlachan syndrome
low-fat diet
low-grade
        l.-g. squamous intraepithelial
            lesion (LGSIL)
low-residue diet
low-salt diet
low-segment transverse incision
low-set ears
low-sodium diet
low-voltage diathermy loop
loxapine
Loxitane
lozenge
        Cough-X l.
Lozol

LP
    lumbar puncture
L-PAM
    melphalan
LPD
    leiomyomatosis peritonealis
      disseminata
L-phenylalanine mustard
LPS
    lipopolysaccharide
L-R
    left to right
LRP
    lichen ruber planus
    lipoprotein receptor-related
      protein
LS
    lichen sclerosus et atrophicus
l/s
    lecithin/sphingomyelin
      L/S ratio
LSA
    left sacroanterior position
LScA
    left scapuloanterior position
LScP
    left scapuloposterior position
LSD
    lysergic acid diethylamide
LSH
    lutein-stimulating hormone
LSP
    left sacroposterior position
LST
    left sacrotransverse position
LTC
    low transverse cesarean
L-transposition
    levotransposition
Lubchenco nomogram
lube
    Sklar l.
Lübke uterine vacuum cannula
lubricant
    AstroGlide personal l.
    Comfort personal l.
    Maxilube personal l.

    Replens l.
    vaginal l.
Lub syndrome
Lucey-Driscoll syndrome
Lucite dilator
Ludiomil
Luer-Lok syringe
Luer retractor
lues
    l. ascites
luetic
LUFS
    luteinized unruptured follicle
      syndrome
Luft disease
Lugol iodine solution
Luikart forceps
luliberin
Lumadex-FSI test
lumbar
    l. artery
    l. epidural anesthesia
    l. puncture (LP)
lumbosacral
    l. plexus injury
    l. plexus lesion
    l. root lesion
lumen, pl. lumina
    urethral l.
Luminal
luminal epithelium
Lumopaque
lump
lumpectomy
LUNA
    laser uterosacral nerve ablation
Lunar DPX dual-energy
  absorptiometer
lung
    aeration of l.
    l. cancer
    capacity of l. (CL)
    l. capacity
    l. carcinoma
    l. compliance
    compliance of l. (CL)
    l. edema

NOTES

lung *(continued)*
    granular l.
    hazy l.
    hypoplastic l.
    junky l.
    l. profile
    SciMed-Kolobow
      membrane l.
    sequestered l.
    l. strip
    l. volume
Lupron
    L. Depot
lupus
    l. anticoagulant
    l. anticoagulant activity
    l. anticoagulant antibody
    l. crisis
    l. erythematosus (LE)
    l. erythematosus
      disseminatus
    gestational l.
    l. nephritis
    l. obstetric syndrome
    l. vulgaris
Lurline PMS
LUST
    lower uterine segment transverse
    L. C-section
luteal
    l. cell
    l. function
    l. ovarian cyst
    l. phase
    l. phase defect
    l. phase inadequacy
luteectomy
luteinalis
    hyperreactio l.
lutein cell
luteinization
    l. inhibition
    l. inhibitor
    l. stimulator
luteinized
    l. thecoma
    l. unruptured follicle
    l. unruptured follicle
      syndrome (LUFS)
luteinizing
    l. hormone (LH)
    l. hormone receptor-binding
      inhibitor

    l. hormone-releasing
      hormone (LH-RH)
    l. hormone-releasing
      hormone analogue
    l. hormone secretion
luteinoma
lutein-stimulating hormone (LSH)
Lutembacher syndrome
luteolysis
luteolytic
    l. action
luteoma
    pregnancy l.
luteoplacental shift
luteum
    corpus l.
Lutheran blood group
Lutrepulse
Lutz-Jeanselme nodules
LV
    left ventricle
LVH
    left ventricular hypertrophy
lwoffi
    Achromobacter l.
    Acinetobacter l.
Lyell
    L. disease
    L. syndrome
Lyme
    L. disease
    L. enzyme-linked
      immunosorbent assay
lymph
    l. node
    l. node biopsy
    l. node drainage
    l. node endometriotic
      adenoacanthoma
    l. node metastasis
    l. node positivity
lymphadenectomy
    inguinal l.
    Meigs pelvic l.
    paraaortic l.
    pelvic l.
    retroperitoneal l.
lymphadenitis
    mediastinal l.
    mesenteric l.

lymphadenopathy
    axillary l.
lymphadenopathy-associated virus
    (LAV)
lymphangiectasia, lymphangiectasis
    congenital pulmonary l.
lymphangiography
lymphangioma
    cavernous l.
    l. circumscriptum
    cystic l.
    l. cysticum
lymphangitis
lymphatic
    l. drainage
    l. drainage of genitalia
    paracervical l.'s
    l. spread
    l. system
lymphedema
lymphoblastoid
    l. cell
    l. interferon
lymphocyst
    l. omentum
lymphocyte
    l. activator
    B l.
    l. dysfunction
    natural killer l.
    T l.
    T_3 l.
    T_4 l.
lymphocyte-activating factor
lymphocytic
    l. adenohypophysitis
    l. choriomeningitis
    l. hypophysitis
    l. leukemia
lymphocytosis
lymphogranuloma
    l. inguinale
    venereal l., l. venereum
lymphography

lymphohistiocytosis
    erythrophagocytic l.
    familial erythrophagocytic l.
    (FEL)
lymphoid
    l. cell
    l. hyperplasia
    l. tissue
lymphokine
lymphokine-activated killer cell
    (LAK)
lymphoma
    Burkitt l.
    Hodgkin l.
    malignant l.
    metastatic l.
    non-Hodgkin l.
    ovarian l.
    recurrent l.
    true histiocytic l. (THL)
lymphonodular pharyngitis
lymphopenia
lymphoproliferative syndrome
lymphoreticulosis
lymphosarcoma
    l. cell leukemia
lymphotoxin antitumor activity
lynestrenol
Lyon hypothesis
lyosomal
    l. storage disease
Lyphocin
lypressin
lysergic
    l. acid
    l. acid diethylamide (LSD)
lysine
lysis
    adhesion l.
lysosomal enzyme disorder
lysosome
lytic lesion
Lytren
    L. formula

NOTES

Maalox
MacDonald sign
macerated fetus
maceration
    fetal m.
Macewen sign
Machado-Joseph disease
Mach band effect
machine
    Berkeley suction m.
    cobalt megavoltage m.
    Mayo-Gibbon heart-lung m.
    megavoltage m.
machinery murmur
MacIntosh
    English M. (E-Mac)
Mackenrodt ligaments
Macleod syndrome
macrencephaly
macroadenoma
    prolactin-secreting m.
macrobeads
    methyltestosterone m.
Macrobid
macrocardius
macrocephaly
macrocrania
macrocrystals
    nitrofurantoin m.
macrocytic anemia of pregnancy
macrodactyly
Macrodantin
macrogamete
macrogenitosomia
    m. precox
macroglobinemia
    Waldenstrom m.
macroglobulin
    α_2-m.
macroglossia
macrogyria
macrolecithal
macromastia, macromazia
macromelus
macrophage
    m. colony-stimulating factor
macrophage-activating factor
  (MAF)
macrophage-inhibition factor
macrophallus

macroprolactinoma
macrosomia
    fetal m.
macrostomia
MACS
    magnetically-activated cell sorter
macular
    m. dystrophy
    m. hemangioma
Madden technique
Madlener operation
Madonna finger
MAF
    macrophage-activating factor
mafenide
Maffucci syndrome
mag
    magnesium
Magan
MAGGI disposable biopsy needle
  guide for ultrasound
magma reticulare
magnesia
    milk of m. (MOM)
magnesium (mag)
    m. citrate
    m. hydroxide
    m. oxide
    m. salicylate
    m. sulfate
magnetic
    m. resonance imaging
    (MRI)
    m. resonance mammography
    (MRM)
magnetically-activated cell sorter
  (MACS)
magnetically responsive microsphere
magnetite (Fe_3O_4)
Magnetrode cervical unit
magnification
    area of interest m. (AIM)
    loupe m.
    m. mammography
    spot m.
Magnus and de Kleijn neck reflex
Mag-Ox 400
Magpi hypospadius repair
Magrina-Bookwalter vaginal
  retractor

Maher disease
maidenhead
maintenance medications
Mainz
    M. pouch
    M. pouch urinary reservoir
Majewski syndrome
major
    m. gene
    m. histocompatibility
      antigen
    thalassemia m.
    β-thalassemia m.
majora
    labia m.
Makler
    M. insemination
    M. insemination device
    M. reusable semen analysis
      chamber
mal
    grand m.
    petit m.
malabsorption
    congenital folate m.
    m. syndrome
    tryptophan m.
malacoplakia
maladie
    m. de Roger
    m. des tics
malaise
malar fat pad
malaria
male
    m. factor
    m. factor infertility
    M. FactorPak seminal fluid
      collection kit
    m. genital duct
    m. genital duct development
    m. infertility
    m. pseudohermaphroditism
    m. reproductive system
    m. sex differentiation
    46,XX m.
    XXY m.
    XYY m.
    ZZ m.
maleate
    ergonovine m.
    methylergonovine m.
    methysergide m.

Malecot catheter
Male-FactorPak
male-pattern hirsutism
malformation
    Arnold-Chiari m.
    arteriovenous m.
    AV m.
    bronchopulmonary m.
    clomiphene fetal m.
    congenital m.
    congenital cystic
      adenomatoid m. (CCAM)
    cystic adenomatous m.
      (CAM)
    faciotelencephalic m.
    fetal m.
    foregut m.
    teratogen-induced m.
    vascular m.
malignancy
    breast m.
    extrapelvic m.
    gastrointestinal m.
    genital tract m.
    metastatic m.
    ovarian m.
    vulvar m.
malignant
    m. calcification
    m. cytotrophoblast
    m. degeneration
    m. effusion
    m. histiocytosis
    m. hypertension
    m. lymphoma
    m. melanoma
    m. mixed müllerian tumor
      (MMMT)
    m. neoplasm
    m. nephrosclerosis
    m. ovarian neoplasm
    m. ovarian teratoma
    m. pleural effusion
    m. syncytiotrophoblast
    m. teratoma
    m. tumor
    m. tumor of cervix
malignum
    adenoma m.
Mallamint
malleable retractor
Mall formula
Mallory-Weiss syndrome

Malmström vacuum extractor
malnutrition
malodorous
Malotuss
malplacement
malposition
    uterine m.
malpresentation
    fetal m.
malrotation
    renal m.
Malström cup
mamma, pl. mammae
    m. accessoria
    m. erratica
    supernumerary m.
mammalgia
mammaplasty, mammoplasty
    augmentation m.
    postreduction m.
    reconstructive m.
    reduction m.
mammary
    m. calculus
    m. duct ectasia
    m. dysplasia
    m. fistula
    m. gland
    m. neuralgia
    m. souffle
mammectomy
mammillaplasty
mammillitis
mammitis
mammogram
    x-ray m.
mammographic
    m. detection
    m. screening
mammography
    Corometrics Model 900SC
     in-office m.
    heavy-ion m.
    magnetic resonance m.
     (MRM)
    magnification m.
    x-ray m.

Mammomat C3 mammography
    system
mammoplasty (var. of
    mammaplasty)
Mammoscan digital imaging
    system
mammose
mammotomy
mammotropic, mammotrophic
mAMSA
    Amsacrine
Man
    Mendelian Inheritance
     in M.
management
    active third-stage m.
    epilepsy m.
    expectant m.
    infertility m.
    laparoscopic m.
    metabolic m.
    noninvasive m.
    physiologic third-stage m.
    pregnancy m.
    risk m.
    surgical m.
Manchester
    M. operation
    M. ovoid
Manchester-Fothergill operation
Mancini plate
Mandelamine
mandelic acid
Mandelurine
mandible
mandibulofacial
    m. dysostosis
    m. dystosis
Mandol
mandrel, mandril
    intrauterine insemination
     cannula with m.
maneuver
    Barlow m.
    Bill m.
    Bracht m.
    Brandt-Andrews m.

NOTES

maneuver *(continued)*
    corkscrew m.
    Credé m.
    DeLee m.
    doll's head m.
    forceps m.
    heel-to-ear m.
    Hillis-Müller m.
    Hodge m.
    key-in-lock m.
    Kristeller m.
    Lecompte m.
    Leopold m.'s
    Levret m.
    Loosett m.
    Lovset m.
    Massini m.
    Mauriceau m.
    Mauriceau-Levret m.
    Mauriceau-Smellie-Veit m.
    McDonald m.
    McRoberts m.
    midforceps m.
    modified Ritgen m.
    Müller-Hillis m.
    Munro-Kerr m.
    Ortolani m.
    Pajot m.
    Pinard m.
    Prague m.
    Ritgen m.
    Rubin m.
    Saxtorph m.
    Scanzoni m.
    Scanzoni-Smellie m.
    scarf m.
    Schatz m.
    Sellick m.
    Thorn m.
    Valsalva m.
    Van Hoorn m.
    Wigand m.
    Woods m.
    Woods screw m.
    Zavanelli m.
manifestation
    ocular m.
    renal m.
manifold
Manipujector
    Kronner M.
manipulation
    gamete m.

manipulator
    uterine m.
manipulator/injector
    Harris-Kronner uterine m.
    (HUMI)
    Kronner Manipujector
    uterine m.
Manning
    M. score
    M. score of fetal activity
Mann isthmic cerclage
mannitol
mannosidosis
Mann-Whitney U test
MANOVA
    multivariate analysis of variance
Mantel-Cox test
M antigen
manual
    Learning to Eat m.
    m. pelvimetry
    m. rotation
MAP
    mean arterial pressure
map
    brain electrical activity m.
    (BEAM)
    chromosome m.
    gene m.
maple
    m. syrup urine
    m. syrup urine disease
    (MSUD)
maplike skull
mapping
    fate m.
    gene m.
maprotiline
Marañón syndrome
marasmus
marble bones
Marchand
    M. adrenals
    M. rest
Marchetti test
March technique
Marcillin
Marckwald operation
Marden-Walker syndrome
Marezine
Marfan syndrome
Margesic A-C

marginal
　　m. insertion
　　m. sinus rupture
marginatum
　　eczema m.
　　erythema m.
Margulies coil
marian lithotomy
Marie syndrome
marijuana
　　m. effect
Marinesco-Garland syndrome
Marinesco-Sjögren syndrome
Marinol
Mariñon syndrome
Marion disease
Marion-Moschcowitz culdoplasty
marital introitus
mark
　　port-wine m.
　　strawberry m.
　　Unna m.
marker
　　adrenal
　　　hyperandrogenism m.
　　Anderson m.
　　assay m.
　　CA 15-3 breast cancer m.
　　CA 72-4 cancer m.
　　CA-125 endometrial
　　　cancer m.
　　CA 19-9 GI cancer m.
　　CA 195 GI cancer m.
　　CA 50 GI cancer m.
　　m. chromosome
　　DNA m.
　　m. gene
　　genetic m.
　　peripheral androgen
　　　activity m.
　　protein m.
　　tumor m.
　　m. X chromosome
Marlex
Marlow
　　M. disposable cannula
　　M. disposable trocar

Marmine
Marmo method
marmorata
　　cutis m.
marmoratus
　　status m.
Maroteaux-Lamy syndrome
Marplan
marrow
　　bone m.
Marshall Hall facies
Marshall-Marchetti-Krantz
　　M.-M.-K. operation
　　M.-M.-K. procedure
Marshall-Marchetti-Kranz (MMK)
Marshall-Marchetti procedure
Marshall-Tanner pubertal staging
Marshall-Taylor vacuum extraction
Marshall test
marsupialization
　　Spence and Duckett m.
　　m. technique
　　transurethral m.
Martius
　　M. bulbocavernosus fat flap
　　M. procedure
Mary Jane breast pump
MAS
　　Maternal Attitude Scale
　　meconium aspiration syndrome
masculine pelvis
masculinization
masculinovoblastoma
mask
　　bag and m.
　　bili m.
　　m. of pregnancy
　　ventilation by m.
　　Venturi m.
mass
　　adnexal m.
　　benign m.
　　bone m.
　　circumscribed m.
　　cortical m.
　　cystic adnexal m.
　　fallopian tube m.

NOTES

mass *(continued)*
    fungating m.
    ill-defined m.
    inner cell m.
    mixed-density m.
    noncalcified nodular m.
    ovarian m.
    pelvic m.
    persistent ovarian m.
    postmenopausal body m.
    stellate m.
    tubal m.
    tumor m.
    uterine m.
    vertebral bone m.
    well-defined m.
massage
    cardiac m.
    closed chest m.
    Shiatsu therapeutic m.
    uterine m.
Massengill douche
Massini maneuver
massive
    m. breast hypertrophy
    m. ovarian cyst
    m. transfusion
Masson-Fontana stain
MAST
    military antishock trousers
    treatment
    MAST suit
    MAST trousers
mast
    m. cell leukemia
mastadenitis
mastadenoma
mastalgia
mastatrophy, mastatrophia
mastectomy
    extended radical m.
    Halsted m.
    McKissick m.
    McWhirter m.
    modified radical m.
    radical m.
    simple m.
    subcutaneous m.
    total m.
    Willy Meyer m.
Masters-Allen syndrome
mastitis
    chronic cystic m.

    gargantuan m.
    glandular m.
    granulomatous m.
    interstitial m.
    lactational m.
    m. neonatorum
    parenchymatous m.
    phlegmonous m.
    plasma cell m.
    puerperal m.
    retromammary m.
    stagnation m.
    submammary m.
    suppurative m.
mastocytosis
mastodynia
Mastodynon
mastoid fontanel
mastoiditis
mastoncus
mastopathy
mastopexy
mastoplasia
mastoplasty
mastoptosis
mastorrhagia
mastoscirrhus
mastotomy
masturbation
Mateer-Streeter ovum
material
    Dextran-70 barrier m.
    FlowGel barrier m.
    genetic m.
    Interceed barrier m.
    metal suture m.
    nylon suture m.
    Poloxamer 407 barrier m.
    polyester suture m.
    polyethylene suture m.
    polypropylene suture m.
    radiocontrast m.
    suture m.
    synthetic suture m.
Materna
    M. prenatal vitamin
maternal
    m. abdominal pressure
    m. age
    m. alcohol consumption
    m. alcoholism
    m. anesthesia
    m. antibody

m. asthma
M. Attitude Scale (MAS)
m. birthing position
m. cholestasis
m. coagulopathy
m. cocaine use
m. condition
m. cortical vein
m. cortical vein thrombosis
m. cotyledon
m. cyanotic heart disease
m. death
m. death rate
m. deprivation syndrome
m. diabetes
m. douche
m. drug abuse
m. dystocia
m. estriol level
m. exercise
m. factor
m. febrile morbidity
m. fracture
m. gonad
m. hemopathy
m. hepatitis
m. HLA haplotype
m. hydration
m. hydrops
m. hydrops fetalis
m. hydrops syndrome
m. hyperparathyroidism
m. hypertension
m. hypotension
m. immune response
m. immunology
m. infection
m. insulin
m. mercury exposure
m. morbidity
m. mortality
m. mortality rate
m. nutrition
m. ocular adaptation
m. outcome
m. parvovirus fetalis
m. peripheral blood

m. phenylketonuria
m. physiology
m. position
m. pulse
m. pyrexia
m. risk
m. screening
m. serum
m. serum alpha-fetoprotein (MSAFP)
m. serum level
m. serum SFP3 screening protocol
m. size
m. stature
m. steroid concentration
m. stress
m. surveillance
m. tissue
m. trauma
m. undernourishment
m. vascular response
m. weight
maternal-fetal
m.-f. histoincompatibility
m.-f. HLA compatibility
m.-f. transmission
maternal-placental-fetal unit
maternal-placental unit
maternity
disputed m.
mating
assortative m.
backcross m.
nonrandom m.
random m.
matrix, pl. matrices
extracellular m.
identity m.
square m.
matter
particulate m.
mattress
apnea alarm m.
maturation
m. of cells
fetal lung m.

NOTES

maturation *(continued)*
    follicular m.
    ovum m.
    premature accelerated
      lung m. (PALM)
    pulmonary m.
    skeletal m.
    m. value
maturation-promoting factor (MPF)
mature
    m. cystic ovarian teratoma
    m. infant
    m. neutrophil
    m. ovarian teratoma
maturity
    fetal m.
    fetal lung m. (FLM)
    neuromuscular m.
    physical m.
Maunoir hydrocele
Mauriac syndrome
Mauriceau-Levret maneuver
Mauriceau maneuver
Mauriceau-Smellie-Veit maneuver
Maxaquin
Maxeran
Maxilube personal lubricant
maximal permissible dose
maximum
    m. breathing capacity
    m. likelihood estimator
    m. oxygen uptake (VO_2max)
    m. temperature (T-max)
    m. urethral closure pressure
      (MUCP)
Maxolon
Mayer pessary
Mayer-Rokitansky-Küster-Hauser
  syndrome
May-Hegglin anomaly
Maylard incision
Mayo
    M. hook
    M. hysterectomy
    M. scissors
Mayo-Fueth inversion procedure
Mayo-Gibbon heart-lung machine
Mayo-Hegar needle holder
Mayor sign
Mazanor
mazindol
mazodynia
mazolysis

mazopathy, mazopathia
mazopexy
mazoplasia
Mazzini test
MB band
MBM
    mother's breast milk
MBP
    modified Bagshawe protocol
McArdle disease
McBurney point
McCall
    M. culdoplasty
    M. stitch
McCall-Schumann procedure
McCaman-Robins test
McCraw gracilis myocutaneous flap
McCune-Albright syndrome
McDonald
    M. cervical cerclage
    M. maneuver
    M. measurement
    M. procedure
McGill forceps
mcg/kg/min
    micrograms per kilogram per
      minute
McGovern nipple
MCH
    mean corpuscular hemoglobin
MCi
    megacurie
McIndoe-Hayes procedure
McIndoe operation
McKissick mastectomy
McKusick-Kaufman syndrome
McLane forceps
MCR
    metabolic clearance rate
McRoberts maneuver
MCT
    M. oil
    M. oil formula
MCV
    mean corpuscular volume
    molluscum contagiosum virus
McWhirter mastectomy
MDI
    mental development index
    metered dose inhaler
M/E
    myeloid/erythrocyte
    M/E ratio

MEA
multiple endocrine abnormalities
Mead-Johnson formula
Meadows syndrome
mean
m. arterial pressure (MAP)
m. corpuscular hemoglobin (MCH)
m. corpuscular volume (MCV)
m. hemoglobin concentration
m. menstrual cycle hematocrit
m. plasma iron concentration
regression of the m.
standard error of the m. (SEM)
measles
German m.
three-day m.
m. vaccine
measles, mumps, rubella (MMR)
measurement
acid-base m.
anthropometric m.
fetal growth m.
intrauterine pressure m.
McDonald m.
optical density m.
pascal unit of pressure m. (Pa)
transcutaneous m.
Measurin
measuring hat
mebanazine
Mebaral
Mebendacin
mebendazole
Mebutar
mecamylamine
mechanical
m. birth injury
m. dysmenorrhea
m. respirator

mechanism
alloimmune m.
autoimmune m.
cellular cytotoxic m.
Douglas m.
Duncan m.
heat transfer m.
host defense m.
host response m.
Schultze m.
two-cell m.
mechlorethamine
m. hydrochloride
Meckel
M. diverticulum
M. syndrome
Meckel-Gruber syndrome
meclizine hydrochloride
meclofenamate
Meclomen
mecometer
meconial colic
meconiorrhea
meconium
m. aspiration
m. aspiration syndrome (MAS)
m. blockage syndrome
m. corpuscle
m. ileus
m. ileus appearance
m. peritonitis
m. plug
m. plug syndrome
m. stain
m.-stained amniotic fluid (MSAF)
m.-stained skin
Medela
M. Dominant vacuum delivery pump
M. manual breast pump
M. membrane regulator
Medevice
M. surgical loop
M. surgical paws

NOTES

Medfusion 1001 syringe infusion
pump
media
    acute otitis m. (AOM)
    Gibco BRL sperm
      preparation m.
    mucoid otitis m. (MOM)
medial oblique view
median
    m. eminence
    m. episiotomy
    m. facial cleft syndrome
    multiples of the m. (mom)
    m. raphe
mediana
    diameter m.
mediastinal
    m. collagenosis
    m. lymphadenitis
mediastinitis
mediastinum
mediating action
mediator
    intracellular m.
medicamentosa
    rhinitis m.
medication
    aerosolized m.
    base m.
    intravenous m.
    iodide-containing m.
    maintenance m.'s
    over-the-counter m.
    parenteral m.
    pressor m.
    prophylactic m.
    teratogenic m.
medicine
    fetal-maternal m.
    neonatal m.
    perinatal m.
Medihaler-Epi
Medihaler-Iso
Medilium
mediolateral
    m. episiotomy
    m. view
Mediterranean anemia
Medi-Trace electrode
Meditran
medium
    sperm capacitation m.
    transmission m.

Med-Neb respirator
medorrhea
medroxyprogesterone
    m. acetate (MPA)
Medscan
medulla oblongata
medullary
    m. carcinoma
    m. cord
    m. cystic disease
medulloblastoma
meduloblastoma
medusae
    caput m.
Meesman dystrophy
mefenamic acid
Mefoxin
megacardia
Megace
megacephaly
megacolon
    aganglionic m.
    congenital m.
    toxic m.
megacurie (MCi)
megacystis-megaureter syndrome
megacystis, microcolon, intestinal
    hypoperistalsis (MMIH)
    MMIH syndrome
Megadyne/Fann E-Z clean
    laparoscopic electrode
megaelectron volt (MeV)
megahertz (MHz)
megakaryocytic leukemia
megalencephaly
megaloblastic anemia
megalocardia
megalocephaly
megaloclitoris
megalocornea
megalodactyly
megalomelia
megalopenis
megalophthalmos
megalosyndactyly
megaloureter, megaureter
megaureter
megavolt (MeV)
megavoltage machine
megestrol acetate
meglumine
    m. diatrizoate
    Hypaque M.

Meigs
    M. pelvic lymphadenectomy
    M. syndrome
Meigs-Kass syndrome
Meigs-Okabayashi procedure
Meigs-Werthein hysterectomy
Meinicke test
meiosis
    diakinesis stage of
      oocyte m.
    dictyate stage of oocyte m.
    diplotene phase of m.
    leptotene phase of m.
    oocyte m.
    pachytene phase of m.
    zygotene phase of m.
meiotic division
Meissner plexus
melancholia
    involutional m.
melaninogenicus
    β m.
melanocyte-stimulating hormone
melanocytic nevus
melanoma
    Clark classification of
      vulvar m.
    cutaneous m.
    malignant m.
    metastatic m.
    nodular m.
    superficial spreading m.
    vulvar m.
melanosis
    neonatal pustular m.
    transient neonatal
      pustular m.
melasma
    m. gravidarum
melatonin
    m. secretion
melena
    m. neonatorum
    m. spuria
Melfiat
Melkersson-Rosenthal syndrome
Mellaril

mellitus
    adult-onset diabetes m.
    (AODM)
    diabetes m.
    gestational diabetes m.
    (GDM)
    insulin-dependent
      diabetes m. (IDDM)
    juvenile diabetes m. (JDM)
    juvenile-onset diabetes m.
    (JODM)
    non-insulin-dependent
      diabetes m. (NIDDM)
    overt insulin-dependent
      diabetes m.
    type I diabetes m.
    type II diabetes m.
Melnick-Needles disease
melorheostosis
melphalan (L-PAM)
membrana granulosa
membrane
    artificial rupture of m.'s
    (ARM, AROM)
    basement m.
    m. bridge
    chorioallantoic m. (CAM)
    cloacal m.
    Descemet m.
    Duralon-UV nylon m.
    dysmenorrheal m.
    egg m.
    erythrocyte m.
    exocelomic m.
    extraembryonic fetal m.
    fetal m.
    germinal m.
    Gore-Tex surgical m.
    Heuser m.
    hyaline m.
    hymenal m.
    intact m.
    Jackson m.
    mucous m.'s
    placental m.
    premature rupture of m.'s
    (PROM)

NOTES

membrane *(continued)*
>preterm premature rupture of m.'s (PPROM)
>preterm rupture of m.'s
>prolonged rupture of m.'s (PROM)
>m. rupture
>Slavianski m.
>spontaneous rupture of m.'s (SROM)
>vernix m.
>vitelline m.
>Wachendorf m.
>yolk m.

membranous
>m. dysmenorrhea
>m. glomerulonephritis
>m. twins

memory
>m. cell
>m. phenomenon

MEN
>multiple endocrine neoplasia, types I, II, III

menacme
menadiol
>m. sodium diphosphate

menadione
menarche
>delayed m.

menarcheal, menarchial
mendelian
>m. genetic disorder
>m. inheritance
>M. Inheritance in Man
>m. trait

mendelizing
Mendel laws
Mendelson syndrome
Menest
Menge pessary
Mengert
>M. index
>M. shock syndrome

meningioma
>acoustic m.

meningismus
meningitis, pl. **meningitides**
>aseptic m.
>cryptococcal m.
>*Listeria m.*
>tuberculous m.

meningocele
>cranial m.
>spinal m.

meningococcal polysaccharide vaccine
meningococcemia
Meningococcus **vaccine**
meningoencephalitis
meningoencephalocele
meningoencephalomyelitis
meningomyelocele
Menkes
>M. disease
>M. syndrome

menocelis
menometrorrhagia
menopausal
>m. estrogen replacement therapy
>m. syndrome

menopause
>iatrogenic m.
>premature m.

menophania
menorrhagia
menorrhalgia
menoschesis
menostasis, menostasia
menostaxis
menotropin
menotropins
menouria
menoxenia
menses
menstrual
>m. age
>m. aspiration
>m. blood loss
>m. colic
>m. cycle
>m. cycle induction
>m. cycle regulation
>m. cycle resumption
>m. edema
>m. endometrium
>m. extraction
>m. extraction abortion
>m. flow
>m. formula
>m. history
>m. irregularity
>m. leukorrhea
>m. molimina

m. period (MP)
m. reflux
m. sclerosis
m. state
menstrual-ovarian cycle
menstruant
menstruate
menstruation
abnormal m.
anovular m.
delayed m.
retained m.
retrograde m.
supplementary m.
suppressed m.
vicarious m.
mental
m. development
m. development index
(MDI)
m. disturbance
m. retardation
m. status evaluation
mentoanterior
left m. position (LMA)
m. position
m. presentation
right m. position (RMA)
mentoposterior
left m. position (LMP)
m. position
m. presentation
right m. position (RMP)
Mentor
M. catheter
M. female self-catheter
mentotransverse
left m. position (LMT)
m. position
right m. position (RMT)
mentum
m. anterior position
m. posterior position
m. transverse position
mepenzolate bromide
mephentermine
mephenytoin

mephobarbital
Mephyton
mepindolol
mepivacaine
meprobamate
conjugated estrogen and m.
Meprospan
mepyramine
mEq
millequivalent
mEq/L
millequivalent per liter
MER
methanol extraction residue
meralgia paraesthetica
2-mercaptoethane sulfonate
(MESNA)
mercaptopurine
6-mercaptopurine
Mercier bar
Merck respirator
Merimack 1040 CO2 laser
Merlis obstetrical excavator
meroacrania
meroanencephaly
merocyte
merogastrula
merogenesis
merogony
diploid m.
meromelia
meromicrosomia
meromorphysis
merorachischisis
merozygote
Mersilene
M. fascial strip
M. gauze hammock
M. mesh
M. suture
Meruvax II
merycism
Mery gland
Merzbacher-Pelizaeus disease
MESA
microsurgical epididymal sperm
aspiration

NOTES

Mesantoin
mesaraica
    tabes m.
mesatipellic pelvis
mesenchymal hamartoma
mesenchyme
    nonspecific m.
mesenteric
    m. adenitis
    m. artery
    m. lymphadenitis
mesenterica
    tabes m.
mesentery
    intestinal m.
mesh
    Mersilene m.
Meshgraft Skin Expander
MESNA
    2-mercaptoethane sulfonate
mesoblast
mesoblastic
    m. nephroma
mesoblastoma
    m. ovarii
    m. vitellinum
mesocephalic
mesoderm
    extraembryonic m.
mesodermal sarcoma
mesomelic dysplasia
mesometanephric carcinoma
mesometric pregnancy
mesometritis
meson
    negative π m.
mesonephric
    m. adenocarcinoma
    m. carcinoma
    m. duct
    m. rest
    m. ridge
    m. tubule
mesonephroi (pl. of mesonephros)
mesonephroid tumor
mesonephroma
mesonephros, pl. mesonephroi
mesoridazine besylate
mesosalpingeal
mesosalpinx
mesothelioma
    benign m. of genital tract
mesovarium, pl. mesovaria

messenger
    m. ribonucleic acid (mRNA)
    m. RNA
    second m.
Mestinon
mestranol
    m. and norethindrone
    m. and norethynodrel
mesylate
    2-Br-alpha-ergocryptine m.
    bromocriptine m.
    dihydroergotamine m.
meta-analysis
metabolic
    m. acidemia
    m. acidosis
    m. alkalosis
    m. clearance rate (MCR)
    m. disorder
    m. error
    m. management
metabolism
    aerobic m.
    amino acid m.
    carbohydrate m.
    estrogen m.
    fat m.
    fetal m.
    inborn error of m.
    m. in intraperitoneal
        chemotherapy
    lipid m.
    lipoprotein-cholesterol m.
    mineral m.
    neonatal m.
    progesterone m.
    prostaglandin m.
    steroid m.
    vitamin m.
    water m.
metabolite
    arachidonic acid m.'s
    steroid m.
metacentric chromosome
metachromatic leukodystrophy
metachromosome
metacyesis
metafemale
metagaster
Metahydrin
metal
    m. coil
    m. metabolism disorder

m. suture material
trace m.
metallic
    m. bead-chain
      cystourethrography
    m. staple
metalloproteinase
    tissue inhibitors of m.
Metandren
metanephric
    m. blastema
    m. bud
    m. duct
metanephros, pl. **metanephroi**
metaphase
metaphoric dysplasia
metaphyseal
    m. dysostosis
    m. dysplasia
    m. dystosis
metaphysis
    rachitic m.
metaplasia
    ciliated m.
    coelomic m.
    squamous m.
    squamous m. of amnion
    tubal m.
    vaginal squamous m.
metaplastic carcinoma
Metaprel
metaproterenol sulfate
metaraminol bitartrate
metastasis, pl. **metastases**
    adnexal m.
    aortic node m.
    bony m.
    fallopian tube m.
    floxuridine in hepatic m.
    hepatic m.
    inguinal lymph node m.
    liver m.
    lymph node m.
    ovarian m.
    ovarian cancer m.
    placental m.
    pulmonary m.

stomach cancer m.
tumor, node, m. (TNM)
uterine sarcoma m.
vascular m.
metastatic
    m. adenocarcinoma
    m. axillary involvement
    m. carcinoma
    m. implant
    m. lesion
    m. lymphoma
    m. malignancy
    m. melanoma
metatarsus varus
metatropic
    m. dysplasia
Metenier sign
met-enkephalin
meter
    Astech m.
    glucose m.
    MiniWright peak flow m.
    Pocketpeak peak flow m.
    US 1005 uroflow m.
    Wright peak flow m.
metered dose inhaler (MDI)
metergoline
methacycline hydrochloride
methadone hydrochloride
methamphetamine exposure
methamphetamine hydrochloride
methandrostenolone
methanol extraction residue (MER)
methantheline bromide
methaqualone
metharbital
methazolamide
methdilazine hydrochloride
methemoglobinemia
methemoglobinuria
methenamine
Methergine
methicillin sodium
methimazole
methionine malabsorption syndrome
methixene hydrochloride

NOTES

method
    Astrand 30-beat
      stopwatch m.
    Attwood staining m.
    barrier m.
    Billings m.
    Bonnaire m.
    brine flotation m.
    Buist m.
    Byrd-Drew m.
    cold knife m.
    contraceptive m.
    Corning m.
    Döderlein m.
    Douglas m.
    encu m.
    ensu m.
    Fick m.
    flush m.
    Gabastou hydraulic m.
    Hamilton m.
    Harrison m.
    Ito m.
    Johnson m.
    Kaplan-Meier m.
    Kluge m.
    Kristeller m.
    Lamaze m.
    laser m.
    Leboyer m.
    life table m.
    Marmo m.
    pilocarpine iontophoresis m.
    Prochownick m.
    Puzo m.
    rhythm m.
    Rodeck m.
    Smellie m.
    Smellie-Veit m.
    sperm washing
      insemination m. (SWIM)
    Stroganoff m.
    symptothermal m.
    Tarkowski m.
    thermodilution m.
    Towako m.
    twin m.
    u-score m.
    Vecchietti m.
    Victor Gomel m.
    Wardill four-flap m.
    Wardill-Kilner advancement
      flap m.

    Watson m.
    Watson-Crick m.
methotrexate
methotrimeprazine
methoxamine hydrochloride
methoxyflurane
methscopolamine
methsuximide
methyclothiazide
Methyl
    Oreton M.
methylbromide
    hyoscine m.
    scopolamine m.
methyl-CCNU
methyldopa
methylene blue
methylergometrine maleate
methylergonovine
    m. maleate
methylmalonic
    m. acidemia
    m. aciduria
methylmercury
methylphenidate hydrochloride
methylprednisolone
15-methyl prostaglandin F$_{2\alpha}$
α-methyl-p-tyrosine
methyltestosterone
    estrogens with m.
    m. macrobeads
    Premarin With M. Oral
methylxanthine
methysergide maleate
metoclopramide hydrochloride
metolazone
Metopirone
    M. test
metopopagus
metoprolol tartrate
Metra
metratonia
metratrophy, metratrophia
metrectomy
metria
metritis
metrizamide
metrizoate sodium
Metrodin
metrodynamometer
metrodynia

MetroGel
    M.-Vaginal
    M.-Vaginal gel
metrography
Metro I.V.
metrolymphangitis
metromalacia
metromalacoma, metromalacosis
metronidazole
    m. vaginal gel
metroparalysis
metropathia
    m. hemorrhagica
metropathic
metropathy
metroperitoneal fistula
metroperitonitis
metrophlebitis
metroplasty
    Strassman m.
metrorrhagia
    m. myopathica
metrorrhea
metrorrhexis
metrosalpingitis
metrosalpingography
metroscope
metrostaxis
metrostenosis
metrotomy
metyrapone
    m. test
metyrosine
Metzenbaum scissors
MeV
    megaelectron volt
    megavolt
MEVA
    M. probe
    M. Probe for endovaginal
       scanning
mexiletine
Mexitil
Meyer-Schwickerath and Weyers
  syndrome
Mezlin

mezlocillin
    m. sodium
MHA
    microhemagglutination assay
MHC antigen
MHz
    megahertz
Miacalcin
Mibelli
    angiokeratoma of M.
    M. angiokeratoma
MIC
    minimum inhibitory
      concentration
Micatin
Michel deformity
miconazole
    m. nitrate
Micral chemstrip
micrencephaly
MICRhoGAM
microadenoma
microangiopathic hemolysis
microangiopathy
    thrombotic m.
microatelectasis
microbial
    m. factor
    m. flora
    m. sensitivity
microbiology
microbrachia
microcalcification
microcephaly
Microcolpohysteroflator
    Hamou M.
microcolpohysteroscopy
microcrania
microcurettage
    Accurette m.
microcurette
    HemoCue m.
microcyst
    milk of calcium m.
microcystica
microcytic anemia
microcytosis

NOTES

microdactyly
microencephaly
microenvironment
microfibrillar collagen
microflora
    vaginal m.
microgastria
microgenitalism
microglandular
    m. adenosis
    m. cervical hyperplasia
micrognathia
micrognathia-glossoptosis syndrome
micrograms per kilogram per
  minute (mcg/kg/min)
microhemagglutination assay
  (MHA)
Micro-Hysteroflator
    Hamou M.-H.
microhysteroscope
    Hamou contact m.
microinjection
microinvasion
    stromal m.
microinvasive
    m. carcinoma
    m. carcinoma classification
    m. cervical cancer
microlithiasis
micromanipulation
micromanipulator
micromazia
micromelia
micromelic dwarfism
Micro-Mist disposable nebulizer
micromyeloblastic leukemia
Micronase
microNefrin
micronized
    m. estradiol
    m. progesterone
Micronor
microorchidism
micropenis
microphallus
microphthalmia
micropodia
microprosopus
microscope
    Optiphot-2UD m.
microscopy
    dark-field m.
microsomia

microspectroscopy
    Fourier transform
    infrared m.
microsphere
    magnetically responsive m.
    radioactive m.'s
microstomia
Microsulfon
microsurgery
    distal tubal m.
    tubal m.
    tubocornual m.
microsurgical
    m. epididymal sperm
      aspiration (MESA)
    m. tubocornual anastomosis
microthelia
microtia
Micro-Touch Platex medical glove
MicroTrak test
microvillus, pl. microvilli
microviscometry
micturition
mid
    midposition
Midamor
midarm circumference
midazolam
midcycle
    m. cervical mucus
    m. surge
middle sacral artery
midfetal testicular regression
  syndrome
midforceps
    m. delivery
    m. maneuver
midgut volvulus
midline incision
Midmark 413 power female
  procedure chair
midmenstrual
midodrine
midpain
midparental height
midpelvis
midplane
midposition (mid)
midsecretory
midstream urine specimen
midwife
midwifery
    Licentiate in M. (L.M.)

MIF
    migration-inhibitory factor
    müllerian inhibiting factor
mifepristone
migraine
    m. headache
migrans
    cutaneous larva m.
    erythema chronicum m.
    (ECM)
    larva m.
migration
    cellular m.
    placental m.
migration-inhibitory factor (MIF)
Mikity-Wilson syndrome
Milex
    M. cervical cup
    M. spatula
milia
    m. neonatorum
milia (*pl. of* milium)
miliaria
    apocrine m.
    m. crystallina
    m. profunda
    m. pustulosa
    m. rubra
miliary tuberculosis
military antishock trousers
  treatment (MAST)
milium, pl. milia
milk
    m. abscess
    atomic m.
    banked breast m.
    breast m.
    m. of calcium microcyst
    m. cyst
    m. ejection
    m. ejection reflex
    evaporated m.
    m. fever
    fluorescein-labeled m.
    m. leg
    m. letdown
    m. of magnesia (MOM)

    mother's breast m. (MBM)
    nem (m. nutritional unit)
    nuclear m.
    m. teeth
    uterine m.
    witch's m.
Millar microtransducer urethral
  catheter
Millen-Read modification
Millen technique
millequivalent (mEq)
    m. per liter (mEq/L)
Miller
    M. blade
    M. ovum
    M. syndrome
Miller-Abbott tube
Miller-Dieker syndrome
milleri
    Streptococcus m.
millijoule (mJ)
millirad (mrad)
milliroentgen (mr)
millivolt (mV, mv)
mill wheel murmur
Milontin
Milophene
Milroy disease
Miltex disposable biopsy punch
Miltown
Mi-Mark
    M.-M. disposable
      endocervical curette
    M.-M. endocervical curette
      set
    M.-M. endometrial curette
      set
β-mimetic
mimetic labor
Minamata disease
mineral
    m. metabolism
    m. oil
    m. requirement
mineralocorticoid
mineralocorticosteroid
minidose heparin

NOTES

269

Mini-Flex
    M.-F. flexible Harris uterine
      injector
    HUI M.-F.
Mini-Gamulin Rh
mini-lap
    mini-laparotomy
mini-laparotomy (mini-lap)
minimal-incision pubovaginal
  suspension
minimally invasive surgical
  technique (MIST)
Minims
minimum
    m. inhibitory concentration
      (MIC)
    m. lethal dose (MLD)
MiniOX I, II, III, 100-IV oxygen
  monitor
Minipress
MiniWright peak flow meter
Minizide
Minkowski-Chauffard syndrome
Minnesota Multiphasic Personality
  Inventory (MMPI)
Minocin
minocycline
minor
    thalassemia m.
    α-thalassemia m.
    β-thalassemia m.
minora
    labia m.
Minot disease
Minot-von Willebrand syndrome
minoxidil
Mintezol
minute
    beats per m. (bpm)
    breaths per m. (bpm)
    liters per m. (L/min)
    micrograms per kilogram
      per m. (mcg/kg/min)
    m. oxygen uptake
    m. ventilatory volume
Minzolum
Miocarpine
miodidymus
miopus
miosis
Miostat
miotic division

mirabilis
    Proteus m.
Miradon
Mirchamp sign
mirror
    Articu-Lase laser m.
    m. image breast biopsy
    m. image interpretation
miscarriage
    recurrent m.
    threatened m.
miscarry
mismatch
    ventilation/perfusion m.
    $\dot{V}/\dot{Q}$ m.
misonidazole
misoprostol
missed
    m. abortion
    m. labor
    m. period
Mission
    M. Prenatal F.A.
    M. Prenatal H.P.
    M. Prenatal Rx
missionary position
MIST
    minimally invasive surgical
      technique
mist
    Ayr saline nasal m.
    Bronitin M.
    Bronkaid M.
    child-adult m. (CAM)
    hood m.
    Primatene M.
    tent m.
    m. tent
Mithracin
mithramycin
mitochondrial
    m. chromosome
    m. DNA
    m. myopathy
mitochondrion, pl. mitochondria
mitogen
    pokeweed m. (PWM)
mitogenic activity
mitomycin
    m. C
mitoplasm
mitosis
    m. phase

mitotic
    m. chromosome
    m. figure
mitoxantrone
    m. hydrochloride
mitral
    m. arcade
    m. atresia
    m. commissurotomy
    m. insufficiency
    m. regurgitation
    m. stenosis
    m. valve
    m. valve insufficiency
    m. valve prolapse
Mitrofanoff principle
mittelschmerz
mitten hand
Mityvac
    M. obstetric vacuum
      extractor cup
    M. reusable vacuum pump
    M. vacuum delivery system
    M. vacuum extractor
mixed
    m. connective-tissue disease
    m. discrete-continuous
      random variable
    m. germ cell tumor
    m. gonadal dysgenesis
    m. lymphocyte reaction
      blocking factor
    m. mesodermal sarcoma
      (MMS)
    m. mesodermal tumor
    m. müllerian sarcoma
    m. ovarian mesodermal
      sarcoma
    m. porphyria
    m. umbilical arterial
      acidemia
    m. uterine tumor
mixed-density mass
mixoploid
mixoploidy
Mixtard

Miya
    M. hook
    M. hook ligature carrier
mJ
    millijoule
MLD
    minimum lethal dose
MLNS
    mucocutaneous lymph node
      syndrome
MM band
MMIH
    megacystis, microcolon,
      intestinal hypoperistalsis
      MMIH syndrome
MMK
    Marshall-Marchetti-Kranz
      MMK procedure
MMMT
    malignant mixed müllerian
      tumor
M-mode
    M.-m. display
    M.-m. echocardiogram
    M.-m. echogram
    M.-m. imaging
    M.-m. ultrasound
MMPI
    Minnesota Multiphasic
      Personality Inventory
MMR
    measles, mumps, rubella
      MMR vaccine
MMS
    mixed mesodermal sarcoma
MMTV
    mouse mammary tumor virus
MOA
    monoamine oxidase
Moban
Mobenol
Mobidin
mobility
    bladder neck m.
Mobiluncus
    M. vaginitis
Möbius syndrome

NOTES

modality
Modane
mode
    delivery m.
Modecate
model
    genetic m.
    pathological m.
    Rossavik growth m.
    statistical m.
modeling
    generalized linear
     interactive m. (GLIM)
modern genetics
Modicon
modification
    Burch m.
    Gesell test with
     Knobloch m.
    Millen-Read m.
modified
    m. Bagshawe protocol
     (MBP)
    m. Ham F-10 solution
    m. Irving-type tubal ligation
    m. Pomeroy technique
    m. radical hysterectomy
    m. radical mastectomy
    m. Ritgen maneuver
modifier
    biologic response m. (BRM)
Moditen
modulation
    antigenic m.
    sex steroid m.
Modumate
Moebius anomaly
Moeller-Barlow disease
Mogen clamp
Mohr syndrome
moiety, pl. **moieties**
molar
    m. degeneration
    Moon m.'s
    m. pregnancy
Molatoc
mold, mould
    Counsellor vaginal m.
molding of head
mole
    amniography in
     hydatidiform m.
    blood m.

    Breus m.
    carneous m.
    complete hydatidiform m.
    cystic m.
    false m.
    fleshy m.
    grape m.
    hydatidiform m.,
     hydatid m.
    invasive m.
    invasive hydatidiform m.
    partial hydatidiform m.
    tuberous m.
    vesicular m.
    vulvar hydatidiform m.
molecular
    m. clone
    m. genetic analysis
    m. genetic technique
molecule
    cell adhesion m. (CAM)
    vascular cell adhesion m.
molestation
    sexual m.
molimen, pl. **molimina**
    menstrual molimina
molindone
molluscum
    m. contagiosum
    m. contagiosum virus
     (MCV)
    m. fibrosum
    m. fibrosum gravidarum
molybdenum
    m. rotating anode x-ray
     tube
    m. target
MOM
    milk of magnesia
    mucoid otitis media
mom
    multiples of the median
MOMP gene
Monaghan respirator
monarticular arthritis
Mondor disease
mongolian
    m. idiot
    m. spot
mongolism
mongoloid
    m. features
Monilia

monilial
  m. esophagitis
  m. rash
  m. vaginitis
moniliasis
Monistat
  M. I.V.
Monistat-3 vaginal suppository
monitor
  Accu-Chek Easy glucose m.
  Accu-Chek II Freedom
    blood glucose m.
  actocardiotocograph fetal m.
  Aequitron 9200 apnea m.
  antepartum m.
  apnea m.
  Arvee model 2400 infant
    apnea m.
  Bear NUM-1 tidal
    volume m.
  CA m.
  cardiac-apnea m.
  Corometrics fetal m.
  Dinamap blood pressure m.
  EdenTec 2000W in-home
    cardiorespiratory m.
  Endotek OM-3 Urodata m.
  Endotek UDS-1000 m.
  fetal m.
  Fetal Dopplex m.
  Fetalert fetal heart rate m.
  fetal heart rate m.
  FetalPulse Plus m.
  Fetasonde fetal m.
  Healthdyne apnea m.
  Holter m.
  intrapartum m.
  MiniOX I, II, III, 100-IV
    oxygen m.
  Nellcor N-499 fetal oxygen
    saturation m.
  neonatal m.
  Neo-trak 515A neonatal m.
  Oxisensor fetal oxygen
    saturation m.
  Press-Mate model 8800T
    blood pressure m.

  Quik Connect fetal m.
  Sonicaid Axis m.
  Sonicaid SYSTEM 8000
    fetal m.
  Toitu MT-810
    cardiographic m.
  transcutaneous m.
  uterine activity m.
monitoring
  blood sugar m.
  critical care m.
  electronic fetal m. (EFM)
  end-tidal CO2 m.
  external fetal m. (EFM)
  fetal m.
  fetal heart rate m.
  heart rate m.
  hemodynamic m.
  home uterine m. (HUM)
  intrapartum m.
  intrauterine fetal m.
  tactile sensory m.
  tissue pH m.
  transcutaneous oxygen
    tension m.
monoamine
  m. oxidase (MOA)
  m. oxidase inhibitor
monoamniotic
  m. twins
monobactam
monobrachius
monocephalus
monochorial twins
monochorionic
  m. diamniotic placenta
  m. monoamniotic placenta
  m. twins
monochromatism
  blue cone m.
  pi cone m.
Monocid
monoclonal
  m. antibody
  m. antibody therapy
monocranius

NOTES

273

Monocryl
    M. suture
monocyte
monocytogenes
    Listeria m.
monodactyly
monodermal tumor
Monodox
monofactorial inheritance
monogamous
monogamy
monogenic
monohybrid
monohydrate
    doxycycline m.
    nitrofurantoin m.
monohydrate/macrocrystals
    nitrofurantoin m.
monokine
monomelic
mononeuropathy
    peripheral m.
mononucleosis
    infectious m.
monoovular twins
4-monooxygenase
    phenylalanine -m.
monophasic
    m. oral contraceptive
    m. regimen
monophosphate
    adenosine m. (AMP)
    cyclic adenosine m. (cAMP)
    cyclic adenosine 3′,5′-m.
    cyclic guanosine 3′,5′-m.
    cytidine m.
monoplegia
monoploid
monopodia
monopolar cautery
monops
monopus
monorchidic
monosome
monosomy
    autosomal m.
    m. G
    m. G syndrome
    m. 7 syndrome
    m. X
Monospot test
Monosticon
    M. Dri-Dot test

Mono-Sure
monosymptomatic delusional
    pseudocyesis
Mono-Test
    M.-T. (FTB)
monotherapy
Mono-VaccTest (O.T.)
monozygosity
monozygotic twins
monozygous
Monro
    foramen of M.
Monsel
    M. gel
    M. paste
    M. solution
mons pubis
monster
    hair m.
monstrosity
Montevideo unit
Montgomery
    M. glands
    M. strap
    M. tubercles
mood state
Moon
    M. molars
    M. teeth
Morand foot
morbidity
    fetal m.
    infant m.
    maternal m.
    maternal febrile m.
    neonatal m.
    perinatal m.
    m. predictor
    puerperal m.
morbilliform
    m. rash
morcellation
    m. operation
Morch respirator
Morel ear
Morgagni
    anterior retrosternal hernia
        of M.
    M. hernia
    hydatid cyst of M.
    M. tubercle
morgagnian

Morganella
    M. morganii
morganii
    Morganella m.
    Proteus m.
moribund
Morison pouch
morning
    m. glory syndrome
    m. sickness
morning-after pill
Moro-Heisler diet
Moro reflex
morphea
morphine
    epidural m.
    m. sulfate
morphogen
morphogenesis
morphologic
    m. assessment
morphological
    m. characteristic
    m. sex
morphology
    adrenal gland m.
    endometrial m.
    kidney m.
    QRS m.
Morquio
    M. disease
    M. syndrome
Morquio-Ulrich syndrome
Morsch-Retec respirator
mortality
    m. data
    fetal m.
    high altitude perinatal m.
    infant m.
    maternal m.
    neonatal m.
    perinatal m.
    m. predictor
    prenatal m.
    m. rate
    reproductive m.
    m. risk factor

mortiferum
    Fusobacterium m.
morula
mosaic
    m. pattern
mosaicism
    chromosomal m.
    erythrocyte m.
    gonadal m.
    trisomy 8 m.
    Turner m.
Moss
    M. classification
    M. tube
mother
    diabetic m.
    D^u-positive m.
    high-risk m.
    hysterical m.
    infant of diabetic m. (IDM)
    rubella-immune m.
    rubella-negative m.
    serology-negative m.
    surrogate m.
motherhood
    surrogate m.
mother-infant bonding
mother's breast milk (MBM)
moth patch
motile sperm
motilin
motility
    sperm m.
motion
    active range of m. (AROM)
    early cardiac m.
    fetal cardiac m.
    limb m.
Motrin
mottling
    m. of skin
mould (*var. of* mold)
mount
    wet m.
mouse
    m. mammary tumor virus
    (MMTV)

NOTES

mouse *(continued)*
    peritoneal m.
    m. uterine unit (MUU)
mouth
    carp m.
    purse-string m.
    tapir m.
mouth-and-hand synkinesia
mouth-to-mouth resuscitation
Movat stain
movement
    cardinal m.'s
    fetal m.
    fetal body m.
    rapid eye m.'s (REM)
    sound-stimulated fetal m.
    tonic-clonic m.'s
    vibroacoustic-induced
      fetal m.
moxalactam
    m. disodium
Moxam
moyamoya disease
Moynahan syndrome
Moynihan respirator
Mozart ear
MP
    menstrual period
MPA
    medroxyprogesterone acetate
MPF
    maturation-promoting factor
M-phase-promoting factor
mr
    milliroentgen
mrad
    millirad
MRI
    magnetic resonance imaging
      GRASS M.
MRM
    magnetic resonance
      mammography
mRNA
    messenger ribonucleic acid
MSAF
    meconium-stained amniotic
      fluid
MSAFP
    maternal serum alpha-
      fetoprotein

MSBP
    Münchhausen syndrome by
      proxy
MS Contin
MSIR Oral
MSUD
    maple syrup urine disease
M-type extractor
Mucat
    M. cervical sampling
    M. cervical sampling device
mucinous
    m. carcinoma
    m. cystadenocarcinoma
    m. ovarian neoplasm
    m. tumor
mucocolpos
mucocutaneous
    m. candidosis
    m. leishmaniasis
    m. lymph node syndrome
      (MLNS)
mucoid
    m. myoma degeneration
    m. otitis media (MOM)
mucolipidosis
mucopolysaccharidosis
    type I H/S m.
    type II m.
    type III m.
    type IS m.
    type IVA, B m.
    type V m.
    type VI m.
    type VII m.
    type VIII m.
mucoprotein
    Tamm-Horsfall m.
mucopurulent cervicitis
mucormycosis
    cutaneous m.
    pulmonary m.
mucorrhea
    cervical m.
mucosa
    endocervical m.
    vaginal m.
mucosal
    m. neuroma syndrome
mucous
    m. discharge
    m. membranes
    m. plug

mucoviscidosis
MUCP
    maximum urethral closure
      pressure
mucus
    cervical m.
    m. extractor
    midcycle cervical m.
    ovulatory m.
    spinnbarkeit (cervical m.)
Mueller (*var. of* Müller)
mulberry ovary
mulibrey nanism
Müller, Mueller
    M. tubercle
Müller-Hillis maneuver
müllerian
    m. abnormality
    m. adenosarcoma
    m. agenesis
    m. anomaly
    m. cyst
    m. duct
    m. duct fusion
    m. duct inhibitory factor
    m. hypoplasia
    m. inhibiting factor (MIF)
    m. inhibiting substance
Mullin system
multicentric carcinoma
multichannel
    m. cystometrogram
    m. recorder
multifactorial inheritance
multifetal
    m. pregnancy
    m. pregnancy reduction
multifetation
multifocal clonic seizure
multifollicular ovary
multigravida
Multiload Cu-375 intrauterine
    device
multiloba
    placenta m.
multilocal genetics
multilocular cyst

multimammae
multinucleation parakeratosis
multipara
    grand m.
multiparity
    grand m.
multiparous
multiplane intracavitary probe
multiple
    m. alleles
    m. births
    m. cervix
    m. congenital anomalies
    m. cyst
    m. endocrine abnormalities
      (MEA)
    m. endocrine neoplasia,
      types I, II, III (MEN)
    m. epiphyseal dysplasia
      tarda syndrome
    m. exostoses
    m. gestation
    m. lentigines syndrome
    m. myeloma
    m. neuroma syndrome
    m. organ failure
    m. pregnancy
    m. resistant cell lines
    m. sclerosis
    m. synostoses
    m. synostosis syndrome
multiple-punch resection
multiples of the median (mom)
multiplex
    arthrogryposis m.
    dysostosis m.
MultiPRO 2000 disposable biopsy
    needle guide for ultrasound
multivariant analysis
multivariate analysis of variance
    (MANOVA)
multivitamin
mummified fetus
mumps
    m. vaccine
    m. virus

NOTES

Mumpsvax
Münchhausen syndrome by proxy (MSBP)
Munro
    M. and Parker classification for laparoscopic hysterectomy
    M. point
Munro-Kerr maneuver
mural pregnancy
MURCS syndrome
Murless
    M. head extractor
    M. head retractor
murmur
    continuous m.
    diamond-shaped m.
    diastolic m.
    functional m.
    Graham Steell m.
    holosystolic m.
    machinery m.
    mill wheel m.
    pansystolic m.
    pulmonary m.
    pulmonic m.
    Still m.
    systolic m.
    systolic ejection m.
Murphy hole
muscarinic
muscle
    bulbocavernosus m.
    coccygeus m.
    detrusor m.
    gracilis m.
    Guthrie m.
    iliococcygeal m.
    ischiocavernosus m.
    levator ani m.
    pectoralis major m.
    pubococcygeal m.
    puborectal m.
    m. relaxant
    smooth m.
    m. splitting
    striated m.
    striated circular m.
    thyroarytenoid m.
muscular
    m. dystrophy
    m. hypertrophy syndrome
    m. injury

musculoskeletal
    m. disorder
    m. system
mushrooming of fimbria
mustard
    nitrogen m.
    phenylalanine m.
    L-phenylalanine m.
    M. procedure
Mustargen
mutagen
mutagenesis
    insertional m.
Mutamycin
mutant
    m. cell
    m. gene
mutation
    gene m.
    point m.
    trinucleotide repeat expansion m.
mutilans
    keratoma hereditarium m.
MUU
    mouse uterine unit
muzzled sperm
mV, mv
    millivolt
MX2-300 xenon quality light source
myalgia
Myambutol
myasthenia gravis
Mycelex
    M.-G
mycelia
mycelium
Mycifradin
    M. Sulfate
Myciguent
mycobacterial
Mycobacterium
    M. avium-intracellulare
    M. leprae
Mycoplasma
    M. hominis
    M. pneumoniae
mycoplasma
    genital m.
mycoplasmal
mycosis
Mycostatin

mycotic
    m. vaginosis
Mydfrin Ophthalmic
myelacephalus
myelitis
    transverse m.
myeloblastic leukemia
myelocele
myelodysplasia
myelodystrophy
myelofibrosis
myelogenous leukemia
myelography
myeloid/erythrocyte (M/E)
myeloma
    multiple m.
    m. protein
myelomeningocele
myelophthisis
myeloproliferative
myeloschisis
myelosuppressive agent
myiasis
Myleran
Mylicon
myoblastoma
    granular cell m.
myocardial
    m. blood flow
    m. function
    m. hypertrophy
    m. infarction
    m. ischemia
myocarditis
myocardium
Myochrysine
myoclonic
    m. seizure
myoclonic-astatic seizure
myoclonus
    Baltic m.
    m. epilepsy
    jaw m.
myocolpitis
myocutaneous flap
myoepithelial cell
myoglobin

myoglobinuria
myognathus
myoma, pl. myomata
    asymptomatic m.
    cervical m.
    degenerating m.
    m. fixation instrument
    intraligamentous m.
    intramural m.
    parasitic m.
    submucosal m.
    submucous m.
    subserosal m.
    subserous m.
    uterine m.
myomectomy
    abdominal m.
    vaginal m.
myometrial contraction
myometritis
myometrium
    hypotonic m.
    uterine m.
myomotomy
myonecrosis
myopathy
    mitochondrial m.
    nemaline m.
    ocular m.
    rod m.
myopia
myosalpingitis
myosalpinx
myosin
    m. filament
    m. light-chain kinase
    m. light-chain
      phosphorylation
myositis
    m. ossificans cirumscripta
    m. ossificans progressiva
myotomy
    Livadatis circular m.
myotonia
    m. congenita
    m. neonatorum
myotonic dystrophy

NOTES

MyoTrac EMG
myringitis
    bullous m.
myrtiform caruncle
Mysoline
mystery syndrome
Mytelase

myxedema
    infantile m.
myxedematous infantilism
myxoma
    familial familial cardiac m.
myxorrhea

nabothian
- n. cyst
- n. follicle
- n. gland
- n. vesicles

N-acetyl-galactosamine
N-acetyl-glucosamine
nadolol
Nadopen-V
Nadrothyron-D
Naegele
- N. forceps
- N. pelvis

Naegeli
- chromatophore nevus of N.
- N. incontinentia pigmenti

nafarelin
- n. acetate

nafazatin
Nafcil
nafcillin
- n. sodium

naftifine hydrochloride
Naftin
Nafucci syndrome
Nägele
- N. obliquity
- N. rule

Nager
- N. acrofacial dysostosis
- N. sign
- N. syndrome

Nager-de Reynier syndrome
nail-patella syndrome
nalbuphine
Nalcrom
Nalfon
Nal-Glu
nalidixic acid
Nallpen
nalorphine
naloxone
- n. hydrochloride

NALS
- neonatal adjuvant life support

naltrexone
nandrolone
nanism
- mulibrey n.

nanocephalic dwarfism

nanocephaly
nanoid
nanomelia
nanosomia
nape nevus
NAPI
- Neurodevelopmental Assessment Procedure for Preterm Infants

nappy test
Naprosyn
naproxen
- n. sodium

Naqua
narasin
Narcan
narcolepsy
narcosis
narcotic
- n. analgesia
- n. analgesic
- n. antagonist
- n. depression
- n. withdrawal syndrome

Nardil
naris, pl. nares
nasal
- n. cannula
- n. CPAP
- n. flaring

nascentium
- trismus n.

nasi
- flaring of ala n.

nasoduodenal feeding
nasogastric (NG)
- n. tube

nasojejunal
nasolabial
- n. fold asymmetry
- n. reflex

nasolacrimal duct
nasopharyngeal
- n. airway obstruction
- n. aspirate
- n. suction

nasopharyngitis
nasotracheal
natal
- n. cleft
- n. teeth

Natalins
    N. Rx
natality
natiform skull
natimortality
National
    N. Collaborative
      Diethylstilbestrol Adenosis
      Project (DESAD)
    N. Institute of Child
      Health and Human
      Development (NICHD)
    N. Surgical Adjuvant Breast
      Project (NSABP)
native squamous epithelium
natriuresis
natural
    n. antibody
    n. childbirth
    n. conception
    n. killer cells (NK cells)
    n. killer lymphocyte
Naturetin
nausea
    n. gravidarum
    n. and vomiting
Navane
navel
    blue n.
    cutis n.
Navratil stirrups
Naxen
NC
    Histussin N.
Nd:YAG
    neodymium:yttrium-aluminum-
      garnet
    Nd:YAG laser
    Nd:YAG laser ablation
Neal insufflator
near-term pregnancy
Nebcin
nebulization ventilator
nebulizer
    Dura Neb portable n.
    Hudson T Up-Draft II
      disposable n.
    Micro-Mist disposable n.
    PulmoMate n.
    Schuco n.
NEC
    necrotizing enterocolitis

neck
    bladder n.
    vesical n.
    webbed n.
neck-righting reflex
necrolysis
    toxic epidermal n.
necrophorum
    Fusobacterium n.
necrosis
    acute tubular n. (ATN)
    cortical n.
    fascial n.
    fat n.
    hepatic n.
    periportal hemorrhagic n.
    pituitary n.
    postsurgical fat n.
    posttraumatic fat n.
    renal cortical n.
    renal tubular n.
    subcutaneous fat n.
    uterine n.
    white matter n.
necrospermia
necrotizing
    n. enterocolitis (NEC)
    n. fasciitis
N.E.E. 1/35
needle
    Adair-Veress n.
    n. aspiration
    Bard Biopty cut n.
    n. biopsy
    Biopty cut n.
    butterfly n.
    Chiba n.
    Cobb-Ragde n.
    CUSALap ultrasonic
      accessory n.
    Dieckmann intraosseous n.
    Euro-Med FNA-21
      aspiration n.
    FNA-21 n.
    insufflation n.
    Kopan n.
    n. localization
    scalp vein n.
    SonoVu US aspiration n.
    stereotactic breast biopsy n.
    Veress n.
    Vim-Silverman n.

Virginia n.
Wolf-Veress n.
needle holder
Crile-Wood n. h.
ENDO-ASSIST
endoscopic n. h.
Heaney n. h.
Mayo-Hegar n. h.
Wangensteen n. h.
Wolf Castroviejo n. h.
NEEP
negative end-expiratory pressure
negative
n. end-expiratory pressure
(NEEP)
n. π meson
negative-pressure
n.-p. box
n.-p. respirator
NegGram
negligence
Neisseria gonorrhoeae
neisserial infection
Nellcor N-499 fetal oxygen saturation monitor
Nelnick-Needles syndrome
Nelova
Nelson
N. sign
N. syndrome
nemaline myopathy
Nemasole
Nembutal
nem (milk nutritional unit)
Neo-Calglucon
Neocate formula
Neo-Codema
neocystostomy
Neo-Durabolic
neodymium:yttrium-aluminum-garnet (Nd:YAG)
NeoFed
neofetus
Neo-fradin
neogala
neomycin
n. sulfate

neonatal
n. adjuvant life support
(NALS)
n. cholestatic jaundice
n. condition
n. conjunctivitis
n. death
n. diagnosis
n. distress
n. encephalopathy
Exosurf N.
n. hepatitis
n. herpes
n. HSV-1 encephalitis
n. HSV-2 encephalitis
n. hypocalcemia
n. hypoglycemia
n. infection
n. intensive care unit
(NICU)
n. line
n. lupus erythematosus
n. medicine
n. metabolism
n. monitor
n. morbidity
n. mortality
n. mortality rate
n. myasthenia gravis
n. neutropenia
n. ocular prophylaxis
n. outcome
n. pustular melanosis
n. respiratory distress
syndrome
n. resuscitation
n. ring
n. screening
n. seizure
n. sepsis
n. small left colon
syndrome
n. teeth
n. tetany
n. thymectomy
neonate
cola-colored n.

NOTES

neonate *(continued)*
    early n.
    n. examination
    preterm n.
neonatologist
neonatology
neonatorum
    acne n.
    adiponecrosis subcutanea n.
    anemia n.
    apnea n.
    asphyxia n.
    diabetes n.
    eczema n.
    edema n.
    erythema n.
    erythema toxicum n.
    erythroblastosis n.
    icterus gravis n.
    impetigo n.
    keratolysis n.
    mastitis n.
    melena n.
    milia n.
    myotonia n.
    ophthalmia n.
    scleredema n.
    sclerema n.
    sepsis n.
    tetania n.
    tetanus n.
    trismus n.
    volvulus n.
Neopap
neoplasia
    anal intraepithelial n. (AIN)
    cervical n.
    cervical epithelial n.
    cervical intraepithelial n.
      (CIN)
    endometrial n.
    endometrial intraepithelial n.
      (EIN)
    estrogen-dependent n.
    gestational trophoblastic n.
      (GTN)
    hematologic n.
    intraepithelial n.
    invasive n.
    lobular n.
    multiple endocrine n., types
      I, II, III (MEN)
    thyroid n.

    trophoblastic n.
    vaginal intraepithelial n.
      (VAIN)
    vulvar intraepithelial n.
      (VIN)
neoplasm
    adrenal n.
    benign ovarian n.
    bilateral ovarian n.
    borderline epithelial
      ovarian n.
    borderline malignant
      epithelial n.
    epithelial stromal ovarian n.
    germ cell ovarian n.
    hepatic n.
    indigenous n.
    isologous n.
    large intestine n.
    lipid cell n.
    lipoid ovarian n.
    malignant n.
    malignant ovarian n.
    mucinous ovarian n.
    ovarian n.
    ovarian lipid cell n.
    ovarian malignant
      epithelial n.
    ovarian sex-cord stromal n.
    serous ovarian n.
    sex-cord stromal n.
    soft tissue ovarian n.
neoplastic
    n. sequela
    n. trophoblastic disease
neosalpingostomy
    terminal n.
Neosar
Neo-Sert umbilical vessel catheter
    insertion set
Neosporin G.U. Irrigant
neostigmine
Neo-Synephrine
Neo-Tabs
Neo-trak 515A neonatal monitor
neovagina
Nephramine
nephrectomy
nephritis, pl. **nephritides**
    n. gravidarum
    interstitial n.
    lupus n.
nephroblastomatosis

Nephro-Calci
nephrocalcinosis
nephrogenic cord
nephrolithiasis
nephroma
  mesoblastic n.
nephron
  cortical n.
Nephronex
nephropathy
  diabetic n.
  reflux n.
  sickle cell n.
nephrophthisis
  familial juvenile n. (FJN)
nephrosclerosis
  malignant n.
nephrosis
  congenital n.
nephrostomy
  percutaneous n.
nephrotic syndrome
nephrotoxicity
nepiology
Neptazane
nerve
  n. block
  facial n.
  femoral n.
  genitofemoral n.
  n. growth factor (NGF)
  hemorrhoidal n.
  n. injury
  obturator n.
  n. palsy
  parasympathetic n.
  pelvic n.
  pelvic floor n.
  perineal n.
  presacral n.
  pudendal n.
  saphenous n.
  sciatic n.
  thoracolumbar
    sympathetic n.
nervi erigentes
Nervine

Nervocaine
nervosa
  anorexia n.
  bulimia n.
nervous system
nesidioblastosis
nest
  cancer n.'s
Nestabs FA
NET-EN
  norethindrone enanthate
Netherton syndrome
netilmicin sulfate
Netromycin
Nettleship syndrome
network
  SEER n.
    Surveillance, Epidemiology
    and End Results network
  Surveillance, Epidemiology
    and End Results n. (SEER
    network)
Neubauer hemocytometer
Neugebauer-LeFort procedure
neural
  n. arch
  n. groove
  n. plate
  n. tube
  n. tube defect (NTD)
neuralgia
  mammary n.
Neuramate
neurectomy
  presacral n.
neurenteric canal
neuritis
  retrobulbar n.
neuroblastoma
neurocutaneous syndrome
neurodermatitis
neurodevelopment
neurodevelopmental
  N. Assessment Procedure
    for Preterm Infants
    (NAPI)
  n. disability

NOTES

neuroectodermal tumor
neuroendocrine system
neuroendocrinology
neurofibroma
neurofibromatosis (NF)
    bilateral acoustic n.
    central type n.
    von Recklinghausen n.
neurofilament
neurogenic
    n. bladder
    n. tumor
neurogram
    pudendal n.
neurohypophysis
neuroleptic
neurologic
    n. abnormality
    n. adverse effect
    n. complication
    n. development
    n. disorder
    n. examination
    n. involvement
neurological injury
neuroma
    acoustic n.
neuromodulator
neuromuscular
    n. blockage
    n. maturity
neuronal
    n. heterotopia
neuron-specific enolase (NSE)
neuropathic
neuropathy
    familial visceral n.
    femoral n.
    nutritional n.
    obstetric n.
    porphyric n.
    retractor n.
neurophysin I, II
neurophysiology
neuroplate
neurosecretion
neurosis, pl. **neuroses**
neurosyphilis
neurotensin
neurotransmitter
    n. release
    substance P pain n.
neurula

neutralization
neutral protamine Hagedorn
    insulin (NPH insulin)
neutron
    fast n.
    n. therapy
neutropenia
    Kostmann n.
    neonatal n.
neutrophil
    mature n.
nevoxanthoendothelioma
nevus, pl. **nevi**
    n. anemicus
    bathing trunk n.
    benign n.
    blue n.
    cutaneous nevi
    n. depigmentosus
    n. elasticus of Lewandowsky
    faun tail n.
    n. flammeus
    halo n.
    n. of Ito
    Ito n.
    Jadassohn-Tieche n.
    melanocytic n.
    nape n.
    Ota n.
    n. of Ota
    port-wine n.
    n. sebaceus
    n. simplex
    spider n.
    Spitz n.
    strawberry n.
    n. unius lateris
    Unna n.
    vulvar n.
    white sponge n.
    wooly-hair n.
newborn
    congenital anemia of n.
    congenital epulis of the n.
    epulis of n.
    n. examination
    genital crisis of n.
    hemolytic disease of the n.
     (HDN)
    hemorrhagic disease of
     the n.
    jaundice of n.
    lamellar desquamation of n.

Parrot atrophy of n.
persistent pulmonary
hypertension of the n.
(PPHN)
physiologic jaundice of
the n.
respiratory distress
syndrome of the n.
n. respiratory distress
syndrome
n. resuscitation
transient tachypnea of
the n. (TTN)
Newport medical instrument
newtonian aberration
New York Heart Association
classification of heart disease
Neyman-Pearson statistical
hypothesis
Nezelof syndrome
Nezhat-Dorsey suction-irrigator
NF
neurofibromatosis
NG
nasogastric
NG tube
NGF
nerve growth factor
Niac
niacin
niacinamide
nialamide
nicardipine
NICHD
National Institute of Child
Health and Human
Development
Nichols
N. procedure
N. sacrospinous fixation
nickel dermatitis
Nickerson Biggy vials
nick translation
Nico-400
Nicobid
Nicoderm
Nicolar

Nicolas-Favre disease
nicotinamide
nicotine
nicotinic acid
nicotinyl alcohol
nicoumalone
NICU
neonatal intensive care unit
nidation
NIDDM
non-insulin-dependent diabetes
mellitus
Niemann-Pick disease
nifedipine
Niferex
niger
Peptococcus n.
Nightingale examining lamp
nigra
lingua n.
nigricans
acanthosis n.
hyperandrogenism, insulin
resistance, acanthosis n.
(HAIR-AN)
Nikolsky sign
Nilstat
Nimbus
N. test
nipple
accessory n.
n. discharge
Duckey n.
n. fed
n. feeding
inverted n.
McGovern n.
out-of-profile n.
Paget disease of n.
n. retraction
n. shield
n. stimulation test
supernumerary n.
nipple-areola complex
nipple-fed baby
nippling
Nipride

NOTES

Nisentil
Nissen fundoplication
Nissl bodies
nit
Nitabuch layer
Nite Train-R enuresis conditioning
   device
nitidus
   lichen n.
nitrate
   butoconazole n.
   miconazole n.
   silver n.
Nitrazine
   fern-positive N.
   N. test
nitrite
   amyl n.
Nitro-Bid
nitroblue tetrazolium dye test
Nitrocap
nitrofurantoin
   n. macrocrystals
   n. monohydrate
   n.
      monohydrate/macrocrystals
nitrogen
   blood urea n. (BUN)
   n. mustard
   n. partial pressure (PN_2)
   n. washout
nitroglycerin
Nitroglyn
nitroimidazole compound
Nitrol
Nitrolingual
Nitronet
Nitrong
nitroprusside
   sodium n.
nitrosourea
Nitrospan
Nitrostat
nitrous oxide
Nix Cream Rinse
Nizoral
NK cells
   natural killer cells
NMGTD
   nonmetastatic gestational
      trophoblastic disease
NMR
   nuclear magnetic resonance

N-multistix
Noack syndrome
Noble-Mengert perineal repair
nocardiosis
Noctec
nocturia
nocturnal epilepsy
nocturnus
   pavor n.
nodal involvement
node
   aortic n.
   atrioventricular n.
   axillary lymph n.
   Cloquet n.
   femoral lymph n.
   gluteal lymph n.
   hypogastric lymph n.
   iliac n.
   inguinal lymph n.
   intramammary lymph n.
   lymph n.
   paraaortic n.
   parauterine lymph n.
   pelvic lymph n.
   periaortic lymph n.
   pericervical n.
   rectal n.
   retroperitoneal n.
   sacral lymph n.
   shotty n.
   signal n.
   subaortic lymph n.
   ureteral n.
   vulvar lymph n.
nodosa
   periarteritis n.
   polyarteritis n.
   trichorrhexis n.
nodular
   n. blueberry lips
   n. embryo
   n. melanoma
   n. renal blastoma
nodule
   Albini n.
   blueberry muffin n.
   Hoboken n.
   Lisch n.
   Lutz-Jeanselme n.'s
   placental site n.
   rheumatoid n.'s

Sister Joseph n.
thyroid n.
NOFT
nonorganic failure to thrive
Noguchi test
Nolvadex
noma
n. pudendi
n. vulvae
nomenclature
FIGO n.
TNM n.
nomogram
body mass index n.
Lubchenco n.
Siggaard-Andersen n.
nonalkylating agent
nonallele
non-A, non-B hepatitis
nonappendiceal carcinoid
noncalcified nodular mass
noncalculous
noncarbonic acid
nonclassic 21-hydroxylase
deficiency
noncommunicating uterine horn
noncovalent
nondeciduous placenta
nondiagnostic culdocentesis
nondisjunction
nonestrogen drug
nonestrogen-regulated growth
nonfenestrated forceps
nonfrosted tip
nongenital pelvic organ
nongonococcal
n. cervicitis
n. urethritis
nongranulomatous salpingitis
nonhemolytic aerobic organism
nonhistone
non-Hodgkin lymphoma
nonhomologous chromosomes
nonimmune fetal hydrops

non-insulin-dependent
n.-i.-d. diabetes mellitus
(NIDDM)
n.-i.-d. diabetic
noninvasive management
nonketotic
n. hyperglycemia
n. hyperglycinemia
nonlactating breast
nonmaternal death
nonmetastatic gestational
trophoblastic disease (NMGTD)
Nonne-Milroy-Meige syndrome
nonnutritive sucking
nonorganic failure to thrive
(NOFT)
nonoxynol-9
n./octoxynol-9
nonpalpable abnormality
nonparous
nonpregnant endometrium
nonradioactive immunoassay
nonrandom mating
nonreactive immunoassay
non-REM sleep
nonsalt-losing adrenogenital
syndrome
non-sex hormone-binding globulin
bound testosterone
nonspecific
n. immunotherapy
n. mesenchyme
n. urethritis
n. vaginitis
nonsteroidal anti-inflammatory drug
(NSAID)
nonstressed fetus
nonstress test (NST)
nonstructural gene
nonviable
n. fetus
nonvolatile acid
Noonan syndrome
noradrenaline
Noradryl
Norcept-E 1/35
Norcuron

NOTES

Nordette
Nordryl
norepinephrine
norethindrone
    n. acetate
    n. acetate and ethinyl
      estradiol
    n. enanthate (NET-EN)
    n. and ethinyl estradiol
    ethinyl estradiol and n.
    mestranol and n.
Norethin 1/35E
Norethin 1/35M
Norethin 1/50M
norethisterone
norethynodrel
    mestranol and n.
Norflex
norfloxacin
norgestimate
    ethinyl estradiol and n.
    n. and ethinyl estradiol
    n. progestin
norgestrel
    ethinyl estradiol and n.
d-norgestrel
norgestrel/ethinyl estradiol
  combination
Norinyl 1+35
Norinyl 1+50
Norisodrine
Norlestrin
    N. 1/50
    N. 2.5/50
    N. Fe
Norlutate
Norlutin
normal
    n. blood loss
    n. ovariotomy
    n. pressure hydrocephalus
    (NPH)
    n. saline
    n. temperature
    n. transformation zone
Norman Miller vaginopexy
Norman-Wood syndrome
Nor-Mil
normoactive bowel sounds
normocephalic
Normodyne
normospermic
Normotest

Noroxin
Norpace
Norpanth
Norplant
    N. implant
    N. system
Norpramin
NOR-Q.D.
Norrie
    N. disease
    N. syndrome
Norris-Carrol criteria
19-nortestosterone
    19-n. derivative
Nor-tet
Northern blot test
Northway staging
Norton operation
nortriptyline
Nortussin
nose-breather
    obligate n.-b.
nosocomial
    n. infection
notencephalia
notochord
notogenesis
notomelus
Novafed
Novafil
Novak curette
Novantrone
Nova Rectal
novo
    stress incontinence de n.
novobiocin
Novobutamide
Novochlorhydrate
Novodimenate
Novo-Flurazine
Novofuran
Novo-Hydrazide
Novolin
    N. 70/30
    N. insulin
    N. L
    N. N
    N. N PenFil
    N. 70/30 PenFil
    N. R
    N. R PenFil
Novomepro
Novonidazol

Novopen
    N.-VK
Novopoxide
Novopramine
Novopropamide
Novo-Ridazine
Novorythro
Novosecobarb
Novosoxazole
Novotetra
Novotriptyn
Noz
    Whoo N.
Nozinan
NPH
    normal pressure hydrocephalus
NPH (insulin)
    neutral protamine Hagedorn
    insulin
        NPH Iletin I
        NPH Iletin II
        NPH Insulin
NPH-N
NSABP
    National Surgical Adjuvant
    Breast Project
NSAID
    nonsteroidal anti-inflammatory
    drug
NSE
    neuron-specific enolase
NST
    nonstress test
NTD
    neural tube defect
Nubain
nuchal
    n. arm
    n. cord
Nuck
    canal of N., N. canal
    N. diverticulum
    N. hydrocele
nuclear
    n. agenesis
    n. antigen
    n. aplasia

    n. jaundice
    n. magnetic resonance
    (NMR)
    n. milk
    n. radiation
    n. sex
nucleatum
    Fusobacterium n.
nucleic acid probe
nucleoid
    Landovski n.
nucleolar
    n. chromosome
nucleoside pair
nucleosome
nucleotide
nucleotidylexotransferase
    DNA n.
nucleotidyltransferase
    DNA n.
    RNA n.
nucleus
    arcuate n.
    steroid n.
nulligravida
nullipara
nulliparity
nulliparous
number
    ovulation n.
    Reynolds n.
nummular eczema
Numorphan
Nunn engorged corpuscles
Nupercainal cream
nurse
    wet n.
nursery
Nursoy formula
nutans
    spasmus n.
Nutramigen formula
Nutr-E-Sol
nutrient requirement
nutrition
    fetal n.
    fluids, electrolytes, n. (FEN)

NOTES

nutrition *(continued)*
    maternal n.
    parenteral n. (PN)
    PediaSure liquid n.
    total parenteral n. (TPN)
    total peripheral
      parenteral n. (TPPN)
nutritional
    n. neuropathy
    n. problem
    n. surveillance
Nutropin
nyctalopia
Nydrazid
nylidrin hydrochloride
nylon suture material
nympha, pl. **nymphae**

nymphectomy
nymphitis
nymphomania
nymphoncus
nymphotomy
Nyquist frequency
nystagmus
nystatin
    n. and triamcinolone cream
    n. and triamcinolone
      ointment
Nystat-Rx
Nystex
Nytilax
Nytone enuretic control unit

O₂

O_2

oxygen

hood O_2

THb O_2

total oxyhemoglobin

OA

occipitoanterior

occiput anterior

OAE

otoacoustic emission test

oat cell carcinoma

OB

obstetrician

obstetrics

Chemstrip 4 The OB

Chromagen OB

OB Gees maternity orthotic

Sil-K OB

Obalan

Obephen

obesity

android o.

o. in endometrial sarcoma

exogenous o.

experimental o.

gynecoid o.

Obeval

Obezine

OB/GYN

obstetrics and gynecology

objective probability

obligate

o. heterozygote

o. nose-breather

oblique

o. diameter

o. lie

o. presentation

obliquity

Litzmann o.

Nagele o.

Nägele o.

Obrinsky syndrome

observation

observer variation

obstetric, obstetrical

o. anesthesia

o. conjugate of outlet

o. history

o. neuropathy

o. position

obstetrician (OB)

high-risk o.

obstetrician-gynecologist

obstetrics (OB)

Association of Professors of Gynecology and O. (APGO)

defensive o.

Federation of International Gynecology and O. (FIGO)

International Federation of Gynecology and O. (FIGO)

obstetrics and gynecology (OB/GYN)

Obstetrique

Federation International de Gynecologie et O. (FIGO)

obstipation

obstruction

bladder neck o.

bowel o.

colonic o.

distal tubal o.

duodenal o.

extramural upper airway o.

fimbrial o.

gastrointestinal o.

intestinal o.

intraluminal upper airway o.

intramural upper airway o.

intrathoracic airway o.

nasopharyngeal airway o.

tubal o.

ureteral o.

ureterovesical o.

urinary outlet o.

urinary tract o.

obstructive

o. dysmenorrhea

o. jaundice

o. uropathy

obturator

o. artery

o. fascia

obturator *(continued)*
    o. nerve
    o. nerve damage
OC
    oral contraceptive
OC-125
occipitoanterior (OA)
    left o. position (LOA)
    o. position
    right o. position (ROA)
occipitofrontal diameter
occipitomental diameter
occipitoposterior (OP)
    left o. position (LOP)
    o. position
    right o. position (ROP)
occipitotransverse (OT)
    left o. position (LOT)
    o. position
    right o. position (ROT)
occiput
    o. anterior (OA)
    o. posterior (OP)
    o. presentation
    o. transverse (OT)
occludens
    zonula o.
occlusion
    distal o.
    proximal o.
    roller o.
    tubal o.
occulta
    spina bifida o.
occult cancer
occultum
    cranium bifidum o.
occupational history
Ochsner forceps
O'Connor-O'Sullivan retractor
OCT
    oxytocin challenge test
Octamide
octaploidy
octoxynol 9
ocular
    o. aspergillosis
    o. bobbing
    o. hypertelorism
    o. hypotelorism
    o. hypotony
    o. involvement
    o. manifestation

    o. myopathy
    o. prophylaxis
oculoauricular dysplasia
oculoauriculovertebral dysplasia
oculocephalic reflex
oculocephalogyric reflex
oculocerebral syndrome
oculocerebrorenal dystrophy
oculocutaneous albinoidism
oculodentodigital (ODD)
    o. dysplasia
    o. syndrome
oculomandibulofacial syndrome (OMF)
oculopharyngeal muscular dystrophy
Ocu-Sol
ODD
    oculodentodigital
odd chromosome
od gene
O'Donnell operation
Oedipus complex
Oestrilin
OFD
    orofaciodigital
    OFD syndrome, type I, II, III
office cystometrics
ofloxacin
OG
    orogastric
Ogden vaginal cream
Ogen
Ogino-Knaus rule
Ohio
    O. bed
    O. humidifier
    O. warmer
Ohmeda Care-Plus incubator
17-OHP
    17-hydroxyprogesterone
Ohtahara syndrome
OI
    osteogenesis imperfecta
    oxygenation index
oil
    camphorated o.
    o. cyst
    o. enema
    ethiodized o.
    glycerin, lanolin and peanut o.

MCT o.
mineral o.
ointment
    nystatin and
      triamcinolone o.
    Pazo hemorrhoid o.
    zinc oxide o.
Okazaki fragment
OKT8
17β-ol-dehydrogenase
oleandomycin phosphate
oligoamnios
oligoasthenospermia
oligoclonal bands
oligodactyly
oligogalactia
oligohydramnios
oligomenorrhea
oligospermia
oligozoospermia
oliguria
Oliver-McFarlane syndrome
Ollier syndrome
Olshausen
    O. procedure
    O. sign
    O. suspension
Olympic Neostraint immobilizer
Olympus
    O. disposable cannula
    O. disposable trocar
    O. hysteroscope
omacephalus (*var. of*
  omocephalus)
Omenn syndrome
omental
    o. cake
    o. cyst
omentectomy
omentum
    lymphocyst o.
omeprazole
OMF
  oculomandibulofacial syndrome
OMI
  oocyte maturation inhibitor

OMM
  ophthalmomandibulomelic
Ommaya reservoir
Omnipen
    O.-N
Omniprobe test
Omni-Tract vaginal retractor
omocephalus, omacephalus
omphal
omphaloangiopagous twins
omphaloangiopagus
omphalocele
omphalomesenteric
    o. cord
    o. cyst
    o. duct
omphalopagus
omphalorrhagia
omphalorrhea
omphalorrhexis
omphalotomy
omphalotripsy
OMPI colposcope
onanism
oncofetal
    o. antigen
    o. fibronectin
oncogene
    o. expression
oncologist
    Society of Gynecologic O.'s
      (SGO)
oncology
    gynecologic o.
    Society of Gynecologic O.
OncoScint test
Oncovin
Ondine
    curse of O.
    O. curse
one-child sterility
one-egg twins
one-horned uterus
one-hour glucose tolerance test
one-tail test
onlay patch anastomosis
ontology

NOTES

onychia
ooblast
oocyesis
oocyte
    o. cryopreservation
    o. culture
    o. donation
    o. donor
    o. extrusion
    o. maturation inhibitor
     (OMI)
    o. meiosis
    primary o.
    o. retrieval
oogenesis
oogonia, sing. **oogonium**
oolemma
oophoralgia
oophorectomy
    prophylactic o.
oophoritic cyst
oophoritis
    autoimmune o.
oophorocystectomy
oophorocystosis
oophorohysterectomy
oophoroma
oophoropathy
oophoropeliopexy
oophoropexy
oophoroplasty
oophororrhaphy
oophorosalpingectomy
oophorosalpingitis
oophorostomy
oophorotomy
oophorrhagia
ooplasm
oozing
    venous o.
OP
    occipitoposterior
    occiput posterior
O&P
    ova and parasites
opacity
    corneal o.
OPD
    otopalatodigital
open
    o. crib
    to keep o. (TKO)
    keep vein o. (KVO)

opening
    urethral o.
    vaginal o.
operation
    Alexander o.
    Bacon-Babcock o.
    Baldy o.
    Band-Aid o.
    Baudelocque o.
    Blalock-Hanlon o.
    Blalock-Taussig o.
    Bozeman o.
    Brunschwig o.
    cesarean o.
    Cotte o.
    Counsellor-Davis artificial
     vagina o.
    Döderlein roll-flap o.
    Donald-Fothergill o.
    Doyle o.
    Emmet o.
    Estes o.
    Falk-Shukuris o.
    Fothergill o.
    Fothergill-Donald o.
    Fothergill-Hunter o.
    Frangenheim-Goebel-
     Stoeckel o.
    Fredet-Ramstedt o.
    Freund o.
    Gigli o.
    Gilliam o.
    Gilliam-Doleris o.
    Giordano o.
    Gittes o.
    Glenn o.
    Goodall-Power o.
    Grant-Ward o.
    Halsted o.
    Haultain o.
    Heaney o.
    Heller-Belsey o.
    Heller-Nissen o.
    Kelly o.
    Kennedy-Pacey o.
    Kocks o.
    Lash o.
    LeFort o.
    LeFort-Neugebauer o.
    Madlener o.
    Manchester o.
    Manchester-Fothergill o.
    Marckwald o.

Marshall-Marchetti-Krantz o.
McIndoe o.
morcellation o.
Norton o.
obstetrical o.
O'Donnell o.
Pomeroy o.
Porro o.
Ramstedt o.
Récamier o.
Saenger o.
Schauta vaginal o.
Schroeder o.
Schuchardt o.
second-look o.
sex change o.
Shirodkar o.
Spinelli o.
Stamey o.
Strap o.
Sturmdorf o.
suprapubic urethrovesical
  suspension o.
suspensory sling o.
switch o.
TeLinde o.
Tessier craniofacial o.
transsphenoidal o.
Urban o.
Vecchietti o.
Waters o.
Way o.
Webster o.
Wertheim o.
Wertheim-Schauta o.
operative
  o. cholangiogram
  o. laparoscopy
  o. site complication
operator
  o. gene
  o. locus
operculum, pl. opercula
operon
Ophthaine
Ophthalgan

ophthalmia
  gonococcal o.
  gonorrheal o.
  o. neonatorum
Ophthalmic
  Mydfrin O.
ophthalmomandibulomelic (OMM)
  o. dysplasia
ophthalmoplegia
  fibrotic o.
Ophthochlor
opiate
  endogenous o.
  o. receptor
opioid
  o. activity
  o. addiction
  o. peptide
  o. receptor antagonist
opioidergic control impairment
opipramol hydrochloride
opisthotonos fetalis
opisthotonus
Opitz-Christian syndrome
Opitz-Frias syndrome
Opitz syndrome
opium
OPMI drape
OPMILAS CO2 laser
opocephalus
opodidymus
Oppenheim
  O. congenital hypotonia
  O. disease
  O. syndrome
opposing wall
opsoclonus
opsomyoclonus
opsonin
opsonization
  o. system
optic
  o. fundus
  o. glioma
optical
  o. density
  o. density measurement

NOTES

Opticrom
Optimal Observation Score
Optimine
Optimox
    O. C-500
    O. Mag 200
Optimyd
Optiphot-2UD microscope
Optivite
    O. PMT
OPUS immunoassay system
ora (*pl. of* os)
Oradexon
Oragrafin
oral
    o. administration
    o. cavity
    o. conjugated estrogen
    o. contraception
    o. contraceptive (OC)
    o. contraceptive efficacy
    o. contraceptive use
    Estratest O.
    o. estrone
    o. hormone replacement
      therapy
    o. hypoglycemic
    o. polio vaccine
    o. sex
    o. steroid contraceptive
    o. temperature
    o. transmucosal fentanyl
      citrate
oral-facial-digital syndrome
orally-administered estrogen
Oramide
Oramorph SR
Orange
    Agent O.
Orap
Orbenin
orbitopagus
orchidoblastoma
orchiopexy
    Fowler-Stephens o.
orchitis
orciprenaline sulfate
order
    high fetal o.
Oretic
Oreton Methyl
organ
    internal generative o.

nongenital pelvic o.
o. of Rosenmüller
sensory o.
o. transplant
o. transplantation
organic acid screen
organism
    Gram-negative o.
    Gram-positive o.
    nonhemolytic aerobic o.
Organization
    World Health O. (WHO)
organogenesis
organomegaly
Organon
    O. percutaneous E2 implant
orgasm
orgasmic
    o. flush
    o. plateau
orientation
    sexual o.
orifice
orificial
origin
    fever of unknown o. (FUO)
    histoimmunological o.
    parental o.
Orimune
Orinase
Ornade
ornithine
    o. decarboxylase
orodigitofacial
    o. dysostosis
    o. dystosis
orofaciodigital (OFD)
    o. syndrome
orogastric (OG)
orogenital syndrome
oromotor function
oropharynx
orphan
    enteric cytopathogenic
      human o. (ECHO)
orphenadrine
Ortho
    O. All-Flex diaphragm
    O. diaphragm kit
    O. Dienestrol
    O. Tri-Cyclen
Ortho-Cept
Ortho-Creme

Ortho-Cyclen
orthogonal lead system
Ortho-Gynol
orthomyxovirus
Ortho-Novum 1/35
Ortho-Novum 1/50
Ortho-Novum 7/7/7
Ortho-Novum 10/11
orthopaedic, orthopedic
    o. anomaly
    o. condition
orthostatic
    o. hypotension
    o. proteinuria
orthotic
    OB Gees maternity o.
orthotopic live transplantation
orthovoltage
    o. radiation
Orthoxine
Ortolani
    O. click
    O. maneuver
    O. sign
    O. test
os, pl. ora, ossa
    cervical o.
    external o.
    internal o.
    parous o.
    o. pubis
    Scanzoni second o.
Os-Cal 500
oscillation amplitude
oscillator
oscillatory
    high-frequency o. (HFO)
    o. ventilation
Osgood-Schlatter
    O.-S. disease
    O.-S. syndrome
Osler-Weber-Rendu disease
Osmoglyn
osmolality
osmolarity
Osmolite formula
osmoregulation

osmotic pressure
ossa (*pl. of* os)
ossicle
    Andernach o.
ossicular
ossification
osteitis
    o. condensans generalisata
    o. fibrosa
    o. pubis
osteoarthropathy
osteoblast
osteoblast-like cell
osteoblastoma
osteocalcin
osteochondritis
    o. deformans juvenilis
    o. dissecans
    o. ischiopubica
osteochondrodystrophia deformans
osteochondrodystrophy
    familial o.
osteochondroma
osteochondrosis deformans tibiae
osteocranium
osteocystoma
osteodystrophia juvenilis
osteodystrophy
    renal o.
osteogenesis
    o. imperfecta (OI)
    o. imperfecta congenita
      syndrome
    o. imperfecta cystica
osteogenic
osteoid
    o. osteoma
osteoma
    osteoid o.
osteomalacia
    juvenile o.
Osteomark agent
Osteomeasure computer-assisted
  image analyzer
osteomyelitis
    o. pubis

NOTES

osteopathia
    o. striata
    o. striata syndrome
osteopedion
osteopenia
    relative o.
osteopetrosis tarda
osteopoikilosis
osteopontin
osteoporosis
    postmenopausal o.
osteoporotic fracture
osteopsathyrosis
osteosarcoma
osteotabes
ostium
    o. primum defect
    o. secundum
    o. secundum defect
Ostrum-Furst syndrome
O'Sullivan-O'Connor retractor
OT
    occipitotransverse
    occiput transverse
O.T.
    Mono-VaccTest O.T.
Ota
    nevus of O.
    O. nevus
otalgia
OTC
    over-the-counter
otitis externa
otoacoustic emission test (OAE)
otocyst
otomycosis
otopalatodigital (OPD)
    o. syndrome
otorrhea
otosclerosis
    o. syndrome
otoscope
    Siegel o.
otospongiosis syndrome
Ototemp 3000 thermometer
Otovent autoinflation kit
Otto pelvis
ouabain
ounce (oz)
    calories per o. (cal/oz)
out
    toeing o.

outcome
    adverse o.
    fetal o.
    maternal o.
    neonatal o.
    obstetrical o.
    perinatal o.
    pregnancy o.
    teratogenic o.
outlet
    conjugate of pelvic o.
    o. forceps delivery
    parous o.
    pelvic o.
    vaginal o.
    vulvovaginal o.
outline
    fetal o.
out-of-phase endometrial biopsy
out-of-profile nipple
output
    cardiac o.
    intake and o. (I&O)
    urine o.
out-toeing
ova (*pl. of* ovum)
    o. and parasites (O&P)
ovale
    foramen o.
ovalocytary anemia
ovaria (*pl. of* ovarium)
ovarialgia
ovarian
    o. ablation
    o. abnormality
    o. abscess
    o. activity
    o. agenesis
    o. amenorrhea
    o. antibody
    o. artery
    o. cancer
    o. cancer metastasis
    o. carcinoma
    o. carcinoma antigen
    o. carcinoma debulking
    o. cautery
    o. clear cell adenocarcinoma
    o. colic
    o. cycle
    o. cycle change
    o. cyst
    o. cystadenocarcinoma

o. cystadenoma
o. cystectomy
o. cystic teratoma
o. disorder
o. dysgenesis
o. dysgerminoma
o. dysmenorrhea
o. embryonal teratoma
o. endometriosis
o. estrogen synthesis
o. factor
o. failure
o. fibroma
o. follicle exhaustion
o. function
o. gametogenesis
o. germinal epithelium
o. gonadoblastoma
o. hormone
o. hyperandrogenism
o. hyperstimulation
o. hyperstimulation
  syndrome
o. hypertrophy
o. leiomyoma
o. ligament
o. lipid cell neoplasm
o. lymphoma
o. malignancy
o. malignant epithelial
  neoplasm
o. mass
o. metastasis
o. neoplasm
o. plexus
o. pregnancy
o. proliferative cystadenoma
o. remnant syndrome
o. seminoma
o. sex-cord stromal
  neoplasm
o. small-cell carcinoma
o. steroid
o. steroidogenesis
o. stroma
o. teratoma
o. thecoma

o. torsion
o. tubular adenoma
o. tumor
o. varicocele
o. vein
o. vein syndrome
o. vein thrombosis
o. wedge resection
ovariectomy
ovarii
  hyperthecosis o.
  mesoblastoma o.
ovarioabdominal pregnancy
ovariocele
ovariocentesis
ovariocyesis
ovariodysneuria
ovariogenic
ovariohysterectomy
ovariolytic
ovarioncus
ovariopathy
ovariorrhexis
ovariosalpingectomy
ovariosalpingitis
ovariosteresis
ovariostomy
ovariotomy
  Beatson o.
  normal o.
ovaritis
ovarium, pl. ovaria
  o. bipartitum
  o. disjunctum
  o. gyratum
  o. lobatum
ovary
  accessory o.
  mulberry o.
  multifollicular o.
  oyster o.
  palpable postmenopausal o.
  polycystic o. (PCO)
  resistant o.
  sclerocystic o.
  Stein-Leventhal type of
    polycystic o.

NOTES

ovary *(continued)*
    strumal carcinoid of o.
    supernumerary o.
    transposition of o.
    wandering o.
ovatus
    Bacteroides o.
Ovcon
overdistention syndrome
overflow incontinence
overhead warmer
overload
    fluid o.
    volume o.
overriding
    o. aorta
    o. of sutures
overt
    o. insulin-dependent diabetes
     mellitus
over-the-counter (OTC)
    o.-t.-c. medication
overt insulin-dependent diabetes
  mellitus
Oves Cervical Cap
ovicidal
oviduct
    ampulla of o.
    angiomyoma of o.
ovigenesis
ovine
    o. trophoblast protein-1
ovoid
    Delclos o.
    Fleming o.
    Manchester o.
    tandem and o.'s (T&O)
ovotestis, pl. ovotestes
Ovral
Ovrette
OvuDate hCG
OvuGen test kit
OvuKIT
    O. Self-Test kit
    O. test
ovular transmigration
ovulation
    contralateral o.
    incessant o.
    o. induction
    o. number
    paracyclic o.
    o. rate

    spontaneous o.
    o. stimulation
ovulational sclerosis
ovulatory
    o. age
    o. cycle
    o. defect
    o. disturbance
    o. mucus
ovulocyclic
    o. porphyria
ovum, pl. ova
    blighted o.
    Bryce-Teacher o.
    o. capture
    fertilized o.
    frozen o.
    hamster o.
    Hertig-Rock o.
    holoblastic o.
    Mateer-Streeter o.
    o. maturation
    Miller o.
    Peters o.
    primitive o.
    primordial o.
    o. transport
    trapped o.
ovum-capture inhibitor
OvuQUICK
    O. Self-Test
    O. Self-Test kit
    O. Self-Test ovulation
     predictor
owl
    o.'s eye cells
    o.'s eye inclusion bodies
Owren disease
oxacillin
    o. sodium
Oxandrin
oxandrolone
oxazepam
Oxford Family Planning
  Association Contraceptive Study
oxidase
    diamine o.
    monoamine o. (MOA)
oxide
    magnesium o.
    nitrous o.
    zinc o.

oximeter
    Accustat pulse o.
    Healthdyne o.
    INVOS 3100 cerebral o.
    OxyShuttle pulse o.
    Oxytrak pulse o.
    pulse o.
oximetry
    pulse o.
    reflectance pulse o.
Oxisensor
    O. fetal oxygen saturation
      monitor
    O. transducer
Ox-Pam
oxprenolol
oxtriphylline
oxybutynin chloride
oxycardiorespirogram
Oxycel cautery
oxycephaly
oxychlorosone sodium
oxycodone
oxy-CR gram
Oxydess II
oxygen (O_2)
    arterial oxygen o. (tension)
      (PaO_2)
    blow-by o.
    o. concentration in
      pulmonary capillary blood
      (CcO_2)
    o. consumption
    o. delivery
    o. dissociation curve
    home o.
    hood o.
    hyperbaric o.
    partial pressure of o. (PO_2)
    partial pressure of
      arterial o. (PaO_2)
    o. saturation (SaO_2)

    o. tension
    tent o.
    o. toxicity lung disease
    transcutaneous partial
      pressure of o. ($tCpO_2$)
oxygenated fetal blood
oxygenation
    extracorporeal membrane o.
      (ECMO)
    fetal o.
    fetal scalp o.
    o. index (OI)
oxygenator
    Lilliput neonatal o.
oxygen-diffusing capacity
oxyhemoglobin
    total o. (THb O_2, THb O_2)
Oxy-Hood oxygen hood
oxymorphone
oxyphenbutazone
oxyphencyclimine
oxyphenonium bromide
OxyShuttle pulse oximeter
oxytetracline HCl
oxytetracycline
oxytoca
    Klebsiella o.
oxytocia
oxytocic
    o. stimulation
oxytocin
    o. analogue
    o. augmentation
    o. challenge test (OCT)
    o. stimulation of labor
oxytocinase
Oxytrak pulse oximeter
Oyst-Cal 500
Oystercal 500
oyster ovary
oz
    ounce

NOTES

P
    phosphorus
    pressure, partial pressure
        P value
2P23
5P15
^{32}P
    phosphorus-32
p24 antigen
P32 intraperitoneal treatment
PA
    alveolar partial pressure
    pernicious anemia
    plasminogen activator
Pa
    arterial partial pressure
    pascal unit of pressure
      measurement
p(A-a)O$_2$
    alveolar-arterial pressure
      difference
Paas disease
PAC
    papular acrodermatitis of
      childhood
PACE-2 test
pacemaker
    artificial p.
Pacey technique
pachygyria
pachyonychia congenita
pachysalpingitis
pachysalpingo-ovaritis
pachytene
    p. phase of meiosis
    p. stage
pachyvaginitis
    p. cystica
Pacific yew
pacifier
pack
    Barrier p.
    Peri-Cold P.
    Peri-Gel P.
    Peri-Warm P.
packed
    p. cells
    p. erythrocyte
    p. red blood cells

packer
    Bernay uterine p.
    Kitchen postpartum
      gauze p.
paclitaxel
PaCO$_2$
    arterial carbon dioxide pressure
      (tension)
    partial pressure of arterial
      carbon dioxide
PAD
    pelvic adhesive disease
pad
    Aquaflex ultrasound gel p.
    buccal fat p.
    LePad breast exam
      training p.
    malar fat p.
    sucking p.
    suctorial p.
Paget
    P. disease
    P. disease of nipple
pagetic
pagetoid
pagophagia
pain
    acyclic pelvic p.
    after-p.'s
    bearing-down p.
    chronic pelvic p. (CPP)
    epigastric p.
    expulsive p.'s
    false p.'s
    flank p.
    hypogastric p.
    intermenstrual p.
    International Association for
      the Study of P.
    labor p.'s
    low-back p.
    lower abdominal p.
    pelvic p.
    periumbilical p.
    pleuritic p.
    psychogenic pelvic p.
    recurrent abdominal p.
    (RAP)
    referred pelvic p.

pain *(continued)*
    splanchnic pelvic p.
    suprapubic p.
pair
    base p.
    chromosome p.
    kb p., kilobase p.
    nucleoside p.
paired allosome
Pajot maneuver
Paks
    Pedi-Boro Soak P.
palate
    cleft p. (CP)
palatognathous
palatopharyngeal incompetence
palatoschisis
palliative surgery
pallor of skin
PALM
  premature accelerated lung
    maturation
palm
    p. leaf pattern
    tripe p.
palmar
    p. crease
    p. erythema
palmaris
    tinea nigra p.
    xanthoma striata p.
palmatae
    plicae p.
palm-chin reflex
Palmer ovarian biopsy forceps
palmitate
    colfosceril p.
palmomandibular sign
palmomental reflex
palpable
    p. cord
    p. postmenopausal ovary
palpation
    spoke-wheel p.
palpebral fissure
palsy
    Bell p.
    brachial birth p.
    brachial plexus p.
    cerebral p. (CP)
    Erb p.
    facial nerve p.
    Klumpke p.

    Landry p.
    nerve p.
    obstetrical brachial
      plexus p.
pamabrom
PAMBA
    para-aminomethylbenzoic acid
Pamelor
Pamine
pamoate
pampiniform plexus
pancreas
pancreatic
    p. insufficiency syndrome
    p. oncofetal antigen (POA)
    p. pseudocyst
pancreatitis
    gallstone p.
pancreatoblastoma
panculture
pancuronium bromide
pancytopenia
    aplastic p.
Pander islands
Panectyl
panencephalitis
Panex
Panhematin
panhysterectomy
Panmycin
Panner disease
panniculectomy
panniculitis
panniculus
pansystolic murmur
pantothenate
    calcium p.
pantothenic acid
pants-over-vest technique
Panwarfin
PaO$_2$
    arterial oxygen pressure (tension)
    partial pressure of arterial
      oxygen
Pap
    Papanicolaou
    Pap smear
Papanicolaou (Pap)
    P. smear
PAPase
    phosphatidic acid
      phosphohydrolase
papaverine

paper-doll fetus
Papette cervical collector
papilla, pl. papillae
    columnar epithelium p.
    p. of columnar epithelium
papillary
    p. adenocarcinoma
    p. carcinoma
    p. endometrial carcinoma
    p. hidradenoma
    p. serous cervical carcinoma
    p. serous
      cystadenocarcinoma
papilledema
papilloma
    choroid plexus p.
    ductal p.
    intraductal p.
papillomatosis
    juvenile p.
    laryngeal p.
    subareolar duct p.
Papillomavirus
papillomavirus
    human p. (HPV)
    p. hybridization
    p. infection
    type 16 p.
Papillon-Léage-Psaume syndrome
Papillon-Léfevre syndrome
Pap-Kaps
papoose board
PAPPA
    pregnancy-associated plasma
      protein A
Pap-Perfect supply system
papular
    p. acrodermatitis of
      childhood (PAC)
    p. dermatitis of pregnancy
    p. urticaria
papule
    pruritic urticarial p.
    urticarial p.
papulonecrotica
    tuberculosis p.

papulosis
    bowenoid p.
PAPVR
    partial anomalous pulmonary
      venous return
papyraceous fetus
papyraceus
    fetus p.
para-aminomethylbenzoic acid
    (PAMBA)
para-aminosalicylate
para-aminosalicylic acid (PAS,
    PASA)
paraaortic
    p. lymphadenectomy
    p. node
    p. node irradiation
    p. positivity
parabiosis
    dialytic p.
    vascular p.
parabolic twins
paracentesis
paracentric inversion
paracervical
    p. anesthesia
    p. block
    p. injection
    p. lymphatics
paracetamol
parachute
    p. mitral valve
    p. reflex
paracolpitis
paracrine
    p. communication
paracyclic ovulation
paracyesis
Paradione
paradoxical incontinence
paraduodenal hernia
Paraflex
ParaGard T380A intrauterine
    copper contraceptive
parainfluenza

NOTES

parakeratosis
    multinucleation p.
paralysis, pl. **paralyses**
    antigenic p.
    birth p.
    congenital abducens
      facial p.
    congenital oculofacial p.
    Duchenne p.
    Erb-Duchenne p.
    facial p.
    facial nerve p.
    hysterical p.
    immunologic p.
    Klumpke p.
    Klumpke-Dejerine p.
    obstetrical p.
    parturient p.
    respiratory p.
    spastic p.
    Werdnig-Hoffmann p.
paralytic ileus
paramedian incision
paramenia
paramesonephric
    p. duct
parameter
    fetal growth p.'s
paramethadione
parametrectomy
    radical p.
parametrial phlegmon
parametric abscess
parametritic
    p. abscess
parametritis
parametrium
paranasal sinus
paraneoplastic syndrome
paraovarian cyst
para, para I, para II, etc.
parapertussis
paraphimosis
Paraplatin
paraplegia
    congenital spastic p.
    infantile spastic p.
parapsoriasis
    guttata p.
parasalpingitis
parasite
    intestinal p.
    ova and p.'s (O&P)

parasitic
    p. fetus
    p. leiomyoma
    p. myoma
    p. pregnancy
parasiticus
    dipygus p.
    janiceps p.
paraspadias
parasympathetic
    p. nerve
    p. nervous system
paratesticular
parathyroid
    p. adenoma
    p. disease
    p. disorder
    p. gland
    p. hormone
parathyromatosis
paratubal cyst
paratyphoid fever
paraurethral
    p. duct
    p. gland
parauterine lymph node
paravaginal
    p. hysterectomy
    p. soft tissue
paravaginitis
paraxial
parchment skin
paregoric
parencephalia
parencephalous
parenchyma
    renal p.
parenchymatous mastitis
parent
    Coping Health Inventory
      for P.'s (CHIP)
parentage
    p. determination
parental origin
parenteral
    p. administration
    p. alimentation
    p. hyperalimentation
    p. medication
    p. nutrition (PN)
    p. progesterone
Parenti-Fraccaro syndrome
paresis

paresthesia
 Berger p.
pargyline
parietal
 p. peritoneum
 p. shunt
parity
Parkinson disease
Parlodel
Parnate
parodynia
 p. perversa
paromomycin sulfate
paronychia
paronychial infection
paroophoritis
paroöphoron
parotid
 p. enlargement
 p. gland
parous
 p. introitus
 p. os
 p. outlet
parovarian
 p. tumor
parovariotomy
parovaritis
parovarium
paroxetine hydrochloride
paroxysmal
 p. nocturnal dyspnea (PND)
 p. nocturnal hemoglobinuria
 p. tachycardia
parrot
 P. artery
 P. atrophy of newborn
 p. jaw
 P. sign
 P. syndrome
Parry-Jones vulvectomy
Parsidol
pars tuberalis
part
 fetal small p.'s
 presenting p.

partial
 p. anomalous pulmonary
  venous return (PAPVR)
 p. breech extraction
 p. hydatidiform mole
 p. pressure of arterial
  carbon dioxide ($PaCO_2$)
 p. pressure of arterial
  oxygen (PaO_2)
 p. pressure of carbon
  dioxide (PCO_2)
 p. pressure of oxygen (PO_2)
 p. thromboplastin time
  (PTT)
 p. zona dissection
particle
 alpha p.
particulate
 p. matter
 p. radiation
partner genes
partograph
parturient
 p. apoplexy
 p. canal
 p. fever
 p. paralysis
parturifacient
parturiometer
parturition
Parvovirus
 P. B19
PAS, PASA
 para-aminosalicylic acid
 PAS stain
**pascal unit of pressure
 measurement (Pa)**
Pasini variant
passage
 transplacental p.
passive
 p. immunity
 p. incontinence
paste
 Monsel p.

NOTES

Pasteur
    P. Institute bacillus
      Calmette-Guérin vaccine
    P. pipette
Pastia sign
Patau syndrome
patch
    blood p.
    moth p.
    Peyer p.
    salmon p.
    transdermal medication p.
patchy infiltrate
patency
    probe p.
    tubal p.
patent
    p. anus
    p. ductus arteriosus (PDA)
    p. processus vaginalis
      peritonei
paternal age
paternity
Pathfinder DFA test
Pathilon
Pathocil
pathogen
pathogenesis
pathognomonic
pathologic
    p. amenorrhea
    p. finding
    p. retraction ring
    p. retraction ring of Bandl
pathological model
pathologist
    Cancer Committee of
      College of American P.'s
pathology
    hilar cell p.
    International Society for
      Gynecologic P. (ISGP)
    perinatal p.
    Society for Gynecologic P.
    uterine p.
pathophysiology
pathway
    Embden-Meyerhof p.
patient
    amenorrheic p.
    anovulatory p.
    antenatal p.
    gynecologic cancer p.

    high-risk p.
    infertile p.
    pregnant cardiac p.
    thalassemic p.
patient-controlled analgesia
pattern
    atypical vessel
    colposcopic p.
    banding p.
    Christmas tree p.
    chromosomal p.
    dysfunctional labor p.
    fern leaf p.
    fetal heart rate p.
    inactivation p.
    mosaic p.
    palm leaf p.
    prominent ductal p.
    silent fetal heart rate p.
    silent oscillatory p.
    snowflake p.
    startle p.
Paul-Bunnell-Davidsohn test
Pavabid
Pavacap
Pavacen
Pavarine
Pavatest
Pavlik harness
pavor
    p. diurnus
    p. nocturnus
Pavulon
PAW
    pulmonary artery wedge
Pawlik fold
PAWP
    pulmonary artery wedge pressure
paws
    Medevice surgical p.
Paxil
Pazo hemorrhoid ointment
Pb4/27
    soft radiation grid P.
PBF
    pulmonary blood flow
PBMC
    peripheral blood mononuclear
     cell
PBS
    phosphate buffered saline
     isotonic PBS
PCAinfuser-Model 310

PCC
Poison Control Center
postcoital contraception
PCE
cis-platinum, cyclophosphamide,
Eldesine
PCO
polycystic ovary
PCO₂
partial pressure of carbon
dioxide
PCOS
polycystic ovary syndrome
PCP
Pneumocystis carinii pneumonia
PCR
polymerase chain reaction
PCR assay
PCR test
PCVC
percutaneous central venous
catheter
PCWP
pulmonary capillary wedge
pressure
PDA
patent ductus arteriosus
bidirectional PDA
PDD
pervasive developmental
disorder
PDI
psychomotor development index
Peacock bromide
peak
Bragg p.
p. expiratory flow rate
(PEFR)
p. inspiratory pressure (PIP)
peak-and-trough levels
Péan forceps
Pearl index
pearls
Bohn epithelial p.
collar of p.
Epstein p.
perineal p.

peau d'orange appearance
p. d. a. of the breast
pectoralis major muscle
pectus
p. carinatum
p. excavatum
p. gallinatum
p. recurvatum
Pederson vaginal speculum
PediaCare
Pedialyte
P. formula
P. oral electrolyte
maintenance solution
PediaPatch
Pediapred
PediaProfen
PediaSure
P. formula
P. liquid nutrition
pediatric
p. bone rongeur
p. bulldog clamp
p. cocktail
P. Early Elemental
Examination (PEEX)
p. gynecology
P. Oncology Group (POG)
p. ovarian teratoma
p. self-retaining retractor
P. Triban
p. vaginoscopy
p. vascular clamp
Pediazole
Pedi-Bath Salts
Pedi-Boro Soak Paks
pedicle clamp
Pedicran with Iron
pedicterus
pediculosis
p. capitis
p. corporis
p. pubis
pedigree chart
Pedi PEG tube
pedis
tinea p.

NOTES

Pedituss Cough
pedologist
pedometer
Pedric
PedTE-Pak-4
Pedtrace-4
    P. hyperalimentation
pedunculated polyp
PedvaxHIB
PEEP
    positive end-expiratory pressure
    PEEP ventilator
PEEX
    Pediatric Early Elemental
    Examination
PEF-24 formula
PEFR
    peak expiratory flow rate
pegademase bovine
Peganone
Peiper reflex
Pelger-Huet anomaly
Pelizaeus-Merzbacher disease
pellagra
pellet
    Testopel P.
    YAG p.
Pellizzi syndrome
pellucida, pl. **pellucidae**
    zona p.
    zonae pellucidae
pellucidum
    septum p.
pelves (*pl. of* pelvis)
pelvic
    p. abscess
    p. adhesive disease (PAD)
    p. architecture
    p. arteriogram
    p. artery
    p. axis
    p. bleeding
    p. boost radiotherapy
    p. brim
    p. cavity
    p. cellulitis
    p. congestion syndrome
    p. contraction
    p. diaphragm
    p. direction
    p. examination
    p. exenteration
    p. exercise

p. exostosis
p. fibromatosis
p. floor
p. floor nerve
p. forceps
p. fracture
p. gutter
p. hematocele
p. inclination
p. index
p. infection
p. inflammation
p. inflammatory disease
  (PID)
p. inlet
p. involvement
p. irradiation
p. joint
p. kidney
p. laparoscopy
p. lymphadenectomy
p. lymph node
p. malignancy in pregnancy
p. mass
p. nerve
p. nerve injury
p. node dissection
p. outlet
p. pain
p. peritonitis
p. plane of greatest
  dimensions
p. plane of inlet
p. plane of least
  dimensions
p. plane of outlet
p. plexus
p. pole
p. presentation
p. recurrence
p. relaxation
p. rest
p. score
p. support index (PSI)
p. surgery
p. tenderness
p. thrombophlebitis
p. vein congestion
p. vein thrombophlebitis
p. version
pelvicephalography
pelvicephalometry
pelvic-floor surgery

pelvifixation
pelvigraph
pelvimeter
Hanely-McDermitt p.
pelvimetry
computed tomographic p.
CT p.
manual p.
planographic p.
stereoscopic p.
x-ray p.
pelvioperitonitis
pelvioplasty
pelvioscopy, pelvoscopy
pelviotomy
pelviperitonitis
pelvis, pl. **pelves**
android p.
anthropoid p.
assimilation p.
axis of p.
beaked p.
bifid p.
contracted p.
cordate p., cordiform p.
Deventer p.
dwarf p.
elephant p.
p. enlargement
flat p.
flying-T p.
frozen p.
funnel-shaped p.
gynecoid p.
heart-shaped p.
inverted p.
p. justo major
p. justo minor
juvenile p.
Kilian p.
kyphotic p.
longitudinal oval p.
masculine p.
mesatipellic p.
Naegele p.
p. nana

Otto p.
p. plana
platypellic p.
platypelloid p.
Prague p.
reniform p.
Robert p.
Rokitansky p.
round p.
sweep the p.
transverse oval p.
pelviscope
pelviscopic intrafascial hysterectomy
pelviscopy
pelvitherm
pelvocephalography
pelvoscopy (*var. of* pelvioscopy)
pemphigoid
bullous p.
pemphigus
benign familial chronic p.
p. vulgaris
Pen A/N
Penbritin
pencil
Valleylab p.
pencil-handled laryngoscope
Pendred syndrome
pendulous abdomen
penetrance
penetrant
p. gene
p. trait
penetration
Penetrex
PenFil
Novolin N P.
Novolin R P.
penicillamine
penicillin
p. G
p. G procaine
p. phenoxymethyl
procaine p.
p. V
penile urethra

NOTES

313

penis
    corona of p.
    hypoplastic p.
penischisis
PEN-Kera moisturizing cream
Penlon infant resuscitator
Penna-Shokeir phenotype
Pennington clamp
penoscrotal transposition
Penrose drain
Pentacef
pentaerythritol tetranitrate
pentalogy syndrome
pentamidine isethionate
penta-X
    p.-X. chromosomal
      aberration
    p.-X. syndrome
Pentazine
pentazocine
Penthrane
Pentids
    P.-P AS
pentobarbital
pentobarbitone
pentology of Fallot
pentosuria
Pentothal
    P. Sodium
pentoxifylline
Pentritol
penumbra
PenVee K
PEP
    progestogen-dependent
    endometrial protein
peptic
    p. ulcer
    p. ulcer disease
peptide
    amino-terminal p.
    atrial natriuretic p.
    brain p.
    carboxyl terminal p. (CTP)
    corticotropin-like
      intermediate lobe p.
    endogenous opioid p.
    gonadotropin-releasing p.
    gonadotropin releasing
      hormone-associated p.
      (GAP)
    gonadotropin-releasing
      hormone-like p.

    opioid p.
    vasoactive intestinal p.
      (VIP)
Peptococcus
    P. anaerobius
    P. asaccharolyticus
    P. niger
Peptostreptococcus
Percocet
Percodan
Percoll technique
percreta
    placenta p.
percussion
    abdominal p.
    p. therapy
percutaneous
    p. blood sampling
    p. central venous catheter
      (PCVC)
    p. drainage
    p. fetal transfusion
    p. line
    p. nephrostomy
    p. nephrostomy catheter
    p. umbilical blood sampling
      (PUBS)
Perduretas Anfetamina
Pereyra
    P. needle suspension
    P. procedure
Perez
    P. reflex
    P. sign
Perez-Castro forceps
perforated bowel
perforation
    ileal p.
    uterine p.
perforator
    Baylor amniotic p.
Performa diagnostic ultrasound
   imaging system
performance
    reproductive p.
perfusion
    placental p.
    renal p.
    uteroplacental p.
pergolide
Pergonal
Periactin
periaortic lymph node

periappendicitis
    p. decidualis
periarteritis nodosa
pericanalicular fibroadenoma
pericardial
    p. puncture
    p. tamponade
pericarditis
pericardium
pericentric inversion
pericervical node
Peri-Cold Pack
pericolpitis
periconceptional rubella
Peridin-C
peridural
    p. analgesia
    p. anesthesia
Peri-Gel Pack
perihepatitis
perihilar streaking
periimplantation
perilobular connective tissue
perimenopausal
    p. woman
perimenopause
perimesonephric cyst
perimetritic
perimetritis
perimortem delivery
perinatal
    p. acidosis
    p. asphyxia
    p. cocaine
    p. death
    p. distress prediction
    p. effect
    p. medicine
    p. morbidity
    p. mortality
    p. mortality rate
    p. outcome
    p. pathology
    p. risk factor
    p. transmission
    p. trauma
perinate

perinatologist
perinatology
perineal
    p. analgesia
    p. anesthesia
    p. body
    p. defect
    p. hygiene
    p. laceration
    p. nerve
    p. pearls
    p. repair
    p. scar
    p. sphincter disruption
perineometer
    Gynos p.
perineorrhaphy
    vaginal p.
perineotomy
perineovaginal fistula
perinephric
    p. abscess
    p. phlegmon
perinephritis
perineum
    dashboard p.
period
    canalicular p.
    effective refractory p.
    embryonic p.
    fertile p.
    intrapartum p.
    last menstrual p. (LMP)
    last normal menstrual p.
     (LNMP)
    menstrual p. (MP)
    missed p.
    postpartum p.
    previous menstrual p.
     (PMP)
    pseudoglandular p.
    puerperal p.
    saccular p.
    terminal saccular p.
periodic
    p. acid-Schiff
    p. auscultation

NOTES

periodic *(continued)*
    p. breathing
    p. fever
    p. patient assessment
periodicity
perioophoritis
perioophorosalpingitis
perioral cyanosis
periostitis
    pubic symphysis p.
periovaritis
peripartum cardiomyopathy
peripheral
    p. androgen activity
    p. androgen activity marker
    p. arterial line
    p. blood mononuclear cell
      (PBMC)
    p. hormone level
    p. hyperalimentation
    p. jaundice
    p. line
    p. mononeuropathy
    p. placental separation
    p. vascular shock
peripherally-inserted central
    catheter (PICC)
periportal hemorrhagic necrosis
perirectal fascia
perisalpingitis
perisalpingoovaritis
perissodactylous
peristalsis
    intestinal p.
peritomy
peritoneal
    p. button
    p. catheter
    p. cavity
    p. cytology
    p. dialysis
    p. envelope
    p. fluid
    p. hernia
    p. implant
    p. insufflation
    p. lavage
    p. mouse
    p. reflection
    p. studding
    p. washings
peritonei
    patent processus vaginalis p.

peritoneum
    abdominal p.
    parietal p.
    visceral p.
peritonitis
    meconium p.
    pelvic p.
    tuberculous p.
Peritrate
peritubal adhesion
periumbilical
    p. incision
    p. pain
periurethral
    p. gland
perivaginitis
perivascular emphysema
periventricular-intraventricular
    hemorrhage
periventricular leukomalacia
perivitelline space
Peri-Warm Pack
Perlutal
Permapen
permethrin
Permitil
pernicious
    p. anemia (PA)
    p. anemia of pregnancy
perocormus
perodactyly
peromelia
peroneal
    p. muscle atrophy
    p. sign
peropus
perosomum
perosplanchnia
peroxide
    hydrogen p.
    zinc p.
perphenazine
Persantine
persistent
    p. anovulation
    p. ectopic pregnancy
    p. estrogen secretion
    p. fetal circulation (PFC)
    p. müllerian duct syndrome
    p. occiput posterior position
    p. occiput posterior
      presentation
    p. ovarian mass

p. pulmonary hypertension
of the newborn (PPHN)
p. trophoblastic tumor
personal probability
Pertofrane
pertubation
pertussis
Bordetella p.
Haemophilus p.
**pervasive developmental disorder
(PDD)**
perversa
parodynia p.
perversus
situs p.
per vias naturales
pes cavus
pessary
Albert-Smith p.
Biswas Silastic vaginal p.
blue ring p.
cube p.
diaphragm p.
doughnut p.
Dumontpallier p.
Dutch p.
Emmert-Gelhorn p.
Findley folding p.
Gariel p.
Gehrung p.
Gellhorn p.
Hodge p.
Mayer p.
Menge p.
Prentif p.
Prochownik p.
prostaglandin p.
ring p.
Smith-Hodge p.
Zwanck p.
pestis
Yersinia p.
petechia, pl. **petechiae**
Peters
P. anomaly
P. ovum
pethidine

petit
P. ligament
p. mal
p. mal epilepsy
petroleum distillate poisoning
petrositis
Peutz-Jeghers syndrome
Peyer patch
**Peyeyra-Lebhertz modification of
Frangenheim-Stoeckel procedure**
Peyronie disease
Pezzer catheter
PF
Astramorph P.
Pfannenstiel incision
Pfaundler-Hurler syndrome
PFC
persistent fetal circulation
Pfeiffer syndrome
P-fimbriae
Pfizerpen
P. AS
Pflüger
cord of P.
PFS
Adriamycin P.
Vincasar P.
PG
prostaglandin
pg
picogram
PGG
prostaglandin G
PGH
prostaglandin H
PGI₂
prostacyclin
PGSI
prostaglandin synthetase
inhibitor
Phaedra complex
phagedenic ulcer
phagocytosis
phakomata
phallus
Phaneuf-Graves repair
Phaneuf uterine artery forceps

NOTES

phantom
p. pregnancy
Schultze p.
pharmacokinetics
quinolone p.
Pharmaseal
P. disposable cervical
dilator
P. disposable uterine sound
pharyngeal
p. diverticulum
p. gonococcal infection
pharyngitis
lymphonodular p.
purulent p.
streptococcal p.
viral p.
phase
active p.
catagen p.
end-expiratory p. (EEP)
fertile p.
follicular p.
hair growth p.
hyperprolactinemia-associated
luteal p.
implantation p.
inadequate luteal p.
latent p.
luteal p.
mitosis p.
proliferative p.
secretory p.
telogen p.
Phazyme infant drops
Ph chromosome
phenacetin
phenanthrene
Phenaphen
Phenazine
Phenazo
phenazocine
Phenazodine
phenazone
phenazopyridine
p. HCl
p. hydrochloride
phencyclidine
phendimetrazine
phenelzine
Phenergan
Phenetron
phenindione

pheniramine
phenobarbital
phenobarbitone
phenocopy
phenogenetics
phenolsulfonphthalein (PSP)
p. test
phenomenon, pl. phenomena
all-or-none p.
Arias-Stella p.
dawn p.
Hata p.
Köbner p.
lip p.
memory p.
piezoelectric p.
rebound p.
recall p.
Rumpel-Leede p.
Somogyi p.
Strassman p.
stuck-twin p.
Wenckebach p.
X-linked p.
phenothiazine
p. poisoning
phenotype
Bombay p.
Penna-Shokeir p.
XX and XY Turner p.
phenotypic
p. sex
p. threshold
phenoxymethyl
penicillin p.
phenoxymethylpenicillin
phenprocoumon
phensuximide
phentanyl
phentermine
phentolamine
phenylalanine
p. hydroxylase
p. 4-monooxygenase
p. mustard
phenylalaninemia
phenylbutazone
phenylephrine
phenylhydantoin
phenylketonuria (PKU)
maternal p.
preconceptionally treated p.
p. test

phenylpropanolamine
phenylpyruvate
phenylpyruvic acid
phenyl salicylate
phenyltoloxamine
phenytoin
pheochromocytoma
Pheryl E
pH (hydrogen ion concentration)
    fetal blood pH
    vaginal pH
Philadelphia chromosome (Ph
  chromosome)
Philip gland
phimosis, pl. phimoses
    p. clitoridis
    p. vaginalis
pHisoHex soap
phlebectasia
phlebitis
    puerperal p.
    suppurative p.
phlebography
phlebometritis
phlebothrombosis
phlegmasia
    p. alba dolens
    cellulitic p.
    p. dolens
    thrombotic p.
phlegmon
    parametrial p.
    perinephric p.
phlegmonous mastitis
Phocas disease
phocomelia
phonocardiography
phorbol ester
phosphatase
    acid p.
    alkaline p.
    placental alkaline p. (PLAP)
phosphate
    p. buffered saline (PBS)
    chromic p.
    Cleocin P.

    clindamycin p.
    polyestradiol p.
phosphatidic acid phosphohydrolase
  (PAPase)
phosphatidylcholine
    disaturated p.
phosphatidylglycerol
phosphatidylinositol (PI)
phosphohydrolase
    phosphatidic acid p.
    (PAPase)
phosphokinase
    creatine p. (CPK)
phospholipase
    p. A_2
    p. activity
    p. C
phospholipid
    p. antibody
phosphorus (P)
    p.-32 (^{32}P)
phosphorylase kinase deficiency
phosphorylation
    myosin light-chain p.
    protein p.
photocoagulation
    laser p.
photodynamic therapy
photometer
    HemoCue hemoglobin p.
    reflectance p.
photomicrograph
photon
photoplethysmography (PPG)
photoretinopathy
photosensitive epilepsy
photostethoscope
phototherapy
    Biliblanket p.
photovaporization
    laser p.
phthalylsulfacetamide
phthalylsulfathiazole
phycomycosis
phygogalactic
Phyllocontin
phylloquinone

NOTES

physical
    p. maturity
    p. therapy (PT)
physician-applied force
physiologic
    p. amenorrhea
    p. anemia
    p. childbirth
    p. follicular regulation
    p. hypogammaglobulinemia
    p. icterus
    p. jaundice
    p. jaundice of the newborn
    p. replacement dose
    p. retraction ring
    p. saline
    p. sclerosis
    p. third-stage management
physiologist
    fetal p.
physiology
    maternal p.
physiotherapy (PT)
physometra
physopyosalpinx
physostigmine
phytanic acid storage disease
phytoagglutinin
phytobezoar
phytomenadione
phytonadione
PI
    phosphatidylinositol
    premature infant
    protease inhibitor
    pulsatility index
        alpha-1 PI
            alpha-1 protease inhibitor
piano-wire adhesion
PICA
    posterior inferior
    communicating artery
pica
PICC
    peripherally-inserted central
    catheter
pickup
    Adson p.'s
    rat tooth p.'s
pickwickian syndrome
picogram (pg)
pi cone monochromatism
picornavirus

PID
    pelvic inflammatory disease
PIE
    postinfectious encephalomyelitis
    preimplantation embryo
    pulmonary infiltrate with
      eosinophilia
    pulmonary interstitial
      emphysema
piebaldness
Pie Medical ultrasound
Pierre Robin syndrome
Piersol point
piezoelectric phenomenon
PIF
    prolactin inhibiting factor
pigeon
    p. breast
    p. toe
pigeon-toed
pigmentation
pigmented lesion
pigmenti
    incontinentia p.
    Naegeli incontinentia p.
pigmentosa
    congenital bullous
      urticaria p.
    retinitis p.
    urticaria p.
pigmentosum
    xeroderma p.
PIH
    pregnancy-induced hypertension
pilaris
    keratosis p.
    pityriasis rubra p.
pileum
pileus
pili
    p. annulati
    p. torti
pill
    birth control p. (BCP)
    combined birth control p.
    morning-after p.
pillar
    Usko p.'s
Pilocar
pilocarpine
    p. iontophoresis method
pilonidal
    p. cyst

p. dimple
p. sinus
Piloptic
pilosebaceous unit
Pilot audiometer
Pima
pimozide
pin
Beath p.
Surgin hemorrhage
occluder p.
Pinard
P. maneuver
P. sign
pincer grasp
pindolol
pineal
p. gland
p. tumor
pinealoma
pingueculum
pink
p. disease
p. tetralogy of Fallot
pinked up
pinna, pl. pinnae
pinworm
p. vaginitis
pion
PIOPED
Prospective Investigation of
Pulmonary Embolus Diagnosis
PIP
peak inspiratory pressure
Pipelle
P. biopsy
P. endometrial suction
curette
piperacetazine
piperacillin
p. sodium
p. sodium/tazobactam
sodium
piperazine
p. dione
p. estrone sulfate
Piper forceps

piperidolate hydrochloride
pipestem urethra
pipette
Pasteur p.
Pipracil
Pirie syndrome
Piskacek sign
Piso test
Pistofidis cervical biopsy forceps
pisum sativum agglutinin (PSA)
Pitocin
P. augmentation
P. induction
Pitressin
pitted (given Pitocin)
pituitary
p. adenoma
p. axis
p. cell
p. desensitization
p. disorder
p. dwarfism
p. gigantism
p. gland
p. gland function
p. gland transplantation
p. gland tumor
p. gonadotropin
p. gonadotropin effect
p. gonadotropin inhibition
p. gonadotropin regulation
p. gonadotropin secretion
p. gonadotropin suppression
p. hormone
p. hormone release
p. necrosis
pituitary-ovarian function
pityriasis
p. alba
p. lichenoides
p. lichenoides et
varioliformis acuta
p. rosea
p. rubra pilaris
PIVKA-II assay
pivot lock

NOTES

321

PK
    pyruvate kinase
PKD
    polycystic kidney disease
PKU
    phenylketonuria
       PKU test
placenta, pl. **placentae**
    ablatio placentae
    abruptio placentae
    accessory p.
    p. accreta
    p. accreta vera
    adherent p.
    amotio placentae
    annular p.
    battledore p.
    bidiscoidal p.
    p. biloba
    p. bipartita
    central p. previa
    chorioallantoic p.
    chorioamnionic p.
    choriovitelline p.
    circummarginate p.
    circumvalate p.
    p. circumvallata
    cotyledonary p.
    deciduate p.
    dichorionic p.
    dichorionic-diamniotic p.
    p. diffusa
    p. dimidiata
    disperse p.
    Duncan p.
    p. duplex
    endotheliochorial p.
    endothelio-endothelial p.
    epitheliochorial p.
    p. extrachorales
    p. fenestrata
    hemochorial p.
    horseshoe p.
    incarcerated p.
    p. increta
    labyrinthine p.
    p. marginata
    p. membranacea
    monochorionic diamniotic p.
    monochorionic
      monoamniotic p.
    p. multiloba
    nondeciduous p.

p. panduraformis
p. percreta
p. previa
p. previa centralis
p. previa creta
p. previa marginalis
p. previa partialis
p. reflexa
p. reniformis
retained p.
Schultze p.
p. spuria
Stallworthy p.
succenturiate p.
supernumerary p.
total p. previa
p. triloba
p. tripartita
p. triplex
twin p.
p. velamentosa
villous p.
zonary p.
placental
    p. abruption
    p. alkaline phosphatase
      (PLAP)
    p. barrier
    p. bleeding site
    p. bruit
    p. cotyledon
    p. dysfunction
    p. dysfunction syndrome
    p. dystocia
    p. extrusion
    p. fragment
    p. giant cell
    p. grade
    p. grading
    p. growth
    p. hemangioma syndrome
    p. hemorrhage
    p. hormone
    p. immunology
    p. implantation
    p. index
    p. infarct
    p. insufficiency
    p. lactogen
    p. leakage
    p. localization
    p. membrane
    p. metastasis

p. migration
p. perfusion
p. polyp
p. presentation
p. protein
p. respiration
p. secretion
p. separation
p. septum
p. sign
p. site
p. site gestational
  trophoblastic disease
p. site nodule
p. site trophoblastic tumor
  (PSTT)
p. souffle
p. stage
p. steroid
p. sulfatase deficiency
p. thickness
p. thrombosis
p. tissue
p. tissue transplant
p. transfer
p. transfusion
p. transfusion syndrome
p. villus
p. weight
placenta, ovary, uterus (POU)
placentascan
placentation
  hemochorioendothelial p.
placentitis
placentography
  indirect p.
placentology
placentoma
placentotherapy
Placidyl
placing reflex
placode
plagiocephaly
plague vaccine
plana
  vertebra p.

plane
  equatorial p.
  first parallel pelvic p.
  fourth parallel pelvic p.
  p. of midpelvis
  p. of pelvic canal
  pelvic p. of greatest
    dimensions
  pelvic p. of inlet
  pelvic p. of least
    dimensions
  pelvic p. of outlet
  second parallel pelvic p.
  third parallel pelvic p.
  wide p.
planning
  family p.
planographic pelvimetry
planovalgus
  talipes p.
plant alkaloid
plantar
  p. crease
  p. dermatosis
  p. reflex
  p. response
  p. wart
plantaris
  keratosis palmaris et p.
planus
  lichen p.
  lichen ruber p. (LRP)
PLAP
  placental alkaline phosphatase
plaque
  pruritic urticarial papules
    and p.'s (PUPP)
  pulmonary p.
plasma
  p. albumin
  p. cell balanitis
  p. cell mastitis
  p. cell pneumonia
  p. cell vulvitis
  p. fibrinogen
  p. fraction
  fresh frozen p. (FFP)

NOTES

plasma *(continued)*
    frozen p.
    p. iron-binding capacity
    p. iron concentration
    p. level
    p. prolactin
    p. prorenin
    p. prorenin increase
    p. protein
    p. testosterone
    p. thromboplastin antecedent (PTA)
    p. thromboplastin antecedent factor
    p. volume
    p. volume expansion
    p. volume regulation
plasmacellularis
    balanitis circumscripta p.
plasmacrit test
Plasmanate
plasmapheresis
plasmid DNA
plasmin
plasminogen
    p. activator (PA)
    p. activator inhibitor type I, II
Plastibell
plastic cup vacuum extractor
plate
    basal p.
    Mancini p.
    neural p.
    trigonal p.
    vaginal p.
plateau
    orgasmic p.
platelet
    p. adhesion
    p. aggregation
    p. antigen
    p. cofactor I
    p. concentrate
    p. count
    p. disorder
    p. function test
    p. neutralization procedure
    p. transfusion
platelet-activating factor
platelet-associated antibody
platelet-derived growth factor
plate-like atelectasis

Platelin Plus Activator
Platinol
    P.-AQ
platinum
platypellic, platypelloid
    p. pelvis
Plegine
pleiotropic gene
pleomastia, pleomazia
pleonosteosis
    Leri p.
plethora hydraemica
plethoric
plethysmography
    impedance p.
    jugular occlusion p.
pleural effusion
Pleur-Evac
pleuritic pain
pleurodesis
    tetracycline p.
pleurodynia
pleuromelus
pleuroperitoneal
    p. foramen
    p. hernia
pleuropulmonic
pleurosomus
plexus
    Auerbach p.
    brachial p.
    cavernous p.
    Frankenhäuser p.
    hypogastric p.
    p. lesion
    Meissner p.
    ovarian p.
    pampiniform p.
    pelvic p.
    submucosal p.
    superior mesenteric p.
    vaginal venous p.
plica, pl. plicae
plicamycin
plication
    Kelly p.
ploidy
plug
    copulation p.
    epithelial p.
    meconium p.
    mucous p.
    silicone p.

plumbism
plume
    electrosurgical p.
    smoke p.
plural pregnancy
Plus
    Answer P.
    Fact P.
PM-60/40
    P. formula
    Similac P.
PMB 200
PMB 400
PMDD
    premenstrual dysphoric disorder
PMP
    previous menstrual period
PMS
    premenstrual syndrome
    Lurline PMS
PMT
    Optivite PMT
PMVP
    pulmonary microvascular
      permeability to protein
PN
    parenteral nutrition
PN_2
    nitrogen partial pressure
PND
    paroxysmal nocturnal dyspnea
pneogaster
pneumatic compression
pneumatocele
pneumatosis cystoides intestinalis
pneumococcal
    p. pneumonia
    p. vaccine
pneumococcus, pl. pneumococci
pneumocystiasis
Pneumocystis carinii pneumonia
  (PCP)
pneumocystography
pneumocystosis
pneumoencephalogram
pneumography
    impedance p.

pneumohydrometra
pneumomediastinum
pneumonia
    acute interstitial p.
    adenoviral p.
    p. alba
    p. alba of Virchow
    aspiration p.
    bacterial p.
    chemical p.
    chickenpox p.
    chlamydial p.
    congenital p.
    eosinophilic p.
    giant cell p.
    Gram-negative p.
    Hecht p.
    hypostatic p.
    interstitial plasma cell p.
    intrauterine p.
    Kaufman p.
    lipoid p.
    lobar p.
    plasma cell p.
    pneumococcal p.
    Pneumocystis carinii p.
    (PCP)
    rheumatic p.
    staphylococcal p.
    streptococcal p.
    thrush p.
    varicella p.
    viral p.
pneumoniae
    Diplococcus p.
    Klebsiella p.
pneumonitis
    aspiration p.
    chemical p.
    viral p.
pneumonocyte
    type II p.
pneumopericardium
pneumoperitoneum
pneumosalpingography
pneumotachography

NOTES

pneumothorax
    tension p.
Pneumovax 23
Pneumo-Wrap
Pnu-Imune 23
PO₂
    partial pressure of oxygen
POA
    pancreatic oncofetal antigen
POC
    products of conception
pocket
    amniotic fluid p.
Pocketpeak peak flow meter
podalic
    p. extraction
    p. version
Pod-Ben-25
podencephalus
podofilox
podophyllin
podophyllum
    p. resin
POEMS
    polyneuropathy, organomegaly,
    endocrinopathy, M protein,
    skin changes
        POEMS syndrome
POG
    Pediatric Oncology Group
poikiloderma
    p. congenitale of Rothmund
poikiloploidy
point
    p. A, subspinale
    p. B, supramentale
    cardinal p.'s
    Halle p.
    Legat p.
    McBurney p.
    Munro p.
    p. mutation
    Piersol p.
    trigger p.
pointes
    torsade de p.
Poiseville-Hagen relationship
Poiseville law
Poison Control Center (PCC)
poisoning
    barbiturate p.
    carbon monoxide p.
    lead p.

petroleum distillate p.
phenothiazine p.
salicylate p.
scopolamine p.
strychnine p.
thallium p.
zinc p.
pokeweed mitogen (PWM)
Poland
    P. anomaly
    P. malformation sequence
    P. syndrome
polar
    p. body
    p. presentation
Polaramine
Polaris
    P. reusable cutters
    P. reusable dissector
    P. reusable forceps
    P. reusable grasper
    P. reusable instrument
polarization
    amniotic fluid
        fluorescence p.
    fluorescent p.
pole
    cephalic p.
    fetal p.
    germinal p.
    pelvic p.
poliodystrophia cerebri progressiva
    infantilis
poliodystrophy
polioencephalitis
    bulbar p.
poliomyelitis
poliovirus hominis
polish
    Sklar p.
Politano-Leadbetter
    ureteroneocystostomy
Poloxamer 407 barrier material
polyamine
polyarteritis nodosa
polyarthritis
polyarticular juvenile rheumatoid
    arthritis
polybutester
polycarbophil
    calcium p.
polycheiria
polychlorinated biphenyl

polychondritis
Polycillin
    P.-N
polyclonal antibody
Polycose formula
Poly CS device
polycyesis
polycystic
    p. fibrous dysplasia
    p. kidney disease (PKD)
    p. ovarian disease
    p. ovary (PCO)
    p. ovary syndrome (PCOS)
    p. renal disease
polycythemia
    p. rubra vera
    p. vera
polydactylism
polydactyly
    short rib-p.
polydimethylsiloxane
polydioxanone
polydipsia
polydysplasia
    hereditary ectodermal p.
polydysspondylism
polydystrophy
    pseudo-Hurler p.
polyembryony
polyester suture material
polyestradiol phosphate
polyethylene suture material
polygalactia
polygalactide suture
Polygam
    P. S/D
polygene
polygenic
    p. disorder
    p. inheritance
polyglandular syndrome
polyglycol suture
polyglyconate suture
polygnathus
Poly-Histine
    P.-H. CS

P.-H. D
P.-H. DM
polyhydramnios
polyhypermenorrhea
polyhypomenorrhea
polymastia, polymazia
polymenorrhea
polymerase
    p. chain reaction (PCR)
    DNA p.
    DNA-directed p.
    DNA-directed RNA p.
    RNA p.
    RNA-directed DNA p.
polymetacarpia
polymetatarsia
polymicrobial bacteremia
polymicrogyria
polymorphic light eruption of
    pregnancy
polymorphism
    restriction fragment
        length p. (RFLP)
polymorphonucleocyte
Polymox
polymyositis
    primary idiopathic p.
polymyxin
    p. B sulfate
polyneuritis
    infantile p.
polyneuropathy
    erythredema p.
polyneuropathy, organomegaly,
    endocrinopathy, M protein, skin
    changes (POEMS)
polyostotic fibrous dysplasia
polyotia
polyp
    adenomatous p.
    cervical p.
    colonic p.
    endocervical p.
    endometrial p.
    fibrinous p.
    hydatid p.
    hyperplastic p.

NOTES

polyp *(continued)*
 pedunculated p.
 placental p.
 retention p.
 sessile p.
polypectomy
polypeptide
 S-methionine-labeled p.
 vasoactive intestinal p.
 (VIP)
polyphosphatidylinositide
polyphospholinostied
polyploidy
polypoid hyperplasia
polyposis
 colonic p.
polypropylene
 p. fascial strip
 p. suture material
polyscelia
polyserositis
 idiopathic p.
polysomia
polysomnogram
 p. with flow-volume loops
polysomy
 sex chromosomal p.
Polysonic ultrasound lotion
polyspermy, polyspermia
polysplenia
 p. syndrome
polysymbrachydactyly
polysyndactyly
polytene chromosome
polytetrafluoroethylene graft
polythelia
polythiazide
Polytrim
polyuria
polyvalent
 p. immunoglobulin therapy
 p. pneumococcal vaccine
Poly-Vi-Flor vitamins
Poly-Vi-Sol vitamins
POMARD anthropomorphic measurement reference chart
POMC
 pro-opiomelanocortin
 propriomelanocortin
Pomeroy
 P. operation
 P. tubal ligation

Pompe
 P. disease
 P. syndrome
ponderal index
Pondimin
Ponstel
Pontén fasciocutaneous flap
pontine
 p. glioma
 p. tumor
Pontocaine
pool
 gene p.
 vaginal p.
pop
 Revital-Ice rehydrating freezer p.
popcorn-like calcification
popliteal
 p. cyst
 p. pterygium syndrome
 p. web syndrome
Porak-Durante syndrome
porcine surfactant
porcupine skin
porencephalic cyst
porencephaly
Porges-Meier test
pork insulin
porokeratosis
porphyria
 acute intermittent p.
 congenital erythropoietic p.
 congenital photosensitive p.
 p. cutanea tarda
 p. cutanea tarda hereditaria
 p. cutanea tarda symptomatica
 cutaneous hepatic p.
 erythrohepatic p.
 erythropoietic p.
 hepatic p.
 hepatoerythropoietic p.
 intermittent p.
 mixed p.
 ovulocyclic p.
 South African genetic p.
 Swedish p.
 symptomatic p.
 p. variegata
 variegate p.
porphyric neuropathy
porphyrin metabolism disorder

Porro
  P. cesarean section
  P. hysterectomy
  P. operation
portable respirator
Portagen formula
portal hypertension
Porter-Silber reaction
portio, pl. **portiones**
  p. vaginalis
Portland
  hemoglobin P.
Portuguese disease
port-wine
  p.-w. hemangioma
  p.-w. mark
  p.-w. nevus
  p.-w. stain
Posiero effect
position (*See also* presentation)
  arm p.
  asynclitic p.
  back-up p.
  batrachian p.
  Bozeman p.
  brow p.
  brow-anterior p.
  brow-down p.
  brow-posterior p.
  brow-up p.
  chin p.
  decubitus p.
  dorsal birthing p.
  dorsal lithotomy p.
  Duncan p.
  Edebohl p.
  en face p.
  English p.
  face-to-pubes p.
  fetal p.
  fetal head p.
  Fowler p.
  frogleg p.
  frontoanterior p.
  frontoposterior p.
  frontotransverse p.
  genucubital p.

  genupectoral p.
  jackknife p.
  knee-chest p.
  knee-elbow p.
  Kraske p.
  lateral recumbent p.
  left frontoanterior p. (LFA)
  left frontoposterior p. (LFP)
  left frontotransverse p.
    (LFT)
  left mentoanterior p. (LMA)
  left mentoposterior p.
    (LMP)
  left mentotransverse p.
    (LMT)
  left occipitoanterior p.
    (LOA)
  left occipitoposterior p.
    (LOP)
  left occipitotransverse p.
    (LOT)
  left sacroanterior p. (LSA)
  left sacroposterior p. (LSP)
  left sacrotransverse p. (LST)
  left scapuloanterior p.
    (LScA)
  left scapuloposterior p.
    (LScP)
  lithotomy p.
  maternal p.
  maternal birthing p.
  mentoanterior p.
  mentoposterior p.
  mentotransverse p.
  mentum anterior p.
  mentum posterior p.
  mentum transverse p.
  missionary p.
  obstetric p.
  occipitoanterior p.
  occipitoposterior p.
  occipitotransverse p.
  persistent occiput
    posterior p.
  right
    acromiodorsoposterior p.

NOTES

position *(continued)*
    right frontoanterior p.
    (RFA)
    right frontoposterior p.
    (RFP)
    right frontotransverse p.
    (RFT)
    right mentoanterior p.
    (RMA)
    right mentoposterior p.
    (RMP)
    right mentotransverse p.
    (RMT)
    right occipitoanterior p.
    (ROA)
    right occipitoposterior p.
    (ROP)
    right occipitotransverse p.
    (ROT)
    right sacroanterior p. (RSA)
    right sacroposterior p.
    (RSP)
    right sacrotransverse p.
    (RST)
    right scapuloanterior p.
    (RScA)
    right scapuloposterior p.
    (RScP)
    sacroanterior p.
    sacroposterior p.
    sacrotransverse p.
    semi-Fowler p.
    semiprone p.
    Simon p.
    Sims p.
    supine p.
    Trendelenburg p.
    Valentine p.
    vertex p.
    Walcher p.
positive
    p. end-expiratory pressure
    (PEEP)
    Hematest p.
    heme p.
positivity
    lymph node p.
    paraaortic p.
postadolescence
postaugmentation
postcoital
    p. bleeding
    p. contraception (PCC)

    p. estrogen
    p. test
postconceptional age
postdate
    p. pregnancy
postdatism
posterior
    anterior and p. (A&P)
    p. asynclitism
    p. commissure
    p. fontanel
    p. fornix
    p. fossa cyst
    p. inferior communicating
    artery (PICA)
    p. lie
    occiput p. (OP)
    p. pelvic exenteration
    p. probability
    p. repair
    p. sagittal diameter
    p. urethritis
    p. vaginismus
posterolateral fontanel
posthetomy
postinfectious encephalomyelitis
  (PIE)
postinflammatory adenopathy
postirradiation syndrome
postischemic stenosis
postlumpectomy
postmature
    p. infant
postmaturity
    p. syndrome
postmembrane
    p. pressure
    p. rupture
postmenarchal
    p. bleeding
    p. cycle
    p. cyclicity
postmenopausal
    p. amenorrhea
    p. atrophy
    p. bleeding
    p. body mass
    p. bone loss
    p. estrogen replacement
    therapy
    p. hirsutism
    p. level
    p. osteoporosis

p. syndrome
p. woman
postmenopause
postmenstrual stress
postmortem
p. delivery
p. study
postnatal
p. year
postoperative
p. bladder dysfunction
p. care
p. chemotherapy
p. complication
p. cystitis
p. pelvic radiation
p. radiation
p. radiotherapy
p. sepsis
p. seroma
p. shock
p. symptom analysis
p. voiding dysfunction
postovulatory age
postpartum
p. amenorrhea
p. attitude
p. blues
p. cardiomyopathy
p. care
p. depression
p. hemolytic uremic
  syndrome
p. hemorrhage
p. hypertension
p. infection
p. period
p. pituitary necrosis
  syndrome
p. pleuropulmonary and
  cardiac disease
p. psychosis
p. tetanus
p. thyroiditis
postperfusion syndrome
postpill amenorrhea

postpuberal, postpubertal
postpuberty
postpubescent
postradiation
p. cystitis
p. fistula
p. periureteral fibrosis
postreduction
p. mammaplasty
postrubella syndrome
postsurgical fat necrosis
postterm
p. infant
p. pregnancy
posttraumatic fat necrosis
posttubal ligation syndrome
postulate
Koch p.'s
postural
p. deformity
p. proteinuria
p. version
posture
fetal p.
postvoid
potassium (K)
p. bromide
p. chloride
p. citrate
p. gluconate
p. hydroxide (KOH)
p. iodide
p. iodide Enseals
potbelly
potential
auditory evoked p.'s (AEP)
brainstem auditory
  evoked p.'s (BAEP)
resting membrane p.
vertex p.
visual evoked p. (VEP)
Potter
P. disease
P. facies
P. syndrome
P. version

NOTES

POU
>placenta, ovary, uterus
>POU theory of Ishihara

pouch
>Broca p.
>continent urinary p.
>copulating p.
>Dennis-Brown p.
>Douglas p.
>Florida p.
>Indiana p.
>intravaginal p.
>kangaroo p.
>Kock p.
>labioperineal p.
>Mainz p.
>Morison p.
>Reality vaginal p.
>rectouterine p.
>Rowland p.
>Seessel p.
>wallaby p.

Poupart ligament
Pourcelot index
povidone-iodine
>p.-i. douche
>p.-i. wipe

powder
>p. pseudocalcification
>Sklar Kleen p.

Pozzi procedure
PPG
>photoplethysmography

PPHN
>persistent pulmonary
>hypertension of the newborn

PPROM
>preterm premature rupture of
>membranes

PPTT
>prepubertal testicular tumor

Practices
>Advisory Committee on
>Immunization P. (ACIP)

practitioner
>Royal College of
>General P.'s (RCGP)

Prader-Gurtner syndrome
Prader-Labhart-Willi syndrome
Prader-Willi syndrome
praevia (*var. of* previa)

Prague
>P. maneuver
>P. pelvis

pralidoxime chloride
Pramet FA
Pramilet FA
PRAMS
>Pregnancy Risk Assessment
>Monitoring System

Pratt dilator
prazosin
preadolescent vaginal bleeding
preantral follicle
precancerous lesion
Precef
precipitable
precipitant
precipitate
>p. labor
>p. labor and delivery

precipitin
precipitous
>p. delivery
>p. labor

Precise
>P. disposable skin stapler
>P. pregnancy test

precision
preclinical carcinoma
precocious
>p. adrenarche
>p. pseudopuberty
>p. puberty
>p. teeth

precocity
preconceptionally treated
>**phenylketonuria**
preconception care
precox
>dentia p.
>icterus p.
>macrogenitosomia p.
>pubertas p.

predecidual
predeciduous teeth
prediction
>perinatal distress p.
>prenatal risk p.
>scar p.

predictive value of test
predictor
>Clearplan Easy ovulation p.
>Conceive Ovulation P.

First Response ovulation p.
morbidity p.
mortality p.
OvuQUICK Self-Test
  ovulation p.
Q-test ovulation p.
prednisolone
prednisone
preeclampsia
  early-onset p.
  p. headache
  superimposed p.
preeclamptic toxemia
preembryo
preemie
Prefill
  Femstat P.
Pregestimil formula
PregnaGen test kit
pregnancy
  abdominal p.
  aborted ectopic p.
  accidental p.
  acute fatty liver of p.
  adolescent p.
  ampullar p.
  at-risk p.
  Besnier prurigo of p.
  bigeminal p.
  bilateral ectopic p.
  bilateral simultaneous
    tubal p.'s
  broad ligament p.
  p. cell
  cervical p.
  chemical p.
  cholestatic hepatosis of p.
  combined p.
  p. complication
  compound p.
  cornual p.
  p. dating
  direct agglutination p.
    (DAP)
  ectopic p.
  epulis of p.
  euploid p.

extraamniotic p.
extrachorial p.
extramembranous p.
extrauterine p.
fallopian p.
false p.
fatty liver of p.
p. fear
full-term p.
gemellary p.
grand p.
hepatic p.
heterotopic p.
high-risk p.
p. hormone
hydatid p.
idiopathic cholestasis of p.
interstitial p.
intrahepatic cholestasis of p.
intraligamentary p.
intramural p.
intraperitoneal p.
intrauterine p. (IUP)
late p.
p. loss
p. luteoma
p. management
mask of p.
mesometric p.
molar p.
multifetal p.
multiple p.
mural p.
near-term p.
p. outcome
ovarian p.
ovarioabdominal p.
parasitic p.
pelvic malignancy in p.
pernicious anemia of p.
persistent ectopic p.
phantom p.
plural p.
polymorphic light eruption
  of p.
postdate p.
postterm p.

NOTES

pregnancy *(continued)*
  previous p.
  prolonged p.
  pruritic urticarial papules
    and plaques of p.
  recurrent jaundice of p.
  refractory anemia of p.
  P. Risk Assessment
    Monitoring System
    (PRAMS)
  sarcofetal p.
  secondary abdominal p.
  singleton p.
  splenic p.
  spurious p.
  successful p.
  SureCell rapid test kit
    for p.
  term p.
  p. test
  toxemia of p.
  toxemic rash of p.
  treatment-associated p.
  treatment-independent p.
  tubal p.
  tuboabdominal p.
  tuboovarian p.
  tubouterine p.
  p. tumor
  twin p.
  unplanned p.
  uterine p.
  uteroabdominal p.
  voluntary interruption of p.
    (VIP)
  p. wastage
  p. zone protein
pregnancy-associated
  p.-a. globulin
  p.-a. hypoplastic anemia
  p.-a. plasma protein
  p.-a. plasma protein A
    (PAPPA)
pregnancy-induced hypertension
  (PIH)
pregnancy-specific protein
pregnancy, uterine, not delivered
  (PUND)
pregnane
pregnanediol
5β-pregnane-3,20-dione
pregnanetriol

pregnant
  p. cardiac patient
  p. diabetic
pregnenolone
Pregnosis
Pregnyl
pregranulosa cells
preimplantation
  p. embryo (PIE)
preinvasive cervical disease
prelabor
  p. membrane rupture
Prelu-2
premalignant
  p. disease
  p. lesion
premammary abscess
Premarin
  P. With Methyltestosterone
    Oral
premature
  p. accelerated lung
    maturation (PALM)
  p. adrenarche
  p. airway closure
  p. amnion rupture
  p. birth
  p. centromere division
  p. delivery
  p. ductus arteriosis closure
  p. ejaculation
  P. formula
  p. infant (PI)
  p. labor
  p. luteal regression
  p. membrane rupture
  p. menopause
  p. pubarche
  p. rupture
  p. rupture of membranes
    (PROM)
  P. Special Care formula
  p. thelarche
  p. uterine contraction
    inhibition
  p. ventricular contraction
    (PVC)
prematurity
  anemia of p.
  apnea of p.
  pulmonary insufficiency
    of p.

retinopapillitis of p.
retinopathy of p. (ROP)
premembrane
p. pressure
p. rupture
premenarchal vulvovaginitis
premenstrual
p. dysphoric disorder
(PMDD)
p. edema
p. salivary syndrome
p. symptoms
p. syndrome (PMS)
p. tension
p. tension syndrome
premenstruum
premutation allele
prenatal
p. care
p. detection
p. diagnosis
p. diethylstilbestrol exposure
p. genetic diagnosis
p. genetics
p. mortality
p. risk factor
p. risk prediction
p. screening
p. selection
p. sex determination
p. treatment
p. ultrasound
Prenate 90
Prentif
P. cavity-rim cervical sap
P. pessary
preovulatory
p. follicle
p. LH surge
prep
preparation
KOH p.
wet p.
Pre-Par
preparation (prep)
bowel p.

International Reference P.
(IRP)
**Preparation-H hydrocortisone 1%
cream**
Prepidil
P. Gel
P. Gel cervical ripener
prepregnancy care
prepuberal, prepubertal
prepubescent
prerenal azotemia
prereproductive
presacral
p. nerve
p. neurectomy
p. sympathectomy
presentation (*See also* position)
acromion p.
arm p.
breech p.
brow p.
brow-down p.
cephalic p.
complete breech p.
compound p.
p. of cord
double-breech p.
double-footling p.
Duncan p.
face p.
face/chin p.
p. of fetus
footling p., foot p.
footling breech p.
frank breech p.
full-breech p.
funic p.
hand and head p.
head p.
incomplete breech p.
incomplete foot p.
incomplete knee p.
knee p.
longitudinal p.
mentoanterior p.
mentoposterior p.
oblique p.

NOTES

presentation *(continued)*
    occiput p.
    pelvic p.
    persistent occiput
      posterior p.
    placental p.
    polar p.
    right occipitoposterior p.
    shoulder p.
    sincipital p.
    single-breech p.
    single-footling p.
    torso p.
    transverse p.
    transverse lie p.
    trunk p.
    umbilical p.
    vertex p.
presenting part
presomite embryo
Press-Mate model 8800T blood
  pressure monitor
pressor
    p. agent
    p. medication
    p. response
pressure
    alveolar partial p. (PA)
    arterial blood p.
    arterial carbon dioxide p.
      (tension) $(PaCO_2)$
    arterial partial p. (Pa)
    blood p.
    central venous p. (CVP)
    colloid osmotic p. (COP)
    continuous distending
      airway p. (CDAP)
    continuous negative
      airway p. (CNAP)
    continuous positive
      airway p. (CPAP)
    end-expiratory p. (EEP)
    esophageal p.
    high-frequency positive p.
      (HFPP)
    intraabdominal p.
    intravesical p.
    jugular venous p. (JVP)
    maternal abdominal p.
    maximum urethral
      closure p. (MUCP)
    mean arterial p. (MAP)

    negative end-expiratory p.
      (NEEP)
    nitrogen partial p. (PN_2)
    osmotic p.
    peak inspiratory p. (PIP)
    positive end-expiratory p.
      (PEEP)
    postmembrane p.
    premembrane p.
    pressure, partial p. (P)
    pulmonary artery wedge p.
      (PAWP)
    pulmonary capillary
      wedge p. (PCWP)
    p. transmission
    urethral p.
    zero end-expiratory p.
pressure-cycled ventilator
pressure-preset ventilator
pressure-separator tubing
preterm
    p. birth
    p. delivery
    p. infant
    p. labor
    p. labor arrest
    p. neonate
    p. premature rupture of
      membranes (PPROM)
    p. rupture of membranes
pretransfusion Hct
prevalence rate
previa, praevia
    central placenta p.
    placenta p.
    vasa p.
previable fetus
previllous embryo
previous
    p. maternal immunity
    p. menstrual period (PMP)
    p. pregnancy
previus blockage at childbirth
Prevotella
    P. biviua
    P. disiens
prezygotic
PRF
    prolactin releasing factor
prickly heat
primaquine
primary
    p. amenorrhea

p. atelectasis
p. bubo
p. cesarean section
p. congenital glaucoma
p. dysmenorrhea
p. embryonic cell
p. empty sella syndrome
p. follicle
p. idiopathic
  dermatomyositis
p. idiopathic polymyositis
p. infertility
p. oocyte
p. uterine inertia
Primatene
  P. Mist
Primaxin
primidone
primigravida
  elderly p.
priming
  cervical p.
primipara
primiparity
primiparous
primitive
  p. (fetal) hemoglobin (HbP)
  p. groove
  p. knot
  p. ovum
  p. reflex
  p. streak
primordial
  p. dwarfism
  p. follicle
  p. germ cell
  p. ovum
  vesicourethral p.
primordium
primum
  foramen p.
  septum p.
Principen
principle
  Doppler p.
  Fick p.

Frank-Starling p.
Mitrofanoff p.
prior probability
Priscoline
Pritchard intramuscular regimen
private blood group
probability
  conditional p.
  joint p.
  objective p.
  personal p.
  posterior p.
  prior p.
  subjective p.
Probalan
Pro-Banthine
probe
  BICAP p.
  BiLAP bipolar
    laparoscopic p.
  biopsy p.
  biplane intracavitary p.
  Bipolar Circumactive P.
    (BICAP)
  blunt p.
  Bruehl-Kjaer transvaginal
    ultrasound p.
  convex p.
  DNA p.
  Endopath needle tip
    electrosurgery p.
  endovaginal p.
  Envision endocavity p.
  gene p.
  IntraDop p.
  MEVA p.
  multiplane intracavitary p.
  nucleic acid p.
  p. patency
  ribonucleic acid p.
  p. sheath
  Spencer p.
  transrectal p.
  transvaginal transducer p.
  Universal vaginal p.
  ViraType p.
  YSI neonatal temperature p.

NOTES

probenecid
problem
   dietary p.
   growth p.
   intersex p.
   nutritional p.
   psychosexual p.
procainamide
procaine
   p. penicillin
   penicillin G p.
procarbazine
Procardia
procedure
   Abbe-McIndoe p.
   Abbe-McIndoe-Williams p.
   Abbe-Wharton-McIndoe p.
   Aldridge sling p.
   Baden p.
   Baldy-Webster p.
   Bastiaanse-Chiricuta p.
   Blair-Brown p.
   Blalock-Hanlon p.
   Blalock-Taussig p.
   Bricker p.
   Burch p.
   Castaneda p.
   Chassar Moir-Sims p.
   Chassar Moir sling p.
   Cole intubation p.
   Cyclops p.
   Danus-Fontan p.
   Davydov p.
   diagnostic p.
   Donald p.
   dot-blot p.
   Duckett p.
   Estes p.
   Evans-Steptoe p.
   Everard Williams p.
   fascial sling p.
   Fontan p.
   Frank p.
   Fredet-Ramstedt p.
   Gepfert p.
   Gittes p.
   Goebell p.
   Goebell-Stoeckel-
     Frangenheim p.
   hemi-Fontan p.
   Heyman-Herndon
     clubfoot p.
   Hood p.

   Ilizarov p.
   Ingelman-Sundberg gracilis
     muscle p.
   interventional p.
   intestinal bypass p.
   Jatene p.
   Kaliscinski ureteral p.
   Kasai p.
   Kelly plication p.
   Kennedy p.
   Kono p.
   Ladd p.
   Lash p.
   Ledbetter-Politano p.
   loop electrosurgical
     excision p. (LEEP)
   Marshall-Marchetti p.
   Marshall-Marchetti-Krantz p.
   Martius p.
   Mayo-Fueth inversion p.
   McCall-Schumann p.
   McDonald p.
   McIndoe-Hayes p.
   Meigs-Okabayashi p.
   MMK p.
   Mustard p.
   Neugebauer-LeFort p.
   Nichols p.
   Olshausen p.
   Pereyra p.
   Peyeyra-Lebhertz
     modification of
     Frangenheim-Stoeckel p.
   platelet neutralization p.
   Pozzi p.
   psoas hitch p.
   Ramstedt p.
   Raz p.
   Raz-Leach p.
   Récamier p.
   Richter and Albrich p.
   Schauffler p.
   Shauta-Aumreich p.
   Shirodkar p.
   sling p.
   Spence p.
   Stamey modification of
     Pereyra p.
   Stanley Way p.
   Swenson pull-through p.
   vaginal wall sling p.
   valvulotomy p.
Pro-Ception

process
- binary p.
- freezing p.
- immune p.
- quality assurance p.

processor
- ThinPrep p.

processus

prochlorperazine

Prochownick method

Prochownik pessary

procidentia
- p. uteri

procollagenase

PRO/Covers ultrasound probe sheath

procreation
- assisted medical p. (AMP)

proctitis

proctocolpoplasty

ProctoCream-HC

proctoelytroplasty

ProctoFoam-HC

proctography
- evacuation p.

proctosigmoiditis

proctosigmoidoscopy

proctotomy

procyclidine

Procytox

Pro-Depo

prodromal labor

Prodrox

product
- P. 80056
- alpha-1 thymosin p.
- blood p.
- p.'s of conception (POC)
- fibrin degradation p.

Pro-Duosterone

prodynorphin

proencephalus

proenkephalin A

proenkephalin B

proenzyme

Profasi HP

profenamine

proficiency
- Bruininks-Oseretsky Test of Motor P.

profile
- biometric p.
- biophysical p. (BPP)
- coagulation p.
- lung p.
- protein p.
- urethral pressure p.
- velocity flow p.
- P. viral probe test

profunda
- miliaria p.

PRO/Gel ultrasound transmission gel

progeria

Progestasert
- P. intrauterine device

progestational
- p. agent
- p. challenge
- p. protection
- p. therapy

progesterone
- p. breakthrough bleeding
- p. challenge test
- p. dermatitis
- p. level
- p. metabolism
- micronized p.
- p. myometrial level
- parenteral p.
- p. receptor
- p. secretion
- serum p.
- p. synthesis
- urinary free p.
- p. withdrawal bleeding

progesterone-releasing T-shaped device

progestin
- C_{21} p.
- norgestimate p.
- p. oral contraceptive

progestin-impregnated vaginal ring

NOTES

progestogen
     p. support therapy
progestogen-dependent endometrial
     protein (PEP)
Proglycem
prognathism
prognosis
     clinical p.
prognostic
     p. factor
     p. indicator
     p. scoring system
Prognosticon Dri-Dot
program
     Early and Periodic
        Screening, Diagnosis, and
        Treatment p. (EPSDT)
progress
     failure to p.
progression
     intraepithelial disease p.
     tumor p.
progressiva
     myositis ossificans p.
progressive
     p. familial scleroderma
     p. systemic sclerosis
Project
     Breast Cancer Detection
        Demonstration P.
        (BCDDP)
     Human Genome P.
     National Collaborative
        Diethylstilbestrol
        Adenosis P. (DESAD)
     National Surgical Adjuvant
        Breast P. (NSABP)
projectile vomiting
prokaryote
prolactin
     p. inhibiting factor (PIF)
     p. level
     plasma p.
     p. regulation
     p. releasing factor (PRF)
     p. secretion
     serum p.
     p. stimulation
     p. suppression
prolactinoma
     bromocriptine-resistant p.
     estrogen-induced p.

prolactin-secreting
     p.-s. adenoma
     p.-s. macroadenoma
prolamine
prolan
prolapse
     cervical p.
     p. of corpus luteum
     first degree p.
     mitral valve p.
     second degree p.
     third degree p.
     p. of umbilical cord
     urethral p.
     uterine p.
     p. of uterus
     vaginal p.
     vaginal stump p.
     vaginal vault p.
Prolene suture
proliferation
proliferative phase
proline amino acid
proline aminopeptidase activity
prolinemia
     encephalopathy with p.
Prolixin
Proloid
prolonged
     p. gestation
     p. labor
     p. pregnancy
     p. Q-T syndrome
     p. rupture
     p. rupture of membranes
        (PROM)
Proloprim
PROM
     premature rupture of membranes
     prolonged rupture of membranes
prometaphase
promethazine
prominence
     Rokitansky p.
prominent ductal pattern
pronate
pronatis
pronephros
Pronestyl
pronucleate stage embryo transfer
     (PROST)
pronucleus
pro-opiomelanocortin (POMC)

pro-oxyphysin
Propacil
Propaderm
propantheline bromide
proparacaine
prophase
prophylactic
    p. antibiotic
    p. aspirin use
    p. chemotherapy
    p. heparin
    p. immunization
    p. medication
    p. oophorectomy
    p. red-cell transfusion
    p. tetracycline
prophylaxis
    aspiration p.
    neonatal ocular p.
    ocular p.
    SBE p.
    silver nitrate eye p.
    vitamin K p.
propionate
    beclomethasone p.
    clobetasol p.
propositus
propoxyphene
propping reflex
propranolol
    p. hydrochloride
pro-pressophysin
propria
    lamina p.
propriomelanocortin (POMC)
proptosis
propylthiouracil
Propyl-Thyracil
prorenin
    plasma p.
prorenin-renin-angiotensin system
Prosed/DS
ProSobee formula
prosogaster
prosopoanoschisis
prosopopagus
prosoposchisis

prosoposternodymus
prosopothoracopagus
Prospective Investigation of Pulmonary Embolus Diagnosis (PIOPED)
PROST
    pronucleate stage embryo transfer
prostacyclin (PGI$_2$)
    p. deficiency
prostaglandin (PG)
    p. biosynthesis
    p. E
    p. E$_2$
    p. E$_2$ gel
    p. F$_{2\alpha}$
    p. F$_2$
    p. G (PGG)
    p. H (PGH)
    p. I$_2$
    p. metabolism
    p. pessary
    p. suppository
    p. synthase
    p. synthesis inhibition
    p. synthetase inhibitor (PGSI)
prostanoid
Prostaphlin
prostatic utricle
Pro-Step hCG
prosthesis, pl. prostheses
    breast p.
    vaginal prolapse p.
    valvular p.
Prostigmin
Prostin F2 alpha
Prostin/15M
protamine
    p. insulin zinc suspension
protease inhibitor (PI)
ProtectaCap cap
protection
    progestational p.
protein
    binding p.
    p. binding

NOTES

341

protein *(continued)*
 carrier p.
 cow's milk p. (CMP)
 C-reactive p. (CRP)
 endometrial p.
 feto-neonatal estrogen-
  binding p.
 follicle regulatory p. (FRP)
 G p.
 gonadotrophin-releasing
  hormone-like p.
 H-ras p21 p.
 p. kinase C
 lipoprotein receptor-
  related p. (LRP)
 p. marker
 myeloma p.
 ovine trophoblast p.-1
 p. phosphorylation
 placental p.
 plasma p.
 pregnancy-associated
  plasma p.
 pregnancy-specific p.
 pregnancy zone p.
 p. profile
 progestogen-dependent
  endometrial p. (PEP)
 pulmonary microvascular
  permeability to p. (PMVP)
 receptor-associated p. (RAP)
 p. standard
 Tamm-Horsfall p.
 thyroxine-binding p. (TBP)
 vitamin D-binding p.
 zona p.
proteinase
proteinosis
 lipoid p.
proteinuria
 gestational p.
 glomerular p.
 orthostatic p.
 postural p.
 tubular p.
proteoglycans
proteolysis
proteolytic enzyme
Proteus
 P. mirabilis
 P. morganii
Prothazine
prothrombin time (PT)

prothrombokinase
protoblast
protocol
 Bagshawe p.
 maternal serum SFP3
  screening p.
 modified Bagshawe p.
  (MBP)
 rape p.
 wean-and-feed p.
protogaster
proton
proto-oncogene
 c-fms p.-o.
 HER-2/neu p.-o.
Protopam
protoporphyria
Protostat
protraction
protriptyline
Protropin
 P. growth hormone
Proval
Proventil
Provera
 P.-Testpac
Providencia rettgeri
proxetil
 cefpodoxime p.
proximal
 p. femoral focal deficiency
 p. occlusion
 p. tubal blockage
proxy
 Münchhausen syndrome
  by p. (MSBP)
Prozac
 P. pulvule
Prozine-50
prune-belly syndrome
prurigo
 p. gestationis
pruritic
 p. urticarial papule
 p. urticarial papules and
  plaques (PUPP)
 p. urticarial papules and
  plaques of pregnancy
pruritus
 p. ani
 p. gravidarum
 p. vulvae
 vulvar p.

PSA
   pisum sativum agglutinin
   PSA test
psammoma body
P450scc
   cytochrome P.
pseudencephalus
pseudoacephalus
pseudoachondroplasia
   p. syndrome
pseudoallele
pseudocalcification
   powder p.
pseudochromosome
pseudocyesis
   monosymptomatic
   delusional p.
pseudocyst
   pancreatic p.
pseudodeciduosis
pseudoephedrine hydrochloride
pseudogene
pseudogestational sac
pseudoglandular period
pseudohermaphrodite
pseudohermaphroditism
   female p.
   male p.
pseudo-Hurler polydystrophy
pseudohypertrophic
pseudohypoparathyroidism
pseudointraligamentous
pseudoleukemia
pseudolymphoma
pseudomembranous
   p. colitis
   p. enterocolitis
pseudomenopause
pseudomenstruation
Pseudomonas
   P. aeruginosa
   P. exotoxin
pseudomosaicism
pseudomucinous tumor
pseudomyxoma peritonei
pseudoovulation
pseudoparalysis

pseudopolyp
pseudoprecocious puberty
pseudopregnancy
pseudopuberty
   precocious p.
pseudosarcoma
   botryoid p.
pseudotoxemia
pseudotuberculosis
   Yersinia p.
pseudotumor
   p. cerebri
   trophoblastic p.
pseudo-Turner syndrome
pseudovagina
PSI
   pelvic support index
psittaci
   Chlamydia p.
psittacosis
psoas hitch procedure
psoriasis
   guttata p.
   vulvar p.
psoriatic arthritis
PSP
   phenolsulfonphthalein
PSTT
   placental site trophoblastic
   tumor
psychiatric
   p. drug
   p. illness
psychoactive drug
psychogenic
   p. pelvic pain
psychological
   p. effect
   p. sex
   p. stress
   p. trauma
psychometric assessment
psychomotor
   p. development index (PDI)
   p. epilepsy
psychoprophylaxis

NOTES

psychosexual problem
psychosis, pl. **psychoses**
    climacteric p.
    gestational p.
    involutional p.
    postpartum p.
    symbiotic p.
psychosocial
    p. adjustment
    p. support
psychosomatic disease
psychotherapy
psychotropic drug
PT
    physical therapy
    physiotherapy
    prothrombin time
PTA
    plasma thromboplastin
    antecedent
pterygium
    p. coli
    p. colli
    congenital p.
Pthirus pubis
ptosis
PTT
    partial thromboplastin time
ptyalism
pubarche
    premature p.
puberal, pubertal
pubertas precox
puberty
    complete precocious p.
    constitutional precocious p.
    delayed p.
    factitious precocious p.
    heterosexual precocious p.
    iatrogenic precocious p.
    idiopathic precocious p.
    incomplete p.
    incomplete precocious p.
    p. initiation
    isosexual idiopathic
     precocious p.
    precocious p.
    pseudoprecocious p.
    true precocious p.
pubescence
pubescent
pubic
    p. arch

    p. hair
    p. ramus
    p. symphysis
    p. symphysis periostitis
    p. triangle
pubiotomy
pubis
    Pthirus p.
pubis
    arcuate ligament of p.
    mons p.
    os p.
    osteomyelitis p.
    pediculosis p.
    symphysis p.
pubococcygeal muscle
pubococcygeus
puborectal
    p. muscle
pubourethral
pubovaginal
PUBS
    percutaneous umbilical blood
    sampling
puddle sign
pudenda (*pl. of* pudendum)
pudendal
    p. anesthesia
    p. apron
    p. artery
    p. block
    p. hematocele
    p. nerve
    p. neurogram
pudendi
    labium majus p.
    noma p.
pudendum, pl. **pudenda**
Pudenz
    P. reservoir
    P. shunt
puerorum
    hydroa p.
puerpera, pl. **puerperae**
puerperal
    p. convulsions
    p. eclampsia
    p. fever
    p. hematoma
    p. infection
    p. mastitis
    p. morbidity
    p. period

p. phlebitis
p. sepsis
p. septicemia
p. tetanus
puerperant
puerperium, pl. **puerperia**
Pulec and Freedman classification
pull-to-sit reflex
Pulmo-Aid ventilator
Pulmocare
    P. diet
    P. formula
PulmoMate nebulizer
pulmonale
    cor p.
pulmonary
    p. agenesis
    p. alveolus
    p. angiography
    p. anthrax
    p. arborization
    p. artery atresia
    p. artery banding
    p. artery catheterization
    p. artery/ductus view
    p. artery sling
    p. artery wedge (PAW)
    p. artery wedge pressure
    (PAWP)
    p. aspergillosis
    p. blood flow (PBF)
    p. capillary wedge pressure
    (PCWP)
    p. complication
    p. diffusing capacity
    p. disease
    p. disorder
    p. dysmaturity syndrome
    p. edema
    p. ejection clicks
    p. emboli
    p. embolism
    p. eosinophilia
    p. fibrosis
    p. function
    p. function tests
    p. gangrene

p. hemosiderosis
p. histoplasmosis
p. hypertension
p. hypoplasia
p. infarction
p. infiltrate with
    eosinophilia (PIE)
p. injury
p. insufficiency of
    prematurity
p. interstitial emphysema
    (PIE)
p. maturation
p. metastasis
p. microvascular
    permeability to protein
    (PMVP)
p. mucormycosis
p. murmur
p. parenchymal disease
p. plaque
p. resection
p. sequestration
p. stenosis
p. suppuration
p. surfactant
p. thromboembolism
p. time constant
p. toilet
p. tuberculosis
p. valve
p. vascular bed
p. venous drainage
pulmonic
    p. murmur
    p. regurgitation
Pulmozyme
pulsatile
    p. discharge
    p. GnRH administration
    p. human menopausal
    gonadotropin
    p. release
pulsatility
    p. index (PI)
    intrinsic p.

NOTES

pulse
    p. frequency
    maternal p.
    p. oximeter
    p. oximetry
pulsed Doppler ultrasound
pulsed-wave ultrasound
pulseless disease
pulvule
    Prozac p.
pump
    Barron p.
    Basis breast p.
    breast p.
    Chicco breast p.
    Chid breast p.
    Clarus model 5169
      peristaltic p.
    Egnell breast p.
    Elmed peristaltic
      irrigation p.
    Grafco breast p.
    insulin p.
    Kendall McGaw
      Intelligent p.
    KM-1 breast p.
    Lactina breast p.
    Mary Jane breast p.
    Medela Dominant vacuum
      delivery p.
    Medela manual breast p.
    Medfusion 1001 syringe
      infusion p.
    Mityvac reusable vacuum p.
    Salem p.
    servocontrolled
      ventilation p.
    suction p.
    Unicare breast p.
punch
    baby Tischler biopsy p.
    p. biopsy
    p. biopsy forceps
    Eppendorfer biopsy p.
    Keyes dermatologic p.
    Keyes vulvar p.
    Miltex disposable biopsy p.
    Tischler-Morgan biopsy p.
    Townsend biopsy p.
    Wittner biopsy p.
puncta (*pl. of* punctum)
punctata
    chondrodysplasia p.

    chondrodystrophia
      congenita p.
    dysplasia epiphysealis p.
punctate
    p. epiphyseal dysplasia
punctum, pl. puncta
puncture
    bone marrow p.
    cisternal p.
    lumbar p. (LP)
    pericardial p.
    subdural p.
PUND
    pregnancy, uterine, not delivered
Punnett square
PUPP
    pruritic urticarial papules and
      plaques
pure
    p. gonadal dysgenesis
    p. random drift
purified hormone
purine
    p. metabolism disorder
Purinethol
Purkinje
    P. cells
    P. fibers
puromycin
purpura
    alloimmune neonatal
      thrombocytopenic p.
    anaphylactoid p.
    autoimmune
      thrombocytopenic p.
    p. fulminans
    p. hemorrhagica
    Henoch-Schönlein p.
    idiopathic
      thrombocytopenic p. (ITP)
    immune
      thrombocytopenic p. (ITP)
    Schönlein-Henoch p.
    thrombocytopenic p.
    thrombotic p.
    thrombotic
      thrombocytopenic p. (TTP)
purse-string
    p.-s. mouth
    p.-s. suture
Purtilo X-linked lymphoproliferative
    syndrome
purulent pharyngitis

Pusey emulsion
pusher
ENDO-ASSIST endoscopic
knot p.
pus tube
pustular varicella
pustulosa
miliaria p.
varicella p.
pustulosis
Juliusberg p.
putrescence
putrescine
Puzo method
PVC
premature ventricular
contraction
P.V. Carpine Liquifilm
PVF K
PWM
pokeweed mitogen
pyelitis
pyelocaliectasis
pyelogram
dragon p.
intravenous p. (IVP)
retrograde p.
washout p.
pyelography
intravenous p. (IVP)
pyelonephritis
p. in exenteration
pygoamorphus
pygodidymus
pygomelus
pygopagus
pyknocytosis
pyknodysostosis syndrome
Pyle
bone age standard of
Greulich and P.
P. syndrome
pyloric
p. atresia
p. stenosis
p. string sign

pyloromyotomy
Ramstedt p.
pyloroplasty
Heineke-Mikulicz p.
pylorospasm
pyocolpocele
pyocolpos
pyogenic
p. abscess
p. arthritis
p. granuloma
p. salpingitis
pyometra
pyometritis
pyomyoma
uterine p.
pyoovarium
Pyopen
pyophysometra
pyosalpingitis
pyosalpingo-oophoritis
pyosalpingo-oothecitis
pyosalpinx
pyrantel pamoate
pyrazinamide
pyrexia
maternal p.
Pyribenzamine
Pyridiate
Pyridium
pyridostigmine
p. bromide
pyridoxine
pyridoxine-responsive anemia
pyrilamine maleate
pyrimethamine
pyrimidine
Pyrinyl
pyrogen
endogenous p.
pyroglutamic acidemia
pyropoikilocytosis
pyrosis
pyruvate
p. decarboxylase
p. kinase (PK)
p. kinase deficiency

NOTES

pyrvinium pamoate · pyuria

pyrvinium pamoate   **pyuria**

Q
quotient
Q band
Q fever
Q̇
blood flow
15q23-24
chromosome 15q23-24
Qa (series of loci)
QCT
quantitative computed
tomography
QDR
quantitative digital radiography
Qf
rate of fluid filtration
QNS
quantity not sufficient for
evaluation
qr
quadriradial
QRS morphology
Qs/Qt
intrapulmonary shunt ratio
right-to-left shunt ratio
Q-test ovulation predictor
Qtest Strep test
Q-T interval
Q-tip test
quadrantectomy
quadrantectomy, axillary dissection,
radiation therapy (QUART)
quadratum
caput q.
quadriplegia
quadriradial (qr)
quadruplet
quality assurance process
quantitation
amniotic fluid q.
quantitative
q. computed tomography
(QCT)
q. digital radiography
(QDR)
q. inheritance
quantity not sufficient for
evaluation (QNS)
quarantine

QUART
quadrantectomy, axillary
dissection, radiation therapy
quarter-strength formula
Quarzan
quasicontinuous inheritance
quasidiploid
quasidominance
Queensland fever
Questionnaire
Family Apgar Q.
Questran
Quetelet index
Queyrat erythroplasia
Quibron
Q.-T
Q.-T/SR
quickening
Quickpac-II OneStep hCG
pregnancy test
Quick test
QuickVue
Q. One-Step hCG-Combo
test
Q. One-Step hCG-urine test
Quidel
QUIDEL Group B strep test
quiescence
uterine q.
Quik Connect fetal monitor
quinacrine
q. banding
q. hydrochloride
Quinaglute
quinalbarbitone sodium
Quinamm
quinate
quinestrol
quinethazone
quingestanol acetate
Quinidex Extentabs
quinidine
quinine
quinolone
q. pharmacokinetics
Quinones-Neubüser uterine-grasping
forceps
Quinones uterine-grasping forceps
Quinora
quintipara

Quinton dual-lumen catheter
quintuplet
Quisling hammer

quotidian fever
quotient (Q)
    ventilation/perfusion q.

R
  radius
  roentgen
    R band
RA
  rheumatoid arthritis
²²⁶Ra
  radium-226
rabies
  r. immune globulin
  r. vaccine
racemic
  r. ephedrine
  r. epinephrine
Racephedrine
rachiopagus
rachischisis
rachitic
  r. metaphysis
  r. rosary
rachitis fetalis
racial difference
RAD
  reactive airway disease
rad
  radiation-absorbed dose
radial
  r. aplasia-thrombocytopenia
    syndrome
  r. arterial catheter
  r. arterial line
  r. artery
  r. clubhand
  r. scar
  r. sclerosing lesion
radiant warmer
radiata
  corona r.
radiation
  r. cystitis
  r. danger
  diagnostic r.
  r. dose
  r. dose limit
  r. dysplasia
  electromagnetic r.
  intraoperative r.
  ionizing r.
  nuclear r.
  orthovoltage r.

  particulate r.
  postoperative r.
  postoperative pelvic r.
  state-of-the-art r.
  supervoltage r.
  r. therapy
  tissue tolerance to r.
  r. tolerance
  whole abdominal r.
radiation-absorbed dose (rad)
radical
  r. excision
  free hydroxyl r.
  r. hysterectomy
  r. mastectomy
  r. parametrectomy
  r. surgery
  r. vulvectomy
radioactive
  r. applicator
  r. cobalt
  r. colloid
  r. gold
  r. immunoassay
  r. implant
  r. isotope
  r. microspheres
  r. ribbons
  r. seed implantation
  r. seeds
  r. tracer
  r. uptake
radioallergosorbent test (RAST)
radiocontrast material
radiocurable
radiofibrinogen uptake scan
radiography
  chest r.
  digital r.
  quantitative digital r.
    (QDR)
radioimmunoassay (RIA)
radioimmunodetection (RAID)
radioimmunosorbent test (RIST)
radioiodination
radioiodine
radioisotope
radiolabeled
radiological examination
radiolucent

radiomutation
radionuclide
    r. venography
radioreceptor assay
radiosensitivity
radiosensitization
radiotherapy
    abdominal strip r.
    adjuvant r.
    pelvic boost r.
    postoperative r.
radium
    r.-226 (^{226}Ra)
    r. implant
    intracavitary r.
radius (R)
    thrombocytopenia-absent r.
    (TAR)
radon
    r.-222 (^{222}Rn)
Radovici
    R. reflex
    R. sign
RAID
    radioimmunodetection
Raimondi catheter
Raji cell
rale
rales
    coarse r.
    crackling r.
    crepitant r.
    wet r.
rami (*pl. of* ramus)
Ramipril
RAMP hCG assay
Ramses
Ramsey-Hunt syndrome
Ramstedt
    R. operation
    R. procedure
    R. pyloromyotomy
ramus, pl. rami
    ischiopubic r.
    pubic r.
Randall
    R. stone forceps
    R. suction curette
random
    r. mating
    r. sampling
    r. variable

range
    cervical tissue impedance r.
range-gated Doppler (RGD)
ranitidine
RAP
    receptor-associated protein
    recurrent abdominal pain
rape
    r. evidence
    r. evidence kit
    r. protocol
    statutory r.
rape-trauma syndrome
raphe
    anococcygeal r.
    median r.
rapid
    r. bone loss
    r. descent
    r. eye movements (REM)
    r. plasma reagin (RPR)
    r. plasma reagin card test
    r. slide test
Rasch sign
rash
    butterfly r.
    ECM r.
    monilial r.
    morbilliform r.
Rashkind balloon
Rasmussen encephalitis
RAST
    radioallergosorbent test
rat-bite fever
rate
    aldosterone excretion r.
    (AER)
    baseline fetal heart r.
    beat-to-beat variability of
    fetal heart r.
    birth r.
    erythrocyte sedimentation r.
    (ESR)
    fertility r.
    fetal death r.
    fetal heart r. (FHR)
    flow r.
    r. of fluid filtration (Qf)
    glomerular filtration r.
    (GFR)
    heart r.
    infant mortality r.
    maternal death r.

maternal mortality r.
metabolic clearance r.
 (MCR)
mortality r.
neonatal mortality r.
ovulation r.
peak expiratory flow r.
 (PEFR)
perinatal mortality r.
prevalence r.
recurrence r.
sedimentation r.
sinusoidal fetal heart r.
survival r.
ventricular response r.
rating
  Apgar r.
ratio
  A/G r.
    albumin/globulin ratio
  albumin/globulin r. (A/G
    ratio)
  amylase-creatinine
    clearance r.
  cerebral-placental r.
  cough-pressure
    transmission r.
  estrogen/progesterone r.
  fetal head:abdominal
    circumference r.
  head:body r.
  head
    circumference/abdominal
    circumference r.
  I/E r.
  intrapulmonary shunt r.
   (Qs/Qt)
  I/T r.
  lecithin/sphingomyelin r.
  left atrial to aortic r.
   (LA:A)
  L/S r.
  M/E r.
  right-to-left shunt r. (Qs/Qt)
  RVPEP/RVET r.
  S/D r.
  sex r.

systolic/diastolic r.
vaginal pool L/S r.
variance r.
ventilation/perfusion r.
V̇/Q̇ r.
waist:hip r.
rat tooth pickups
Rauber layer
Raussly disease
ray
  beta r.
  gamma r.
Raz
  R. double-prong ligature
   carrier
  R. procedure
Raz-Leach procedure
Razoxane
RCA test
RCGP
  Royal College of General
   Practitioners
RD1000 resuscitator
RDS
  respiratory distress syndrome
reaction
  acetowhite r.
  acrosome r.
  anorectic r.
  Arias-Stella r.
  Arthus r.
  cortical r.
  decidual r.
  graft-versus-host r.
  harlequin r.
  Jarisch-Herxheimer r.
  laser r.
  polymerase chain r. (PCR)
  Porter-Silber r.
  Shwartzman r.
  startle r.
  wheal-and-flare r.
  zona r.
reactive airway disease (RAD)
reactivity
  fetal heart rate r.
  vascular r.

NOTES

reagin
    rapid plasma r. (RPR)
Reality vaginal pouch
real-time
    r.-t. B-scanner
    r.-t. imaging on ultrasound
    r.-t. sonography
    r.-t. ultrasonography
    r.-t. ultrasound
reanastomosis
    tubocornual r.
rebound phenomenon
recall phenomenon
Récamier
    R. operation
    R. procedure
receptor
    activated estrogen r.
    adrenergic r.'s
    α-adrenergic r.'s
    β-adrenergic r.'s
    androgen r.
    r. assay
    class I, II r.
    r. coupling
    endogenous opiate r.
    endometrial r.
    E-rosette r.
    estradiol r.
    estrogen r.
    G-protein-coupled r.
    hormone r.
    hormone complex r.
    r. internalization
    J pulmonary r.'s
    opiate r.
    progesterone r.
    steroid hormone r.
β-receptor agonist
receptor-associated protein (RAP)
receptor-mediated endocytosis
recessive
    autosomal r. (AR)
    r. disorder
    r. gene
    r. inheritance
    r. trait
rechallenge
reciprocal
    r. genes
    r. translocation
Recklinghausen
    R. disease

    R. disease type 1
    R. tumor
Reclomide
Reclus disease
recoil
    arm r.
recombinant
    r. DNA
    r. DNA technology
    r. human growth hormone
Recombivax HB
recommendation
    screening r.
recommended dietary allowance
reconstruction
    Abbe-McIndoe vaginal r.
    Dibbell cleft lip-nasal r.
reconstructive mammaplasty
record
    daily fetal movement r.
    Infant Behavior R. (IBR)
recorder
    Dopcord r.
    multichannel r.
recovery
    bacterial r.
    labor, delivery, and r. (LDR)
    r. score
    r. time
    ultrasonic egg r.
recreational drug
rectal
    r. cancer
    r. examination
    r. node
    r. postradiation ulcer
    r. suppository
    r. temperature
recti (*pl. of* rectus)
rectocele
    r. repair
rectolabial fistula
rectoscopic endometrial ablation
rectosigmoid
    r. colon
    r. colon endometriosis
rectouterine
    r. cul-de-sac
    r. fold
    r. pouch
rectovaginal
    r. examination

r. fistula
r. septum
rectovestibular fistula
rectovulvar fistula
rectum
rectus, pl. **recti**
diastasis recti
recurrence
pelvic r.
r. rate
r. risk
recurrent
r. abdominal pain (RAP)
r. abortion
r. anaphylaxis
r. aneuploidy
r. carcinoma
r. euploidic abortion
r. infection
r. jaundice of pregnancy
r. lymphoma
r. miscarriage
r. pregnancy loss
r. premenstrual lithium
serum concentration
decline
r. spontaneous abortion
(RSA)
r. vaginitis
recurvatum
genu r.
pectus r.
red
r. blood cell
r. cell antigen
r. cell enzyme deficiency
r. cell volume
r. degeneration
r. reflex
Redi-kit
LEEP R.-k.
Redisol
reducible hernia
reductase
5α-r.
dihydrofolate r.
17-ketosteroid r. deficiency

reduction
chromosome r.
embryo r.
fetal r.
funic r.
limb r.
r. mammaplasty
multifetal pregnancy r.
selective r.
weight r.
redundant hymen
reel foot
referred pelvic pain
reflectance
r. photometer
r. pulse oximetry
reflection
peritoneal r.
reflex
acoustic r.
acoustic blink r.
anal r.
asymmetric tonic neck r.
(ATNR)
autonomic walking r.
Babinski r.
Babkin r.
bowing r.
bregmocardiac r.
Breuer-Hering inflation r.
bulbocavernous r.
crossed adductor r.
crossed extension r.
darwinian r.
dazzle r.
deep tendon r. (DTR)
diving r.
doll's eye r.
embrace r.
fencing r.
Ferguson r.
forced grasping r.
gag r.
Gallant r.
Gamper bowing r.
gastrocolic r.
Gerace r.

NOTES

reflex *(continued)*
    grasp r.
    Grünfelder r.
    Head r.
    Hering-Breuer r.
    labial r.
    labyrinthine r.
    Landau r.
    letdown r.
    lip r.
    Magnus and de Kleijn
      neck r.
    milk ejection r.
    Moro r.
    nasolabial r.
    neck-righting r.
    oculocephalic r.
    oculocephalogyric r.
    palm-chin r.
    palmomental r.
    parachute r.
    Peiper r.
    Perez r.
    placing r.
    plantar r.
    primitive r.
    propping r.
    pull-to-sit r.
    Radovici r.
    red r.
    rooting r.
    snout r.
    startle r.
    stepping r.
    sucking r.
    swallow r.
    r. sympathetic dystrophy
      (RSD)
    tonic neck r.
    white pupillary r.
reflexic apnea
reflux
    esophageal r.
    r. esophagitis
    gastroesophageal r. (GER)
    intrarenal r.
    menstrual r.
    r. nephropathy
    ureterovesical r.
    vesicoureteral r.
refractory anemia of pregnancy

Refsum
    R. disease
    R. syndrome
regeneration
    tissue r.
regimen
    feeding r.
    monophasic r.
    Pritchard intramuscular r.
    Yuzpe r.
    Zuspan r.
region
    sex-determining r. (SRY)
regional
    r. analgesia
    r. anesthesia
    r. enteritis
registry
    Herbst r.
    Teratogen R.
Regitine
Reglan
Regonol
regression
    Galton law of r.
    r. of the mean
    premature luteal r.
    tumor r.
regressive infantilism
Regular
    R. (Concentrated) Iletin II
      U-500
    R. Iletin I
    R. Iletin II
    R. Insulin
    R. Purified Pork Insulin
regulation
    Baby Doe r.'s
    gonadotropin r.
    menstrual cycle r.
    physiologic follicular r.
    pituitary gonadotropin r.
    plasma volume r.
    prolactin r.
regulator
    r. gene
    Medela membrane r.
regurgitation
    aortic r.
    mitral r.
    pulmonic r.
    tricuspid r.
Regutol

Rehydralyte
    R. formula
Reichel cloacal duct
Reifenstein syndrome
reimplantation
Reiner-Beck snare
Reiner-Knight forceps
reinfusion
    autologous bone marrow r.
Reinke crystalloids
reinsemination
Reis-Wertheim vaginal
  hysterectomy
rejection
    fetal r.
relapsing fever
related
    alcohol r. (AR)
relation
    Frank-Starling r.
relationship
    Poiseville-Hagen r.
relative
    r. osteopenia
    r. risk
    r. sterility
relaxant
    muscle r.
relaxation
    pelvic r.
    uterine r.
relaxin
    r. serum level
release
    GnRH-facilitated FSH r.
    GnRH-facilitated LH r.
    gonadotropin r.
    gonadotropin pulsatile r.
    growth hormone r.
    neurotransmitter r.
    pituitary hormone r.
    pulsatile r.
REM
    rapid eye movements
    REM PolyHesive II patient
    return electrode

remission
    complete r.
    induced r.
    spontaneous r.
remnant
    branchial cleft r.
removal
    extracorporeal CO_2 r.
    (ECOR)
Renaissance spirometry system
renal
    r. acidification
    r. agenesis
    r. artery stenosis
    r. biopsy
    r. calculi
    r. cell carcinoma
    r. clearance test
    r. colic
    r. cortex
    r. cortical necrosis
    r. disease
    r. duplication
    r. dysgenesis
    r. dysplasia
    r. ectopia
    r. failure
    r. function
    r. function test
    r. infarction
    r. insufficiency
    r. malrotation
    r. manifestation
    r. osteodystrophy
    r. parenchyma
    r. perfusion
    r. plasma flow
    r. stone
    r. transplantation
    r. tuberculosis
    r. tubular acidosis (RTA)
    r. tubular function
    r. tubular necrosis
    r. vascular thrombosis
    r. vein thrombosis
Rendu-Osler-Weber syndrome
Renese

NOTES

reniform pelvis
renin
    r. substrate
renin-angiotensin-aldosterone system
renin-angiotensin system
Renografin
Renoquid
Renpenning syndrome
Reovirus
repair
    anterior r.
    anterior and posterior r.
    A&P r.
    cystocele r.
    Danus-Stanzel r.
    episiotomy r.
    LeFort-Wehrbein-Duplay
     hypospadias r.
    Magpi hypospadius r.
    Noble-Mengert perineal r.
    perineal r.
    Phaneuf-Graves r.
    posterior r.
    rectocele r.
    Senning r.
    sphincter r.
    surgical r.
    vaginal r.
    vaginal wall r.
    vesicovaginal r.
    York-Mason r.
    Zancolli clawhand
     deformity r.
repeat
    r. cesarean section
    r. curettage
repeated abortion
repetitive pregnancy loss
replacement
    cephalic r.
    estrogen r.
    fluid r.
    heart valve r.
replenishment
Replens
    R. lubricant
replication fork
Replogle tube
report
    Janus r.
    Walton r.
repressed gene
repressor gene

reproduction
    assisted r.
    vegetative r.
reproductive
    r. cycle
    r. disorder
    r. endocrinology
    r. failure
    r. function
    r. genetics
    r. history
    r. mortality
    r. performance
    r. system
    r. system development
    r. technology
    r. tract
    r. tract abnormality
    r. tract embryology
    r. wastage
requirement
    iron r.
    mineral r.
    nutrient r.
    sodium r.
    vitamin r.
rescue
    abdominal r.
    r. surfactant
resectability
resection
    en bloc r.
    endometrial r.
    laparoscopic multiple-
     punch r.
    low rectal r.
    multiple-punch r.
    ovarian wedge r.
    pulmonary r.
    segmental r.
    surgical r.
    Torpin cul-de-sac r.
    transcervical r.
    transsphenoidal
     microsurgical r.
    wedge r.
Resercen
reserpine
reservatus
    coitus r.
reservoir
    double-bubble flushing r.
    Mainz pouch urinary r.

Ommaya r.
Pudenz r.
residual
   r. ductal tissue
   r. ovary syndrome
   r. urine
   r. volume
residue
   methanol extraction r.
    (MER)
resin
   podophyllum r.
resistance
   airway r.
   androgen r.
   bromocriptine r.
   dicumarol r.
   differential vascular r.
   r. index (RI)
   insulin r.
   systemic vascular r.
   total pulmonary r.
   vascular r.
resistant
   r. ovary
   r. ovary syndrome
resolution
   axial r.
   lateral r.
resonance
   nuclear magnetic r. (NMR)
resorption
   bone r.
   fetal r.
Respbid
respiration
   agonal r.'s
   Bouchut r.
   Cheyne-Stokes r.
   grunting r.'s
   Kussmaul r.
   placental r.
   vicarious r.
respirator (ventilator)
   Ambu r.
   BABYbird II r.
   Bath r.

Bear r.
Bennett r.
Bird Mark 8 r.
Bourns infant r.
Bragg-Paul r.
Breeze r.
Clevedan positive
   pressure r.
cuirass r.
Dann r.
Drinker r.
Emerson r.
Engstrom r.
Gill r.
Huxley r.
Kirmisson r.
mechanical r.
Med-Neb r.
Merck r.
Monaghan r.
Morch r.
Morsch-Retec r.
Moynihan r.
negative-pressure r.
portable r.
Sanders jet r.
respiratory
   r. acidosis
   r. alkalosis
   r. arrest
   r. complication
   r. depression
   r. distress
   r. distress syndrome (RDS)
   r. distress syndrome of the
    newborn
   r. insufficiency
   r. paralysis
   r. syncytial virus (RSV)
   r. system
   r. toilet
   r. tract
   r. tract infection
response
   abnormal r.
   amnestic r.
   anamnestic r.

NOTES

359

response *(continued)*
  antibody r.
  auditory brainstem r. (ABR)
  auditory evoked r.
  baroreflex r.
  brainstem auditory
    evoked r.'s (BAER)
  cortisol r.
  First R.
  immune r.
  infantile breath-holding r.
  lactation letdown r.
  maternal immune r.
  maternal vascular r.
  plantar r.
  pressor r.
  Rh immune r.
  righting r.
  startle r.
  target organ r.
  visual evoked r. (VER)
rest
  bed r.
  Marchand r.
  mesonephric r.
  pelvic r.
  Walthard cell r.
  wolffian r.
resting membrane potential
restless legs syndrome
Restoril
restriction
  r. endonuclease
  r. endonuclease analysis
  fetal growth r. (FGR)
  r. fragment length
    polymorphism (RFLP)
  salt r.
  r. site
  sodium r.
resumption
  menstrual cycle r.
resuscitation
  cardiopulmonary r. (CPR)
  intrauterine r.
  mouth-to-mouth r.
  neonatal r.
  newborn r.
resuscitator
  Ambu infant r.
  Fisher and Paykel
    RD1000 r.
  Laerdal r.

  Penlon infant r.
  RD1000 r.
Resyl
retained
  r. menstruation
  r. placenta
retardation
  deafness, onycho-
    osteodystrophy, mental r.
    (DOOR)
  fetal growth r.
  FRAXE-associated mental r.
  growth r.
  intrauterine growth r.
    (IUGR)
  mental r.
  Wilms tumor, aniridia,
    gonadoblastoma, mental r.
    (WAGR)
retarded fetal growth
rete
  r. cords
  r. cyst of ovary
  r. testis
retention
  fetal r.
  r. polyp
  r. suture
  urinary r.
reticulare
  magma r.
reticulocyte count
reticulocytosis
reticuloendotheliosis
reticulum
Retin-A
retinal
  r. aplasia
  r. change
  r. detachment
retinitis
  gravidic r.
  r. pigmentosa
retinoblastoma
retinoblastoma-mental retardation
  syndrome
retinoic acid
retinoid
retinol
retinopapillitis of prematurity
retinopathy
  diabetic r.
  eclamptic r.

gravidic r.
r. of prematurity (ROP)
r. punctata albescens
toxemic r. of pregnancy
retinoschisis
retraction
intercostal r.'s
nipple r.
r. ring
subcostal r.'s
r. syndrome
retractor
Allport r.
Army-Navy r.
Aufricht nasal r.
Balfour r.
bladder r.
Bookwalter r.
Breisky-Navratil r.
Brown uvula r.
Cottle-Neivert r.
Deaver r.
DeLee Universal r.
Ferris Smith-Sewall r.
Gelpi-Lowrie r.
Gelpi perineal r.
Gott malleable r.
Goulet r.
Haight baby r.
Harrington r.
Heaney-Hyst r.
Iron interne r.
Jackson right-angle r.
Kelly r.
lateral wall r.
Latrobe r.
Luer r.
Magrina-Bookwalter
vaginal r.
malleable r.
Murless head r.
r. neuropathy
O'Connor-O'Sullivan r.
Omni-Tract vaginal r.
O'Sullivan-O'Connor r.
pediatric self-retaining r.
Richardson r.

right-angle r.
Roberts thumb r.
Schuknecht r.
self-retaining r.
Senn-Dingman r.
Shambaugh r.
thumb r.
vaginal r.
Weitlaner r.
Wullstein r.
retraining
bladder r.
retrieval
oocyte r.
ultrasound-directed egg r.
retrobulbar neuritis
retrocecal hernia
retrocession
retrodeviation
retrodisplacement
retroesophageal abscess
retroflexion, retroflection
uterine r.
retrograde
r. menstrual flow
r. menstruation
r. pyelogram
retrolental fibroplasia
retromammary mastitis
retroperitoneal
r. drain
r. endometriosis
r. fetus
r. infection
r. lymphadenectomy
r. node
r. soft tissue
r. soft tissue sarcoma
retroperitoneum
retropharyngeal abscess
retroplacental clot
retroposed
retroposition
retropubic
r. colpourethrocystopexy
r. sling
r. urethropexy

NOTES

retrosternal hernia
retrotonsillar abscess
retroversioflexion
retroversion
      uterine r.
retroverted
retrovirus
rettgeri
      Providencia r.
Rett syndrome
return
      partial anomalous
      pulmonary venous r.
      (PAPVR)
      total anomalous pulmonary
      venous r.
returning-soldier effect
Reuter tube
reversal
      gender r.
      hyperandrogenism r.
      sex r.
      vasectomy r.
reverse
      r. banding
      r. genetics
      r. transcriptase
      r. transcription
      r. triiodothyronine
reverse-last shoes
revision
      Dibbell cleft lip-nasal r.
Revital-Ice rehydrating freezer pop
Reye syndrome
Reynolds number
RF
      White class, B through RF
RFA
      right frontoanterior position
RFLP
      restriction fragment length
      polymorphism
RFP
      right frontoposterior position
RFT
      right frontotransverse position
RGD
      range-gated Doppler
Rh
      rhesus
      Rh antigen
      Rh blood group
      Rh blood group system

Rh disease
Rh factor
Gamulin Rh
Rh hemolytic disease
Rh immune response
Rh immunization
Rh immunoglobulin
Rh incompatibility
Rh isoimmunization
Mini-Gamulin Rh
Rh-negative
Rh-positive
Rh sensitization
rhabdomyoblast
rhabdomyoma
rhabdomyosarcoma
      embryonal r.
rhabdosphincter
rhaebocrania
rhagades
Rh$_o$(D) imaging
rhesus (Rh)
      r. D disease
      r. hemolytic disease
rheumatic
      r. disease
      r. fever
      r. heart disease
      r. pneumonia
rheumaticosis
rheumatoid
      r. arthritis (RA)
      r. factor
      r. nodules
      r. vasculitis
rheumatologic disorder
Rhinall
Rhindecon
rhinitis medicamentosa
rhinocephaly
Rhinocort
rhinoprobe
Rhino Triangle brace
rhinovirus
rhizomelia syndrome
rhizomelic
      r. chondrodysplasia punctata
      syndrome
      r. dwarfism
Rh-null syndrome
Rho (D)
      R. imaging
      R. immune globulin

RhoGAM
rhonchus, pl. **rhonchi**
Rh-positive
    R.-p. infant
    R.-p. red cell stroma
rhythm
    circadian r.
    junctional r.
    r. method
RI
    resistance index
RIA
    radioimmunoassay
Rias-Stella change
ribavirin
ribbon
    radioactive r.'s
riboflavin
    r. deficiency
ribonuclease (RNase)
ribonucleic
    r. acid (RNA)
    r. acid probe
ribosomal RNA
ribosome
Ricelyte
Rice-Lyte formula
Rich
    Rolaids Calcium R.
Richardson retractor
Richards-Rundle syndrome
Richner-Hanhart syndrome
Richter
    R. and Albrich procedure
    R. hernia
ricin
ricinus communis agglutinin
rickets
    hypophosphatemic r.
    vitamin D-resistant r.
Rickettsiae
rickettsial
ridge
    cervicovaginal r.
    genital r.
    germ r.
    gonadal r.

    mesonephric r.
    transverse r.
    wolffian r.
Ridpath curette
Riechert-Mundinger stereotactic
    system
Rieger syndrome
Rifadin
rifampicin
rifampin
rifamycin, rifomycin
Riga-Fede disease
right
    r. acromiodorsoposterior
      position
    r. to be well-born
    r. frontoanterior position
      (RFA)
    r. frontoposterior position
      (RFP)
    r. frontotransverse position
      (RFT)
    left to r. (L-R)
    R. Light examination light
    r. mentoanterior position
      (RMA)
    r. mentoposterior position
      (RMP)
    r. mentotransverse position
      (RMT)
    r. occipitoanterior position
      (ROA)
    r. occipitoposterior position
      (ROP)
    r. occipitoposterior
      presentation
    r. occipitotransverse position
      (ROT)
    r. ovarian vein syndrome
    r. sacroanterior position
      (RSA)
    r. sacroposterior position
      (RSP)
    r. sacrotransverse position
      (RST)
    r. scapuloanterior position
      (RScA)

NOTES

right *(continued)*
    r. scapuloposterior position
    (RScP)
right-angle
    r.-a. retractor
    r.-a. scissors
righting response
right-to-left
    r.-t.-l. shunt
    r.-t.-l. shunt ratio (Qs/Qt)
Riley-Day syndrome
Riley-Schwachman syndrome
Riley-Smith syndrome
Rimactane
ring
    amnion r.
    r. applicator
    Bandl r.
    r. chromosome
    r. 18 chromosome
    r. 22 chromosome
    r. chromosome 18 syndrome
    r. chromosome 22 syndrome
    constriction r.
    contraceptive r.
    double r.
    Falope r.
    gestational r.
    Graefenberg r.
    hymenal r.
    Imlach r.
    Kayser-Fleischer r.
    neonatal r.
    pathologic retraction r.
    r. pessary
    physiologic retraction r.
    progestin-impregnated
      vaginal r.
    retraction r.
    Silastic r.
    trigonal r.
    T-shaped constriction r.
    tubal r.
    zipper r.
Ringer
    lactated R.
    R. solution
ringworm
Rinman sign
Rinne test
Rinse
    Nix Cream R.

ripener
    Prepidil Gel cervical r.
ripening
    Bishop score of cervical r.
    cervical r.
risk
    r. factor
    fetal r.
    r. management
    maternal r.
    recurrence r.
    relative r.
    teratogenic r.
RIST
    radioimmunosorbent test
Ritalin
Ritgen maneuver
ritodrine
    r. hydrochloride
Ritter disease
Rivotril
RMA
    right mentoanterior position
RMP
    right mentoposterior position
RMT
    right mentotransverse position
^{222}Rn
    radon-222
RNA
    ribonucleic acid
      messenger RNA
      RNA nucleotidyltransferase
      RNA polymerase
      ribosomal RNA
      soluble RNA
      transfer RNA (tRNA)
RNA-directed DNA polymerase
RNase
    ribonuclease
ROA
    right occipitoanterior position
Robert pelvis
Roberts
    R. syndrome
    R. thumb retractor
robertsonian
    r. fusion
    r. translocation
Robicillin VK
Robimycin

Robin
    R. anomalad
    R. syndrome
Robinow
    R. dwarfism
    R. mesomelic dysplasia
    R. syndrome
Robinul
Robitet
Robitussin
Rocaltrol
Rocephin
Roche Diagnostics
Rochester-Ochsner forceps
Rochester-Péan forceps
rockerbottom
    r. feet
    r. foot
Rockey-Davis incision
Rock-Mulligan hood
Rocky Mountain spotted fever
rod
    Gram-negative r.'s
    Gram-positive r.'s
    r. myopathy
Rodeck method
roentgen (R)
roentgenography
Roe v. Wade
Roferon-A
Rofsing test
Rogaine
Roger
    R. forceps
    maladie de R.
Rohr stria
Rokitansky
    R. pelvis
    R. prominence
    R. tubercle
Rokitansky-Küster-Hauser syndrome
Rolaids Calcium Rich
rolandic
    r. epilepsy
    r. sharp waves
rolandometer

role
    gender r.
rollerball
    r. electrode
    r. endometrial ablation
    r. technique
roller-bar electrode
roller occlusion
roll-over test
Rolserp
Romaña sign
Ronase
Rondomycin
rongeur
    pediatric bone r.
    Tobey ear r.
room
    birthing r.
    LDR r.
    r. temperature
rooming-in
rooting reflex
ROP
    retinopathy of prematurity
    right occipitoposterior position
rosary
    rachitic r.
Rosch-Thurmond fallopian tube catheterization set
rosea
    pityriasis r.
Rose equation
Rosenmüller
    organ of R.
roseola infantum
Rosewater syndrome
Rossavik growth model
Ross growth chart
ROT
    right occipitotransverse position
rotation
    r. and descent
    external r.
    forceps r.
    internal r.
    manual r.
rotational delivery

NOTES

rotavirus
Rotazyme test
Rothmann-Makai syndrome
Rothmund
    poikiloderma congenitale
      of R.
    R. syndrome
Rothmund-Thomson syndrome
Rothmund-Werner syndrome
Rotor syndrome
Rotunda treatment
Rouget bulb
round
    r. ligament
    r. ligament syndrome
    r. pelvis
round-headed acrosomeless
  spermatozoa
roundworm
Roussy-Lévy syndrome
routine
    r. antenatal diagnostic
      imaging ultrasound study
    r. preoperative test
Roux-en-Y choledochojejunostomy
Rowland pouch
Roxanol
    R. SR
Royal
    R. College of General
      Practioners' Oral
      Contraception Study
    R. College of General
      Practitioners (RCGP)
RPR
    rapid plasma reagin
RPS4X
RPS4Y
RSA
    recurrent spontaneous abortion
    right sacroanterior position
RScA
    right scapuloanterior position
RScP
    right scapuloposterior position
RSD
    reflex sympathetic dystrophy
RSP
    right sacroposterior position
RST
    right sacrotransverse position

RSV
    respiratory syncytial virus
RS virus
RTA
    renal tubular acidosis
RU 486
rubella
    congenital r.
    r. embryopathy
    r. immune
    measles, mumps, r. (MMR)
    periconceptional r.
    r. scarlatinosa
    r. vaccine
    r. virus
rubella-immune mother
rubella-negative mother
rubeola
    r. scarlatinosa
Rubex
Rubin
    R. maneuver
    R. test
Rubinstein syndrome
Rubinstein-Taybi syndrome
rubor
rubra
    miliaria r.
ruddy
rudimentary
    r. testis syndrome
    r. uterine horn
Rud syndrome
ruga, pl. rugae
rugal fold
rugation
rule
    Arey r.
    Budin r.
    four-hour r.
    Haase r.
    His r.
    informed consent
     disclosure r.'s
    Lossen r.
    Nägele r.
    r. of 60s
    Ogino-Knaus r.
    r. of outlet
    Sandberg r.
    Weinberg r.
rumination

Rum-K
Rumpel-Leede phenomenon
Runeberg anemia
runt
> r. disease

runting
rupture
> amnion r.
> hepatic r.
> marginal sinus r.
> membrane r.
> postmembrane r.
> prelabor membrane r.
> premature r.
> premature amnion r.
> premature membrane r.
> premembrane r.
> prolonged r.
> splenic r.
> total perineal r.
> tubal r.
> uterine r.

ruptured
> r. cerebral aneurysm
> r. episiotomy
> r. uterus

Rusconi
> anus of R.

Russell
> R. syndrome
> R. viper venom time

Russell-Silver
> R.-S. dwarfism
> R.-S. syndrome

Russian tissue forceps
Rutledge classification of extended
> **hysterectomy**

RVPEP/RVET ratio
Rx
> Mission Prenatal R.
> Natalins R.

Rynacrom

NOTES

SA
sacroanterior
SAB
spontaneous abortion
Sabbagha formula
Sabin-Feldman dye test
Sabin vaccine
sabre shin deformity
Sabril
sac
allantoic s.
amniotic s.
chorionic s.
embryonic s.
gestational s.
pseudogestational s.
vitelline s.
yolk s.
saccular
s. aneurysm
s. period
sacculation
sacral
s. agenesis
s. dimple
s. lymph node
sacroanterior (SA)
left s.
s. position
sacrococcygeal teratoma
sacroiliac joint
sacropexy
abdominal s.
sacroposterior (SP)
left s. position (LSP)
s. position
right s. position (RSP)
sacrospinous
s. ligament suspension
sacrotransverse (ST)
left s. position (LST)
s. position
right s. position (RST)
sacrotuberous
sacrum
SAD
source-to-axis distance
saddle
s. block
s. block anesthesia

Saenger
S. operation
S. ovum forceps
Saethre-Chotzen syndrome
SAFE
sexual assault forensic evidence
SAFE kit
sagittal
s. fontanel
s. suture
s. suture line
sagrada
cascara s.
sail sign
Sakati-Nyhan syndrome
sal ammoniac
Salazopyrin
salbutamol
Saldino-Noonan
S.-N. dwarfism
S.-N. syndrome
Salem pump
salicylate
choline s.
magnesium s.
phenyl s.
s. poisoning
sodium s.
salicylism
salicylsalicylic acid
saline
s. abortion
s. cathartic
Dulbecco phosphate
buffered s.
hypertonic s.
s. implant
normal s.
phosphate buffered s. (PBS)
physiologic s.
s. solution
salivary gland
salivation, lacrimation, urination, defecation, gastrointestinal distress and emesis (SLUDGE)
Salk vaccine
salmeterol xinafoate
salmon
s. patch
Salmonella typhi

salmonellosis
Salmon sign
salpingectomy
salpingemphraxis
salpinges (*pl. of* salpinx)
salpingioma
salpingitic
salpingitis
    chronic interstitial s.
    foreign body s.
    gonorrheal s.
    granulomatous s.
    s. isthmica nodosa (SIN)
    leperous s.
    nongranulomatous s.
    pyogenic s.
    tuberculous s.
salpingocele
salpingocentesis
salpingocyesis
salpingography
salpingolysis
salpingoneostomy
salpingo-oophorectomy
    abdominal s.-o.
    bilateral s.-o. (BSO)
    unilateral s.-o.
salpingo-oophoritis
salpingo-oophorocele
salpingo-ovariectomy
salpingo-ovariolysis
salpingoperitonitis
salpingopexy
salpingoplasty
salpingorrhagia
salpingorrhaphy
salpingoscopy
salpingostomatomy
salpingostomy
    linear s.
salpingotomy
    abdominal s.
salpinx, pl. salpinges
salsalate
salt
    gold s.
    Pedi-Bath S.'s
    s. restriction
    s. wasting
salt-losing adrenogenital syndrome
  (SLAS)
Saluron
salutary effect

salvage therapy
sample
    arterial blood s. (ABS)
    venous blood s. (VBS)
sampler
    Cervex-Brush cervical cell s.
    Cordguard umbilical cord s.
    Cytobrush Plus endocervical
      cell s.
    Wallach Endocell
      endometrial cell s.
sampling
    biological s.
    blood s.
    capillary blood s.
    chemical s.
    chorion s.
    chorionic villus s. (CVS)
    endocervical s.
    endometrial s.
    fetal blood s.
    fetal scalp blood s.
    fetal skin s.
    Mucat cervical s.
    percutaneous blood s.
    percutaneous umbilical
      blood s. (PUBS)
    random s.
    scalp blood s.
    trophoblast s.
    umbilical blood s.
Sampson cyst
Sanchez-Salorio syndrome
Sandberg rule
Sanders jet respirator
Sandhoff disease
Sandifer syndrome
Sandimmune
Sandoglobulin
Sandostatin
sandwich assay
Sanfilippo syndrome
Sanger incision
sanguinolentis
    fetus s.
sanguinopurulent
Sani-Spec vaginal speculum
Sanorex
Sansert
Santavuori-Haltia syndrome
Santavuori syndrome
SaO₂
    oxygen saturation

SAP-35
sap
 Prentif cavity-rim cervical s.
saphenous nerve
sarcofetal pregnancy
sarcoidosis
sarcoma
 alveolar soft part s.
 botryoid s.
 cervical s.
 clear cell s.
 embryonal s.
 endometrial s.
 endometrial stromal s. (ESS)
 Ewing s.
 heterologous uterine s.
 homologous uterine s.
 Kaposi s.
 Kaposi varicelliform s.
 mesodermal s.
 mixed mesodermal s.
  (MMS)
 mixed müllerian s.
 mixed ovarian
  mesodermal s.
 obesity in endometrial s.
 retroperitoneal soft tissue s.
 secretory s.
 uterine s.
 uterine müllerian s.
 vulvar s.
sarcomatous myoma degeneration
sarcomere
Sarcoptes scabiei
sarcosinemia
SART
 Society for Assisted
 Reproductive Technology
S.A.S.-500
Sassone score
satellite lesion
saturation
 s. analysis
 oxygen s. (SaO$_2$)
 s. strip
satyr ear
satyriasis

Saunders
 S. disease
 S. sign
Savage syndrome
Save-A-Tooth
saw
 Gigli s.
Saxonius
 coitus S.
Saxtorph maneuver
SB-6 antiserum
SBE
 subacute bacterial endocarditis
 SBE prophylaxis
ScA
 scapuloanterior
scabies
scalded-skin syndrome
scale
 Albert Einstein Neonatal
  Developmental S.
  (AENNS)
 Apgar s.
 Borg Physical Activity S.
 Brazelton Neonatal
  Behavioral Assessment S.
  (BNBAS)
 Cattell Infant Intelligence S.
 Conners S.
 Cranley Maternal-Fetal
  Attachment S.
 Dyadic Adjustment S.
 Family Adaptability and
  Cohesion S.-III (FACES-
  III)
 Family Environment S.
  (FES)
 Flint Infant Security S.
  (FISS)
 Gesell Developmental S.
 Graham-Rosenblith s.
 HSC S.
 Kent Infant Development S.
  (KIDS)
 Maternal Attitude S. (MAS)
 Toddler Temperament S.

NOTES

371

scale *(continued)*
  Vineland Adaptive
    Behavior S.'s
scalp
  s. blood sampling
  s. pH determination
  s. vein needle
scalpel
  Bowen double-bladed s.
  ENDO-ASSIST retractable s.
  Harmonic s.
  Shaw I s.
scan
  abdominopelvic s.
  iodine 125-labeled
    fibrinogen s.
  longitudinal s.
  radiofibrinogen uptake s.
  time position s.
  transverse s.
  S. ultrasound gel
  ventilation/perfusion s.
  V̇/Q̇ s.
Scanlon Assessment
scanner
  Aloka 650 s.
  Aloka SSD-720 real-time s.
  EUB-405 ultrasound s.
scanning
  duplex s.
  iodomethyl-norcholesterol s.
  isotope s.
  MEVA Probe for
    endovaginal s.
Scanzoni
  S. maneuver
  S. second os
Scanzoni-Smellie maneuver
scaphocephaly
scaphoid fontanel
scapula
  congenital elevation of
    the s.
scapuloanterior (ScA)
  left s. position (LScA)
  right s. position (RScA)
scapuloposterior (ScP)
  left s. position (LScP)
  right s. position (RScP)
scar
  lower-segment s.
  perineal s.

  s. prediction
  radial s.
  s. tissue
scarf
  s. maneuver
  s. sign
scarification
scarlatina
scarlatinosa
  rubella s.
  rubeola s.
scarlet fever
SCARMD
  severe childhood autosomal
    recessive muscular dystrophy
Scarpa fascia
scarred womb
scattered echo
S-C disease
  sickle cell-hemoglobin C disease
Schafer syndrome
Schatz maneuver
Schauffler procedure
Schaumann bodies
Schauta vaginal operation
Scheie syndrome
Scheuermann
  S. disease
  S. juvenile kyphosis
Scheuthauer-Marie-Sainton
  syndrome
Schick
  S. sign
  S. test
Schilder
  S. disease
  S. encephalitis
Schiller
  S. solution
  S. test
  S. tumor
Schiller-Duvall body
Schilling test
Schimmelbusch disease
schistocelia
schistocephalus
schistocormia
schistocystis
schistoglossia
schistomelia
schistoprosopia
schistorrachis

schistosomal cercariae
schistosomia
schistosomiasis
schistosomus
schistosternia
schistothorax
schistotrachelus
schizencephaly
schizocyte
schizocytosis
schizophrenia
Schlusskoagulum
Schmidt syndrome
Schmorl jaundice
Scholz disease
Schönlein-Henoch purpura
Schroeder
    S. operation
    S. tenaculum forceps
    S. tenaculum loop
    S. uterine tenaculum
    S. vulsellum forceps
Schubert uterine biopsy forceps
Schuchardt
    S. incision
    S. operation
Schuco nebulizer
Schuffner dots
Schuknecht
    S. classification
    S. retractor
Schultze
    S. mechanism
    S. phantom
    S. placenta
Schwachman-Diamond syndrome
Schwachman syndrome
schwannoma
Schwartz-Jampel-Aberfeld syndrome
Schwartz-Jampel syndrome
sciatic nerve
SCID
    severe combined
    immunodeficiency disease
SciMed-Kolobow membrane lung
scimitar syndrome

scintigraphy
    ventilation s.
scirrhous carcinoma
scissoring
scissors
    Adson ganglion s.
    bandage s.
    Braun episiotomy s.
    Evershears bipolar
     laparoscopic s.
    Jorgenson s.
    Lister s.
    Mayo s.
    Metzenbaum s.
    right-angle s.
    Seilor s.
    Smellie s.
    Spencer stitch s.
    straight s.
    umbilical s.
sclera, pl. sclerae
    blue s.
scleral hemorrhage
scleredema neonatorum
sclerema
    s. neonatorum
sclerocystic
    s. disease of the ovary
    s. ovary
scleroderma
    progressive familial s.
sclero-oophoritis
sclerosing
    s. adenitis
    s. adenosis
    s. agent
    s. lesion
sclerosis, pl. scleroses
    glomerular s.
    menstrual s.
    multiple s.
    ovulational s.
    physiologic s.
    progressive systemic s.
    Sholz s.
    tuberous s.
sclerosteosis

NOTES

sclerotherapy
scoliosis
    Adams test for s.
Scopemaster contact hysteroscope
scopolamine
    s. methylbromide
    s. poisoning
score
    abstinence s.
    Amiel-Tison s.
    Apgar s.
    biophysical profile s.
    Bishop s.
    BPP s.
    cervical s.
    Charlson s.
    Dubowitz s.
    Ferriman-Gallwey
     hirsutism s.
    Manning s.
    Manning s. of fetal activity
    Optimal Observation S.
    pelvic s.
    recovery s.
    Sassone s.
    Silverman s.
    Wood-Downes asthma s.
    Yale Optimal
     Observation S.
Scotch-tape test
Scott cannula
ScP
   scapuloposterior
screen
    antigen s.
    Glucola s.
    organic acid s.
    toxicology s.
    urine toxicology s.
screener
    Algo newborn hearing s.
screening
    Amniostat fetal lung
     maturity s.
    antenatal s.
    antibody s.
    colposcopic s.
    cytologic s.
    Denver Developmental S.
    genetic s.
    hepatitis s.
    s. laboratory tests
    mammographic s.

    maternal s.
    neonatal s.
    prenatal s.
    s. recommendation
    ultrasound s.
    uterine s.
screwdriver teeth
scrofula
scrofuloderma
scrofulosorum
    lichen s.
scroll ear
scrotal tongue
scrotum
    bifid s.
    shawl s.
scrub
    Sklar s.
Scully tumor
scultetus binder
scurvy
    hemorrhagic s.
    infantile s.
SD
   standard deviation
S/D
   systolic/diastolic
    Gammagard S/D
    Polygam S/D
    S/D ratio
S-D disease
   sickle cell-hemoglobin D disease
sea-blue histiocyte syndrome
Seabright bantam syndrome
seal finger
sebaceous
    s. cyst
    s. hyperplasia
    s. nevus syndrome
sebaceum
    adenoma s.
sebaceus
    nevus s.
seborrheic
    s. dermatitis
    s. keratosis
sebum
    s. preputiale
Sechrist neonatal ventilator
Seckel
    bird-headed dwarf of S.
    S. dwarfism
    S. syndrome

secobarbital
Seconal
second
cycles per s. (cps)
s. degree prolapse
S. International Standard (SIS)
s. messenger
s. parallel pelvic plane
s. stage of labor
s. trimester
s. twins
secondary
s. abdominal pregnancy
s. amenorrhea
s. atelectasis
s. dysmenorrhea
s. infertility
s. sex characteristic
s. uterine inertia
second-hand smoke
second-look
s.-l. laparoscopy
s.-l. laparotomy
s.-l. operation
secretion
abnormal cortisol s.
adrenal androgen s.
androgen s.
follicle-stimulating hormone s.
follicular phase gonadotropin s.
gonadotropin s.
impaired s.
luteinizing hormone s.
melatonin s.
persistent estrogen s.
pituitary gonadotropin s.
placental s.
progesterone s.
prolactin s.
steroid s.
syndrome of inappropriate antidiuretic hormone s.
vaginal s.

secretory
s. adenocarcinoma
s. carcinoma
s. disease
s. IgA
s. phase
s. sarcoma
section
cesarean s. (C-section)
frozen s.
Kerr cesarean s.
low cervical cesarean s.
lower uterine segment transverse cesarean s. (LUST C-section)
low transverse cesarean s.
Porro cesarean s.
primary cesarean s.
repeat cesarean s.
vaginal birth after cesarean s. (VBAC)
Sectral
secundigravida
secundina, pl. **secundinae**
secundines
secundipara
secundum
foramen s.
ostium s.
septum s.
Sedabamate
sedation
sedative
s. effect
Sedatuss
sediment
urinary s.
sedimentation rate
seed
gold s.'s
radioactive s.'s
SEER network
Seessel pouch
segment
uterine s.
segmental resection

NOTES

SEH
  subependymal hemorrhage
Seilor scissors
Seip-Lawrence syndrome
Seitelberger disease
Seitzinger tripolar cutting forceps
seizure
  absence s.
  atonic s.
  autonomic s.
  benign familial neonatal s.
  s. control
  s. disorder
  eclamptic s.
  epileptic s.
  febrile s.
  gelastic s.
  hysterical s.
  infantile myoclonic s.
  jackknife s.
  lightning s.
  multifocal clonic s.
  myoclonic s.
  myoclonic-astatic s.
  neonatal s.
  sylvian s.
  tonic s.
  tonic-clonic s., tonoclonic
    seizure
  vertiginous s.
selection
  prenatal s.
  truncate s.
selective
  s. abortion
  s. inguinal node dissection
  s. no-fault system
  s. reduction
  s. termination
self-breast examination
self-catheter
  Mentor female s.-c.
self-catheterization
  clean intermittent s.-c.
self-examination
  breast s.-e. (BSE)
self-monitoring
self-priming action
self-retaining retractor
Self-Test
  OvuQUICK S.-T.
sellar enlargement
sella turcica

Sellheim incision
Sellick maneuver
SEM
  standard error of the mean
semen
  s. analysis
  frozen s.
  s. liquefaction
  viscous s.
  s. volume
Semicid
semi-Fowler position
seminal vesicle
semination
seminiferous
  s. tubule
seminoma
  ovarian s.
semiprone position
Semm
  S. Pelvi-Pneu insufflator
  S. uterine vacuum cannula
  S. Z technique
Sengstaken-Blakemore tube
senile vaginitis
senna
  s. concentrate/docusate
    sodium
  S. X-Prep
Senn-Dingman retractor
Senning repair
Senokot
  S.-S
sensitivity
  assay s.
  culture and s. (C&S)
  microbial s.
sensitization
  Kell s.
  Rh s.
sensitizer
  hypoxic cell s.
Sensorcaine
**Sensorimedics Horizon Metabolic
  Cart**
sensorineural change
sensory
  s. deficit
  s. loss
  s. organ
  s. stimulation
Senter syndrome

SEPA
superficial external pudendal
artery
separation
blastomere s.
peripheral placental s.
placental s.
uterine scar s.
separator
Benson baby pylorus s.
Sephadex binding test
sepsis, pl. sepses
Chlamydia s.
Escherichia coli s.
neonatal s.
s. neonatorum
postoperative s.
puerperal s.
sepsis-pneumonia syndrome
septa (*pl. of* septum)
septal hypertrophy
septate
s. hymen
s. uterus
septectomy
balloon s.
septic
s. abortion
s. arthritis
s. pelvic thrombophlebitis
s. shock
septicemia
puerperal s.
septimetritis
septostomy
atrial s.
balloon s.
Septra DS
septum, pl. septa
aortopulmonary s.
atrioventricular s.
s. pellucidum
placental s.
s. primum
rectovaginal s.
s. secundum

transverse vaginal s.
uterine septa
septuplet
sequela, pl. sequelae
neoplastic s.
sequence
DNA s.
fetal brain disruption s.
Poland malformation s.
Y chromosome-specific
DNA s.
sequencing
chromosome s.
gene s.
sequential
s. administration
s. oral contraceptive
sequestered lung
sequestration
pulmonary s.
sera (*pl. of* serum)
Serax
Sereen
Serentil
Serevent
series
gastrointestinal s.
seriography
biplane s.
sermorelin acetate
serologic test
s. t. for syphilis (STS)
serology
serology-negative mother
seroma
postoperative s.
Seromycin
Serono
S. SR1 FSH analyzer
S. test
Serophene
serosanguineous fluid
serostatus
serotonin
s. reuptake inhibitor
serous
s. adenocarcinoma

NOTES

serous *(continued)*
    s. carcinoma
    s. cystadenoma
    s. ovarian neoplasm
    s. tumor
Serpalan
Serpasil
serpiginosa
    elastosis performans s.
Sertoli
    S. cell
    S. cell tumor
Sertoli-cell-only syndrome
Sertoli-Leydig
    S.-L. cells
    S.-L. cell tumor
sertraline
    s. HCl
    s. hydrochloride
serum, pl. **sera**
    s. albumin
    s. amylase
    s. antibody
    s. assay
    s. concentration
    s. estrogen
    fetal s.
    s. free hemoglobin
    s. hepatitis
    s. iron
    s. level
    s. lithium concentration
    maternal s.
    s. progesterone
    s. prolactin
    s. sickness
    s. testosterone
    s. transaminase
Services
    Child Protective S. (CPS)
    Department of Children
      and Youth S. (DCYS)
servocontrolled ventilation pump
Servo 900C ventilator
servomechanism
sessile polyp
set
    haploid s.
    Janacek reimplantation s.
    Mi-Mark endocervical
      curette s.
    Mi-Mark endometrial
      curette s.

    Neo-Sert umbilical vessel
      catheter insertion s.
    Rosch-Thurmond fallopian
      tube catheterization s.
setting-sun sign
severe
    s. childhood autosomal
      recessive muscular
      dystrophy (SCARMD)
    s. combined
      immunodeficiency disease
      (SCID)
sex
    s. assignment
    s. cell
    s. change operation
    s. chromatin
    chromosomal s.
    s. chromosomal abnormality
    s. chromosomal anomaly
    s. chromosomal polysomy
    s. chromosome
    s. cord
    s. determination
    endocrinologic s.
    genetic s.
    gonadal s.
    s. hormone
    s. hormone-binding globulin
      (SHBG)
    illicit s.
    morphological s.
    nuclear s.
    oral s.
    phenotypic s.
    psychological s.
    s. ratio
    s. reversal
    social s.
    s. steroid
    s. steroid modulation
    s. surrogate
sex-conditioned gene
sex-cord
    s.-c. stromal germ cell
      tumor
    s.-c. stromal neoplasm
    s.-c. stromal tumor
sex-determining region (SRY)
sex-influenced gene
sex-limited gene
sex-linked
    s.-l. chromosome

s.-l. gene
s.-l. heredity
s.-l. inheritance
sextuplet
sexual
s. abuse
s. activity
s. ambiguity
s. asphyxia
s. assault
s. assault forensic evidence
(SAFE)
s. derivation
s. deviation
s. differentiation
s. dimorphism
s. dwarfism
s. dysfunction
s. function
s. habits
s. hair
s. history
s. infantilism
s. intercourse
s. molestation
s. orientation
s. response curve
s. response cycle
s. transmission
sexually transmitted disease (STD)
SG
Chemstrip 10 with S.
SGA
small for gestational age
Sgambati test
SGO
Society of Gynecologic
Oncologists
shadow
acoustic s.
cardiothymic s.
thymic s.
shaggy heart border
shaken baby syndrome
shake test
Shambaugh retractor

Shapleigh curette
**Sharplan USA ultrasonic surgical
aspirator**
Shauta-Aumreich procedure
Shaw I scalpel
shawl scrotum
SHBG
sex hormone-binding globulin
Shearer forceps
shears
ADC Medicut s.
sheath
fibrin s.
Insul-Sheath vaginal
speculum s.
probe s.
PRO/Covers ultrasound
probe s.
Sheathes ultrasound probe cover
shedding
asymptomatic viral s.
endometrial s.
s. syndrome
viral s.
Sheehan syndrome
sheet
amniotic s.
impervious s.
Ioban 2 iodophor
cesarean s.
shelf
Blumer s.
Shenton line
Shepard equation
Shiatsu therapeutic massage
shield
Dalkon s.
Fuller s.
Lea S.
nipple s.
Surety S.
shift
Doppler s.
luteoplacental s.
Shigella
shigellosis

NOTES

Shimadzu
- S. ultrasound
- S. ultrasound system

shingles

Shirodkar
- S. cervical cerclage
- S. operation
- S. procedure

shock
- anaphylactic s.
- bacteremic s.
- cardiogenic s.
- endotoxic s.
- hemorrhagic s.
- hypovolemic s.
- insulin s.
- peripheral vascular s.
- postoperative s.
- septic s.
- toxic s.

shoe
- reverse-last s.'s

Shohl solution

Sholz sclerosis

Shone anomaly

Shorr stain

short
- s. arm of chromosome
- s. frenulum linguae
- s. limbs
- s. rib-polydactyly
- s. rib-polydactyly syndrome (SRPS)

short-axis view

short-bowel syndrome

short-increment sensitivity index (SISI)

short-limb
- s.-l. dwarfism
- s.-l. dystrophy

short-rib dwarfism

shotty node

shoulder
- s. dystocia
- s. presentation

show
- bloody s.

Shprintzen syndrome

Shug male contraceptive device

shunt, shunting
- aortopulmonary s.
- arteriovenous s.
- atrioventricular s.
- AV s.
- Blalock-Taussig s.
- Codman Accu-Flow s.
- Denver hydrocephalus s.
- fetoamniotic s.
- H-H neonatal s.
- intrapulmonary s.
- Kasai peritoneal venous s.
- left-to-right s.
- LeVeen s.
- parietal s.
- Pudenz s.
- right-to-left s.
- ventriculoperitoneal s.
- VP s.
- Waterston s.

Shur-Seal

Shute forceps

Shutt suture punch system

Shwartzman reaction

Shy-Drager syndrome

Shy-Magee syndrome

SIADH
- syndrome of inappropriate antidiuretic hormone

sialic acid

sialidosis

sialorrhea

Siamese twins

sicca syndrome

sicchasia

sickle
- s. cell
- s. cell anemia
- s. cell crisis
- s. cell dactylitis
- s. cell disease
- s. cell hemoglobin (HbS)
- s. cell hemoglobin C (HbsC)
- s. cell-hemoglobin C disease (S-C disease)
- s. cell-hemoglobin D disease (S-D disease, S-D disease)
- s. cell-hemoglobin S disease
- s. cell nephropathy
- s. cell thalassemia
- s. cell-β-thalassemia disease
- s. cell-thalassemia disease
- s. cell trait
- s. thalassemia (HbS-Thal)

Sickledex test

sicklemia

sickness
    morning s.
    serum s.
SID
    sudden infant death
sideroblastic anemia
siderophagic cyst
SIDS
    sudden infant death syndrome
Siegel otoscope
Siegert sign
Siemens-Elema Servo 900C
    ventilator
Siemens SI 400 ultrasound
Siemens Sonoline SI-400
    ultrasound system
Sierra-Sheldon tracheotome
Siggaard-Andersen nomogram
sigmoid colon
sigmoiditis
sigmoidoscopy
sign
    Ahlfeld s.
    Alstrom s.
    Arnoux s.
    Babinski s.
    banana s.
    Beccaria s.
    Béclard s.
    Biederman s.
    Blumberg s.
    Bolt s.
    Borsieri s.
    Braxton Hicks s.
    Brudzinski s.
    Calkins s.
    Chadwick s.
    chandelier s.
    cherub s.
    Chvostek s.
    Comby s.
    Coopernail s.
    crenation s.
    Cullen s.
    Dalrymple s.
    Danforth s.
    Darrier s.

    double-bubble s.
    dovetail s.
    dragon s.
    Elliot s.
    fadir s.
    Federici s.
    flag s.
    Foerster s.
    fontanel s.
    Galeazzi s.
    Gauss s.
    Golden s.
    Goldstein s.
    Goodell s.
    Gowers s.
    Granger s.
    Grisolle s.
    groove s.
    Hahn s.
    halo s.
    halo s. of hydrops
    harlequin s.
    Hartman s.
    Hegar s.
    Hellendall s.
    Higoumenakia s.
    Hoehne s.
    Homans s.
    Hutchinson s.
    Jacquemier s.
    jello s.
    Kanter s.
    Kantu s.
    Kergaradec s.
    Kernig s.
    Kleppinger envelope s.
    Krisovski s.
    Küstner s.
    Ladin s.
    lemon s.
    MacDonald s.
    Macewen s.
    Mayor s.
    Metenier s.
    Mirchamp s.
    Nager s.
    Nelson s.

NOTES

sign *(continued)*
    Nikolsky s.
    Olshausen s.
    Ortolani s.
    palmomandibular s.
    Parrot s.
    Pastia s.
    Perez s.
    peroneal s.
    Pinard s.
    Piskacek s.
    placental s.
    puddle s.
    pyloric string s.
    Radovici s.
    Rasch s.
    Rinman s.
    Romaña s.
    sail s.
    Salmon s.
    Saunders s.
    scarf s.
    Schick s.
    setting-sun s.
    Siegert s.
    Simon s.
    Sisto s.
    Spalding s.
    square window s.
    Stellwag s.
    Sumner s.
    Tanyoz s.
    Tenney-Parker s.
    Toriello-Carey s.
    Tresilian s.
    Trousseau s.
    turtle s.
    Vipond s.
    vital s.
    Von Fernwald s.
    von Graefe s.
    Weill s.
    Wreden s.
    Zaufal s.
signal
    abnormal feedback s.'s
    s. node
signet ring cell carcinoma
significance
    atypical glandular cells of
        undetermined s.
    atypical squamous cells of
        undetermined s. (ASCUS)

Siker laryngoscope
SIL
    squamous intraepithelial lesion
SIL/ASCUS lesion
Silastic
    S. band
    S. cup extractor
    S. ring
    S. silo reduction of
        gastroschisis
Silc extractor
silent
    s. allele
    s. amnionitis
    s. fetal heart rate pattern
    s. gene
    s. oscillatory pattern
    s. pelvic inflammatory
        disease
silicone
    s. implant
    s. implant leakage
    s. injection
    s. plug
silicosis
Sil-K
    S.-K. OB
    S.-K. OB barrier
silk suture
Silon tent
silver
    s. cell
    S. dwarfism
    s. nitrate
    s. nitrate conjunctivitis
    s. nitrate eye prophylaxis
    S. syndrome
    s. wire suture
Silverman-Anderson index
Silverman score
Silver-Russell syndrome
Silverskiöld syndrome
Sim
    S. SC-20 formula
    S. SC-24 formula
simethicone
simian crease
Similac
    S.-20
    S.-24-LBW with whey and
        iron
    S. formula
    S. PM-60/40

S. Special Care-24
S. Special Care formula
S. 24 with iron
similar twins
Simmonds
S. disease
S. syndrome
Simon
S. position
S. sign
Simonton technique
simple
s. colloid goiter
s. cyst
s. mastectomy
s. urethritis
s. vulvectomy
simplex
herpes s.
lichen s.
nevus s.
toxoplasmosis, other agents,
rubella, cytomegalovirus,
herpes s. (TORCH)
Simpson
S. forceps
S. uterine sound
Sims
S. curette
S. position
S. uterine sound
S. vaginal speculum
Sims-Huhner test
SIMV
synchronized intermittent
mandatory ventilation
SIN
salpingitis isthmica nodosa
sincipital presentation
Sinequan
single
s. intrauterine death
s. kidney
single-breech presentation
single-dose methotrexate therapy
single-energy photon absorptiometry
single-footling presentation

single-gene defect
single-photon absorptiometry
singleton
s. fetus
s. pregnancy
single-tooth tenaculum
single-use diagnostic system
(SUDS)
Singley forceps
sinistrocardia
sinistrocerebral
sinistrotorsion
sinobronchitis
sinovaginal bulb
Sinufed
sinus, pl. sinus, sinuses
s. arrest
s. arrhythmia
s. bradycardia
s. histiocytosis
paranasal s.
pilonidal s.
s. tachycardia
urogenital s.
uterine s.
uteroplacental s.
Valsalva s.
s. of Valsalva
s. venosus defect
sinusoid
sinusoidal fetal heart rate
Sioux alarm
Sipple syndrome
Sirecust 404N neonatal monitoring
system
sireniform fetus
sirenomelia
SIS
Second International Standard
SISI
short-increment sensitivity index
SISI test
sister
s. chromatid
s. chromatid exchange
Sister Joseph nodule
Sisto sign

NOTES

site
    antibody reaction s.
    antigen binding s.
    binding s.
    bleeding s.
    placental s.
    placental bleeding s.
    restriction s.
situ, in situ
    carcinoma in s. (CIS)
    vulvar carcinoma in s.
      (VIN III)
situs
    s. inversus
    s. inversus totalis
    s. inversus viscerum
    s. perversus
    s. solitus
    s. transversus
sitz bath
Siver disease
sixth disease
size
    corpus luteum s.
    focal spot s.
    maternal s.
    tumor s.
    uterine s.
size-date discrepancy
Sjögren-Larsson syndrome
Sjögren syndrome
SK-Amitriptyline
skeletal
    s. abnormality
    s. calcium deficiency
    s. dysplasia
    s. growth
    s. maturation
skeleton
    gill arch s.
Skene
    S. duct
    S. gland
skin
    alligator s.
    s. atrophy
    s. calcification
    collodion s.
    congenital localized absence
      of s. (CLAS)
    crocodile s.
    s. disease

    dusky s.
    fish s.
    s. fold
    gelatinous s.
    India rubber s.
    s. lesion
    meconium-stained s.
    mottling of s.
    pallor of s.
    parchment s.
    porcupine s.
    s. staple
    s. tag
    s. temperature
    s. test
    s. thickening
    s. trigger theory
    vulvar s.
skinning
    s. colpectomy
    s. vulvectomy
skip area
Sklar
    S. asceptic germicidal
      disinfectant
    S. aseptic germicidal cleaner
    S. cream
    S. foam
    S. Kleen liquid
    S. Kleen powder
    S. lube
    S. polish
    S. scrub
Sklarasol
Sklarsoak disinfectant
SK-pramine
skull
    bregma of s.
    cloverleaf s.
    coronal suture line of s.
    s. fracture
    hot cross bun s.
    lacunar s.
    maplike s.
    natiform s.
    sutures of s.
    tower s.
    West-Engstler s.
Sky-Boot stirrup system
SLA
    superficial linear array
    SLA transducer

SLAS
  salt-losing adrenogenital
    syndrome
Slavianski membrane
SLE
  systemic lupus erythematosus
sleep
  s. apnea
  non-REM s.
  twilight s.
sleeping habits
SLI
  subdermal levonorgestrel
    implant
slick-gut syndrome
slide
  Testsimplets prestained s.
sliding
  s. hernia
  s. lock
sling
  Aldridge rectus fascia s.
  levator s.
  s. procedure
  pulmonary artery s.
  retropubic s.
  suburethral s.
Slo-bid
Slo-Niacin
Slo-Phyllin
Slo-Salt
Slo-Salt-K
Slotnick-Goldfarb syndrome
Slow Fe
  S. F. with folic acid
Slow-Fe
Slow-K
Slow-Mag
slow-release sodium fluoride
Slow-Trasicor
SLUDGE
  salivation, lacrimation,
    urination, defecation,
    gastrointestinal distress and
    emesis

Sly
  S. disease
  S. syndrome
S-M-A formula
small
  s. bowel
  s. bowel endometriosis
  s. bowel strangulation
  s. cell carcinoma
  s. chromosome
  s. for gestational age (SGA)
  s. intestine decompression
  s. left colon syndrome
small-for-dates
small-for-gestational-age infant
smallpox
  s. vaccine
Smead-Jones closure
smear
  ASCUS s.
  cervical s.
  Pap s.
  Papanicolaou s.
  vaginal s.
  vaginal irrigation s. (VIS)
  wet s.
smegma
  s. clitoridis
  s. embryonum
  s. preputii
Smellie
  S. method
  S. scissors
Smellie-Veit method
S-methionine-labeled polypeptide
smiling incision
Smith-Hodge pessary
Smith-Lemli-Opitz syndrome
smoke
  s. evacuator
  s. inhalation
  s. plume
  s. removal tube (SRT)
  second-hand s.
smooth
  s. muscle
  s. muscle contraction

NOTES

SMZ-TMP
    trimethoprim-sulfamethoxazole
snapshot GRASS technique
snare
    Reiner-Beck s.
snout reflex
snowflake pattern
snowstorm appearance
Sn-protoporphyrin
snuffles
soak
    Cidex s.
soap
    Basis s.
    pHisoHex s.
    TLC antiseptic s.
soapsuds enema
social
    s. drug
    s. factor effect
    s. issue
    s. sex
Social Support Scale for Children
    test (SSSC)
Society
    American Fertility S. (AFS)
    S. for Assisted Reproductive
        Technology (SART)
    S. of Gynecologic
        Oncologists (SGO)
    S. of Gynecologic Oncology
    S. for Gynecologic
        Pathology
socioeconomic status
sodium
    ampicillin
        sodium/sulbactam s.
    s. balance
    s. bicarbonate
    s. bromide
    cefazolin s.
    cefoperazone s.
    cefotaxime s.
    cefoxitin s.
    ceftriaxone s.
    cephalothin s.
    s. chloride
    s. citrate with citric acid
    cromolyn s.
    s. cyclamate
    1D s. dodecyl sulfate gel
    s. diatrizoate
    diclofenac s.

Diphenylan S.
docusate s.
s. equilin sulfate
estramustine phosphate s.
s. estrone sulfate
s. excretion
s. fluoride
heparin s.
imipenem-cilastaten s.
s. iodide
s. iodide I-125
s. iodide I-131
methicillin s.
mezlocillin s.
nafcillin s.
naproxen s.
s. nitroprusside
oxacillin s.
oxychlorosone s.
Pentothal S.
piperacillin s.
piperacillin
    sodium/tazobactam s.
s. requirement
s. restriction
s. salicylate
senna
    concentrate/docusate s.
thiopental s.
s. thiosulfate
s. valproate
zobactam s.
zomepirac s.
sodium-free formula
sodomize
sodomy
soft
    s. radiation grid Pb4/27
    s. tissue abnormality
    s. tissue ovarian neoplasm
softener
    stool s.
Soft-Wand atraumatic tissue
    manipulator balloon
Sohval-Soffer syndrome
Solar Beam medical examination
    light
Solatene
Solazine
sole crease
Solfoton
Solganal
solid-phase enzyme immunoassay

solitary
    s. dilated duct
    s. kidney
solitus
    situs s.
Solium
Solos
    S. disposable cannula
    S. disposable trocar
soluble
    s. antigen excess
    s. gas technique
    s. RNA
solution
    Bouin s.
    Burow s.
    clindamycin phosphate
      topical s.
    Cornoy s.
    Denhardt s.
    Dianeal dialysis s.
    DuraPrep surgical s.
    Hartmann s.
    lacmoid staining s.
    lactated Ringer s.
    Locke s.
    Lugol iodine s.
    modified Ham F-10 s.
    Monsel s.
    Pedialyte oral electrolyte
      maintenance s.
    Ringer s.
    saline s.
    Schiller s.
    Shohl s.
    sperm viability staining s.
    Transeptic cleansing s.
    Tyrode s.
somamammotropin
    chorionic s.
somatic
    s. cell
    s. cells
    s. chromosome
    s. nervous system feedback
      loop
somatoliberin

somatomedin C
somatomedin level
Somatom Plus computed
    tomography
somatopagus
somatoschisis
somatostatin
somatotridymus
somatotrope
somatotropinoma
somatrem
    s. growth hormone
somatropin
    s. growth hormone
Somer uterine elevator
somite
    s. embryo
    s. formation
somnambulism
somnogram
Somogyi phenomenon
Somophyllin
Sonicaid
    S. Axis monitor
    S. SYSTEM 8000 fetal
      monitor
    S. Vasoflow Doppler system
Sonoclot
    S. coagulation analyzer
    S. test
Sono-Gram fetal ultrasound image
    card
sonographic finding
sonography
    Acuson computed s.
    real-time s.
    transvaginal s. (TVS)
    vaginal s.
sonolucency
sonolucent
    s. tissue
sonomicroscopy
SonoVu US aspiration needle
S.O.P.
    Genoptic S.
Sopher ovum forceps
Sorbitrate

NOTES

387

Sorsby syndrome
sorter
    fluorescence-activated cell s.
      (FACS)
    magnetically-activated cell s.
      (MACS)
sorting
Sotos syndrome
souffle
    fetal s.
    funic s., funicular s.
    mammary s.
    placental s.
    umbilical s.
    uterine s.
sound
    active bowel s.'s
    bowel s.'s
    cracked pot s.
    fetal heart s.'s
    grating s.
    heart s.'s
    hyperactive bowel s.'s
    hypoactive bowel s.'s
    normoactive bowel s.'s
    Pharmaseal disposable
      uterine s.
    Simpson uterine s.
    Sims uterine s.
    urethral s.
    uterine s.
    Waring blender s.
sound-stimulated fetal movement
source
    cesium s.
    dummy s.
    MX2-300 xenon quality
      light s.
source-to-axis distance (SAD)
source-to-skin distance (SSD)
South
    S. African genetic porphyria
    S. African tick fever
Southern
    S. blot
    S. blot technique
    S. blot test
Soyacal
    S. IV fat emulsion
Soyalac formula
SP
    sacroposterior

space
    Bogros s.
    intervillous s.'s
    perivitelline s.
    subchorial s.
    vesicocervical s.
    volume of dead s.
    yolk s.
spacer
    dummy s.
spacing
    third s.
Spalding sign
span
    fertilizable life s.
Spanish fly
Sparine
sparing
    brain s.
spasm
    infantile s.
    levator ani s.
    urethral s.
spasmodic dysmenorrhea
spasmus nutans
spastic
    s. diplegia
    s. diplegia syndrome
    s. paralysis
spasticity
spatula
    Ayre s.
    Cytobrush s.
    s. foot
    Milex s.
Spearman-Brown prediction formula
Special Care formula
species
species-specific antibody
specific
    s. immunotherapy
    s. urethritis
specificity
    assay s.
specimen
    catheter s.
    clean-catch urine s.
    hemolyzed s.
    midstream urine s.
    xanthochromic s.
Speck test
Spect-Align laser system
spectinomycin

spectra (*pl. of* spectrum)
Spectra-Diasonics ultrasound
Spectra 400 extended surveillance
  and alert system
spectral Doppler
Spectrobid
spectrophotometry
  atomic absorption s.
spectrum, pl. spectra
  Doppler shift spectra
  electromagnetic s.
Spectrum stethoscope
specular echo
speculum, pl. specula
  Amko vaginal s.
  Auvard s.
  bivalve s.
  blackened s.
  duckbill s.
  s. examination
  Graves bivalve s.
  Halle infant nasal s.
  Holinger infant
   esophageal s.
  Huffman infant vaginal s.
  Kogan endocervical s.
  Pederson vaginal s.
  Sani-Spec vaginal s.
  Sims vaginal s.
  SRT vaginal s.
  weighted s.
speech reception threshold (SRT)
Spee embryo
spell
  A & B s.
Spemann induction
Spence
  axillary tail of S.
  S. axillary tail
  S. and Duckett
   marsupialization
  S. procedure
Spencer
  S. probe
  S. stitch scissors
sperm
  acrosome-intact s.

s. agglutination test
s. allergy
anonymous donor s. (ADS)
s. antibody
s. attrition
s. bank
s. capacitation
s. capacitation medium
s. chromatin decondensation
s. count
s. donation
donor s.
s. donor
epididymal s.
frozen s.
haploid s.
s. immobilization test
motile s.
s. motility
muzzled s.
s. penetration assay
S. Select sperm recovery
  system
s. transport
s. viability staining solution
washed s.
s. washing insemination
  method (SWIM)
Spermac stain
spermagglutination
sperm-aster
spermatic
  s. cord
spermatin
spermatocide
spermatogenesis
spermatogonia
spermatotoxin
spermatozoon, pl. spermatozoa
sperm-counting fluid
sperm-egg adhesion
sperm-free ejaculate
spermicide
spermidine
spermine
sperm-mediated
sperm-oocyte interaction

NOTES

Spersacarpine
S phase fraction
sphenocephaly
sphenoid fontanel
sphenopagus
spherocytosis
  hereditary s.
sphincter
  anal s.
  esophageal s.
  s. repair
  urethral s.
sphingolipidosis
sphingomyelin
spiculated lesion
spider
  s. angioma
  s. finger
  s. nevus
  vascular s.
Spiegelberg criteria
Spielmeyer-Vogt disease
spigelian hernia
spina
  s. bifida
  s. bifida cystica
  s. bifida occulta
spinal
  s. analgesia
  s. anesthesia
  s. angioma
  s. blockade
  s. bone loss
  s. compression fracture
  s. cord
  s. cord injury
  s. headache
  s. injury
  s. meningocele
spine
  cleft s.
  cloven s.
  dysraphia of s.
Spinelli operation
spinnbarkeit
  s. (cervical mucus)
spinning-top deformity
spinocerebellar degenerative disease
spinosa
  ichthyosis s.
spinulosus
  lichen s.

spiral
  s. artery
  s. electrode
spiramycin
Spirette
  CCD S.
spirochete
spironolactone
Spitz nevus
splanchnic
  s. fold
  s. pelvic pain
splanchnocystica
  dysencephalia s.
splanchnopathy
splanchnopleuric
spleen
  accessory s.
splenectomy
splenic
  s. flexure
  s. pregnancy
  s. rupture
  s. sequestration syndrome
  s. tissue
  s. torsion
splenomegaly
splenosis
splicing
  gene s.
splint
  Denis Browne s.
  Denis Browne clubfoot s.
  Freidman s.
  Ilfeldt s.
  talipes hobble s.
split
  cricoid s.
split-thickness graft
splitting
  blastocyst s.
  embryo s.
  muscle s.
spoke-wheel palpation
spondylitis
  ankylosing s.
spondylocostal dysplasia syndrome
spondyloepiphyseal
  s. dysplasia
  s. dysplasia congenita
    syndrome
spondylolisthesis
spondylolysis

spondylometaphyseal dysplasia
spondylothoracic dysplasia
  syndrome
sponge
    absorbable gelatin s.
    contraceptive s.
    s. forceps
    intravaginal s.
    Lapwall s.
    s. stick
    Today vaginal
      contraceptive s.
    vaginal s.
    Weck-sel s.
sponge-holding forceps
spongiform encephalopathy
spongioblastoma
spongy degeneration of infancy
spontaneous
    s. abortion (SAB)
    s. amputation
    s. breech extraction
    s. cephalic delivery
    s. evolution
    s. gangrene of newborn
    s. labor
    s. menstrual cycle
    s. ovulation
    s. preterm delivery
    s. remission
    s. rupture of membranes
    (SROM)
    s. version
sporotrichosis
spot
    blood s.
    blue s.
    blueberry muffin s.
    Brushfield s.
    café au lait s.
    s. compression
    s. compression view
    Fordyce s.
    Koplik s.
    s. magnification
    mongolian s.
    strawberry s.

spotlight
    KDC-Healthdyne
      nonfluorescent s.
spotted fever
Sprangeler-Wiedemann syndrome
spray
    butorphanol tartrate nasal s.
    DDAVP nasal s.
    Itch-X s.
spread
    halstedian concept of
      tumor s.
    lymphatic s.
    vessel s.
Sprengel
    S. anomaly
    S. deformity
sprout
    syncytial s.
sprue
    celiac s.
spun
    s. hematocrit
    s. urine
spuria
    melena s.
    placenta s.
spurious pregnancy
Spurway syndrome
sputum, pl. sputa
    s. culture
    s. cytology
squama
squamocolumnar junction
squamous
    s. cell
    s. cell carcinoma
    s. epithelium
    s. intraepithelial lesion (SIL)
    s. metaplasia
    s. metaplasia of amnion
square
    chi-s. (χ^2)
    s. matrix
    Punnett s.
    s. window
    s. window sign

NOTES

squirming Valsalva
SR
    Indocin S.
    Oramorph S.
    Roxanol S.
Sα-reductase
SRI automated immunoassay analyzer
SROM
    spontaneous rupture of membranes
SRPS
    short rib-polydactyly syndrome
SRT
    smoke removal tube
    speech reception threshold
        SRT vaginal speculum
SRY
    sex-determining region
SSC-20 formula
SSC-24 formula
SSCVD
    sterile, spontaneous, controlled vaginal delivery
SSD
    source-to-skin distance
SSKI
SSSC
    Social Support Scale for Children test
SSVD
    sterile, spontaneous vaginal delivery
ST
    sacrotransverse
St.
    St. Clair-Thompson curette
    St. Louis encephalitis
    St. Vitus dance
stabilization
stable access cannula
stab wound
staccato cough
stadiometer
    Harpenden s.
Stadol
stage
    cortical supremacy s.
    delayed first s.
    developmental s.'s
    diakinesis s.
    dictyate s.

    indifferent gonadal s.
    s.'s of labor
    leptotene s.
    pachytene s.
    placental s.
    Tanner s.
    zygotene s.
staging
    American Joint Committee for Cancer S. (AJCC)
    clinical s.
    FIGO s.
    Marshall-Tanner pubertal s.
    Northway s.
    surgical s.
    Tanner s. (Grade I, II, III, IV)
stagnation mastitis
STAI-I
    State-Trait-Anxiety Index-I
stain, staining
    Betke s.
    blood pigment s.
    Feulgen s.
    Giemsa s.
    Gram s.
    Gram-Weigert s.
    Grimelius s.
    iodine s.
    Kinyoun s.
    Kleihauer-Betke s.
    KOH s.
    Leder s.
    Masson-Fontana s.
    meconium s.
    Movat s.
    PAS s., PASA s.
    port-wine s.
    Shorr s.
    Spermac s.
    Wright s.
stainless steel suture
stalk
    allantoic s.
    body s.
    infundibular s.
    yolk s.
stalking
    celery s.
Stallworthy placenta
Stamey
    S. catheter

S. modification of Pereyra procedure
S. operation

stammering
s. bladder

stance
Buddha s.

standard
s. curve
s. deviation (SD)
s. error of the mean (SEM)
protein s.
Second International S. (SIS)

Stanley Way procedure
Staphcillin
staphylococcal pneumonia
staphylococcal-scalded skin syndrome
Staphylococcus
S. *aureus*
S. *epidermidis*
S. *saprophyticus*

staphylococcus, pl. **staphylococci**
staple
absorbable s.
metallic s.
skin s.
titanium s.

stapler
EEA s.
Endo-GIA s.
Endo-GIA30 suture s.
Endopath endoscopic articulating s.
Precise disposable skin s.
Vista disposable skin s.

star
s. effect
S. ventilator

Stargardt disease
Starling
S. equation
S. equilibrium
S. law of transcapillary exchange

startle
s. disease
s. pattern
s. reaction
s. reflex
s. response

starvation
accelerated s.
s. ketosis

stasis
urinary s.

state
accompanying mood s.
fugue s.
gradient recalled acquisition in a steady s. (GRASS)
menstrual s.
mood s.

state-of-the-art radiation
State-Trait-Anxiety Index-I (STAI- I)
static ß-scanner
station
0 s.
complete/complete/+ s.
fetal s.

statistical model
Stat-Lab Technologies
Statobex
stature
constitutional short s.
idiopathic short s.
maternal s.

status
acid-base s.
s. asthmaticus
s. dysmyelinisatus
s. epilepticus
Karnofsky performance s.
s. lymphaticus
s. marmoratus
socioeconomic s.
s. thymicolymphaticus
s. thymicus

statutory rape
STD
sexually transmitted disease

NOTES

steatorrhea
    idiopathic s.
steely-hair syndrome
Steiner
    S. canals
    S. tumor
Steinert
    S. disease
    S. myotonic dystrophy
    S. syndrome
Stein-Leventhal
    S.-L. syndrome
    S.-L. type of polycystic
      ovary
Stelazine
stellate mass
Stellwag sign
stem cell assay
Stemetil
stenosis
    anorectal s.
    antral s.
    aortic s.
    aqueductal s.
    bladder neck s.
    cervical s.
    esophageal s.
    hypertrophic s.
    idiopathic hypertrophic
      subaortic s.
    infundibular s.
    mitral s.
    postischemic s.
    pulmonary s.
    pyloric s.
    renal artery s.
    subaortic s.
    tracheal s.
    tubular s.
    urethral s.
    valvular pulmonic s.
Stensen duct
stent
    double-J s.
    urinary s.
step-down cannula
stepping reflex
stereocolpogram
stereocolposcope
stereoscopic pelvimetry
stereotactic
    s. breast biopsy
    s. breast biopsy needle

stereotaxis
Steri-Drape 2
Steri-Drape drape
sterile
    s. pyuria syndrome
    s. specimen trap
    s., spontaneous, controlled
      vaginal delivery (SSCVD)
    s., spontaneous vaginal
      delivery (SSVD)
    s. vaginal examination
      (SVE)
sterility
    absolute s.
    adolescent s.
    one-child s.
    relative s.
sterilization
    intermittent s.
    involuntary s.
    tubal s.
    voluntary s.
sterilize
Steri-Strip skin closure
sternocleidomastoid hemorrhage
sternodymus
sternopagus
sternoschisis
sternoxiphopagus
steroid
    adrenal s.
    adrenocortical s.
    s. biosynthesis
    s. cell
    s. concentration
    s. contraceptive
    endogenous s.
    s. hormone
    s. hormone receptor
    17-ketogenic s.
    long-acting contraceptive s.
    low-dose s.'s
    s. metabolism
    s. metabolite
    s. nucleus
    ovarian s.
    placental s.
    s. secretion
    s. secretion inhibition
    sex s.
    s. sulfatase
    s. sulfatase deficiency
    s. therapy

steroidogenesis
    adrenocortical s.
    fetal-placental s.
    follicle s.
    ovarian s.
    testicular s.
steroidogenic
stethoscope
    Allen fetal s.
    Doptone fetal s.
    Spectrum s.
    ultrasound s.
Stevens-Johnson syndrome
Stewart-Treves syndrome
stick
    sponge s.
Sticker disease
Stickler syndrome
stiff-baby syndrome
stigma, pl. stigmata
stilbestrol
Still
    S. disease
    S. murmur
stillbirth
stillborn infant
Stilling-Türk-Duane syndrome
Stillman cleft
Stilphostrol
stimulant
stimulation
    ACTH s.
    cervical carcinoma s.
    endometrial s.
    exogenous gonadotropin s.
    follicle maturation s.
    ovulation s.
    oxytocic s.
    prolactin s.
    sensory s.
    tactile s.
    s. test
    vibroacoustic s.
    visual s.
stimulator
    adrenergic s.
    alpha-adrenergic s.

hematopoietic system s.
Innova pelvic floor s.
long-acting thyroid s.
    (LATS)
luteinization s.
stimulus, pl. stimuli
    tactile s.
stirrups
    Allen laparoscopic s.
    candy-cane s.
    Lloyd-Davies s.
    Navratil s.
stitch
    s. abscess
    McCall s.
stochastic independence
stockinette
    impervious s.
stocking
    antiembolism s.
    elastic s.
    Juzo-Hostess two-way stretch
        compression s.'s
    leg-compression s.'s
    TED s.'s
Stock-Spielmeyer-Vogt syndrome
stomach cancer metastasis
stomatitis
    aphthous s.
    herpetic s.
stomatocytosis
stomatomy
stomatoschisis
stomatotomy
stomocephalus
stone
    kidney s.
    renal s.
    womb s.
stool
    acholic s.
    s. colonization
    currant jelly s.
    s. examination
    s. softener
STORCH test
stork bite

NOTES

storm
   thyroid s.
Stormby brush
Stortz
   S. disposable cannula
   S. disposable trocar
Storz
   S. endoscope
   S. infant bronchoscope
   S. laparoscope
Stoxil
strabismus
straight
   s. catheter test
   s. scissors
straight-back syndrome
strait
   inferior s.
   superior s.
strangulated hernia
strangulation
   small bowel s.
strangury
strap
   Montgomery s.
   S. operation
Strassman
   S. metroplasty
   S. phenomenon
   S. technique
   transverse fundal incision
      of S.
strata (*pl. of* stratum)
stratification
stratified squamous epithelium
stratum, pl. strata
   s. basale
   s. compactum
   s. functionale
strawberry
   s. appearance
   s. cervix
   s. hemangioma
   s. mark
   s. nevus
   s. spot
   s. tongue
streak
   gonadal s.
   s. gonads
   primitive s.
streaking
   perihilar s.

streaky infiltrate
streblodactyly
Streeter
   S. bands
   S. dysplasia
   S. horizon
Strema
Strength
   Tums Extra S.
Streptase
streptococcal
   s. group
   s. infection
   s. pharyngitis
   s. pneumonia
   s. vaginitis
Streptococcus
   S. agalactiae
   S. milleri
   S. pneumoniae
   S. viridans
streptococcus, pl. streptococci
   fecal streptococci
   group A s.
   group B s.
   group D streptococcus
   β-hemolytic s.
streptogenes
   erythema s.
streptokinase
   s.-urokinase
streptomycin
stress
   s. incontinence de novo
   life s.
   maternal s.
   postmenstrual s.
   psychological s.
   s. reaction in exenteration
   s. test
   s. urinary incontinence
      (SUI)
   visual analog scale for s.
stressed fetus
stria, pl. striae
   abdominal s.
   striae atrophicae
   striae cutis distensae
   striae gravidarum
   Langhans s.
   Rohr s.
striata
   osteopathia s.

striated
- s. circular muscle
- s. muscle

striatus
- lichen s.

stridor
- inspiratory s.
- laryngeal s.

strip
- fascial s.
- leucocyte detection s.
- lung s.
- Mersilene fascial s.
- polypropylene fascial s.
- saturation s.

Stroganoff method
stroke
stroma
- cervical s.
- fibromuscular cervical s.
- gonadal s.
- ovarian s.
- Rh-positive red cell s.
- uterine endolymphatic s.
- uterine endometrial s.
- uterine epithelial s.

stromal
- s. adenomyosis
- s. cell
- s. development
- s. endometriosis
- s. hyperthecosis
- s. microinvasion

stromal-epithelial interaction
stromatosis
stromelysin
strongyloidiasis
strontium bromide
strophocephaly
strophulus
structural gene
struma, pl. **strumae**
- s. ovarii

strumal carcinoid of ovary
Strumpell-Lorrain disease
strychnine poisoning

STS
- serologic test for syphilis

Stuart
- S. factor
- S. index
- S. Prenatal vitamins

Stuartnatal 1+1
Stuart-Prower factor
stuck-twin phenomenon
studding
- peritoneal s.

Student t test
study
- acoustic stimulation s.
- acute-phase serum s.
- barium s.
- biochemical s.
- Cancer and Steroid Hormone s.
- CASH s.
- cytogenetic s.
- fetal blood s.
- histopathological s.
- Intergroup Rhabdomyosarcoma S. (IRS)
- Oxford Family Planning Association Contraceptive S.
- postmortem s.
- routine antenatal diagnostic imaging ultrasound s.
- Royal College of General Practioners' Oral Contraception S.
- tissue s.
- transesophageal electrophysiologic s.
- urodynamic s.

stunted
- s. embryo
- s. fetus

Sturge-Kalischer-Weber syndrome
Sturge syndrome
Sturge-Weber syndrome

NOTES

Sturmdorf
    S. hemostatic suture
    S. operation
stuttering
sty, stye
stylopodium
stype
    s. tampon
subacute bacterial endocarditis (SBE)
subaortic
    s. lymph node
    s. stenosis
subarachnoid
    s. block
    s. hemorrhage
subareolar duct papillomatosis
subchorial
    s. lake
    s. space
subchorionic hemorrhage
subclinical hypothyroidism
subcostal retractions
subcutanea
    lipogranulomatosis s.
subcutaneous
    s. fat necrosis
    s. mastectomy
subdermal
    s. implant
    s. levonorgestrel implant (SLI)
subdural
    s. hematoma
    s. hemorrhage
    s. puncture
subependymal hemorrhage (SEH)
subfertility
subfragment-1
subinvolution
subjective probability
sublethal gene
Sublimaze
sublingual
    s. gland
    s. hematoma
submammary mastitis
submaxillary gland
submental hematoma
submetacentric chromosome
submucosal
    s. myoma

    s. plexus
    s. urethral augmentation
submucous
    s. leiomyoma
    s. myoma
subnormal temperature
suboccipitobregmatic diameter
suboptimal surgery
subpectoral implant
subphrenic
    s. abscess
subseptate uterus
subsequent fertility
subserosal myoma
subserous
    s. fascia
    s. myoma
subset
    T-cell s.'s
substance
    müllerian inhibiting s.
    s. P pain neurotransmitter
    s. X
substrate
    renin s.
subunit
suburethral sling
subzonal insemination (SUZI)
succedaneum
    caput s.
succenturiate placenta
successful pregnancy
succinate
    sumatriptan s.
succinylcholine
succinylsulfathiazole
sucking
    s. cushion
    nonnutritive s.
    s. pad
    s. reflex
suckle
suckling
sucralfate
sucrose-free formula
suction
    airway s.
    s. catheter
    s. curettage
    s. drainage
    nasopharyngeal s.
    s. pump
    Vabra s.

suctioning
  bulb s.
  DeLee s.
suction-irrigator
  Nezhat-Dorsey s.-i.
suctorial pad
Sudafed
sudanophilic leukodystrophy
sudden
  s. infant death (SID)
  s. infant death syndrome
    (SIDS)
Sudrin
SUDS
  single-use diagnostic system
  SUDS HIV-1 antibody test
sufentanil citrate
sugar
  blood s.
  fasting blood s.
SUI
  stress urinary incontinence
suicide
suis
  Herpesvirus s.
suit
  MAST s.
sulbactam
Sulf-10
sulfa
sulfacarbamide
sulfacetamide
sulfachlorpyridazine
sulfacytine
sulfadiazine
sulfadimethoxine
sulfadimidine
sulfadoxine
sulfaethidole
sulfafurazole, sulphafurazole
sulfaguanidine
sulfalene
sulfamerazine
sulfameter
sulfamethazine
sulfamethizole

sulfamethoxazole
sulfamethoxazole/phenazopyridine
  hydrochloride
sulfamethoxydiazine
sulfamethoxypyridazine
Sulfamylon
sulfanilamide
sulfaphenazole, sulphaphenazole
sulfapyridine
sulfasalazine
sulfatase
  steroid s.
sulfate
  amikacin s.
  bleomycin s.
  dehydroepiandrosterone s.
    (DHEAS)
  dehydroisoandrosterone s.
  DHEA s.
  ephedrine s.
  estrone s.
  ferric s.
  ferrous s. (FeSO$_4$)
  gentamicin s.
  hexoprenaline s.
  magnesium s.
  metaproterenol s.
  morphine s.
  Mycifradin S.
  neomycin s.
  netilmicin s.
  orciprenaline s.
  piperazine estrone s.
  polymyxin B s.
  sodium equilin s.
  sodium estrone s.
  terbutaline s.
  trimethoprim s.
  vincristine s.
sulfathiazole
sulfathiourea
sulfisomidine
sulfisoxazole
sulfisoxazole/phenazopyridine
  hydrochloride
sulfonamide

NOTES

sulfonate
   2-mercaptoethane s.
   (MESNA)
sulfonylurea
sulfotransferase
   estrogen s.
sulfur granule
sulindac
sulphafurazole (*var. of*
   sulfafurazole)
sulphaphenazole (*var. of*
   sulfaphenazole)
sulpiride
Sultrin
sumatriptan succinate
Sumner sign
Sumycin
sunken fontanel
sunny-side up delivery
superfecundation
superfetation
superficial
   s. external pudendal artery
   (SEPA)
   s. linear array (SLA)
   s. spreading melanoma
   s. thrombophlebitis
superimposed
   s. eclampsia
   s. preeclampsia
superimpregnation
superinvolution
superior
   s. mesenteric artery
   s. mesenteric plexus
   s. strait
   s. vena cava
   s. vena caval syndrome
superlactation
supernumerary
   s. chromosome
   s. digit
   s. mamma
   s. nipple
   s. ovary
   s. placenta
superovulation
   s. induction
supervoltage
   s. radiation
supine
   s. hypotensive syndrome

   s. position
   s. pressor test
supplement, supplementation
   Aminosyn-PF s.
   calcium s.
   Fer-In-Sol s.
   vitamin s.
supplementary
   s. genes
   s. menstruation
supply
   iodine s.
support
   s. group
   neonatal adjuvant life s.
   (NALS)
   psychosocial s.
   ventilator s.
suppository
   AVC s.
   glycerin s.
   Monistat-3 vaginal s.
   prostaglandin s.
   rectal s.
   Terazol vaginal s.
   vaginal s.
Supprelin
suppressed menstruation
suppression
   endogenous gonadotropin
   activity s.
   estradiol s.
   gonadal steroid s.
   immunologic s.
   pituitary gonadotropin s.
   prolactin s.
   testosterone s.
suppressor
   s. cell
   s. gene
   s. T cell
Supprettes
   Aquachloral S.
suppuration
   pulmonary s.
suppurative
   s. appendicitis
   s. mastitis
   s. phlebitis
supracervical hysterectomy
supraciliary tap
suprapubic
   s. catheter

s. cystotomy
s. pain
s. urethrovesical suspension
  operation
supraumbilical incision
supraventricular
s. tachyarrhythmia (SVT)
s. tachycardia (SVT)
s. tachydysrhythmia
Suprax
SureCell
S. Chlamydia Test kit
S. Herpes (HSV) Test
S. rapid test kit
S. rapid test kit for
  pregnancy
Surety Shield
surface
s. antigen
s. epithelium
s. epithelium vascular
  channel
s. immunoglobulin
s. irradiation
s. tension
surfactant
beractant s.
bovine s.
s. deficiency syndrome
heterologous s.
Human Surf s.
Infrasurf s.
porcine s.
pulmonary s.
rescue s.
Survanta s.
surf test
surge
estrogen s.
LH s.
midcycle s.
preovulatory LH s.
surgery
bypass s.
conservative s.
cytoreductive s.
fetal s.

gastric reduction s.
hysteroscopic s.
intraabdominal s.
laser s.
palliative s.
pelvic s.
pelvic-floor s.
radical s.
suboptimal s.
tubal reconstruction s.
vaginal s.
surgical
s. infection
s. management
s. repair
s. resection
s. staging
s. weight loss
surgically-induced abortion
Surgicenter 40 CO2 laser
Surgilase 55W laser
Surgilene
Surgin hemorrhage occluder pin
Surgiport
Surmontil
surrogacy
surrogate
gestational s.
s. mother
s. motherhood
sex s.
Survanta
S. surfactant
surveillance
S., Epidemiology and End
  Results network (SEER
  network)
fetal s.
immunologic s.
maternal s.
nutritional s.
s. technique
s. tracheal aspirate
ultrasound s.
survival
actuarial s.
allograft s.

NOTES

survival *(continued)*
    life table s.
    long-term s.
    s. rate
susceptibility
    genetic s.
suspected pituitary adenoma
suspension
    Aldridge-Studdefort
      urethral s.
    Alexander-Adams uterine s.
    Baldy-Webster uterine s.
    bladder neck s.
    Coffey s.
    endoscopic bladder neck s.
      (EBNS)
    Gilliam-Doleris uterine s.
    minimal-incision
      pubovaginal s.
    Olshausen s.
    Pereyra needle s.
    protamine insulin zinc s.
    sacrospinous ligament s.
    uterine s.
suspensory sling operation
Sus-Phrine
Sustacal
    S. formula
Sustagen
    S. formula
Sustaire
sutural calcification
suture
    absorbable s.
    apposition of skull s.
    catgut s.
    continuous running
      monofilament s.
    cranial s.
    Dexon s.
    Endoloop s.
    frontal s.
    gut s.
    interrupted s.
    s. material
    Mersilene s.
    Monocryl s.
    overriding of s.'s
    polygalactide s.
    polyglycol s.
    polyglyconate s.
    Prolene s.
    purse-string s.

    retention s.
    sagittal s.
    silk s.
    silver wire s.
    stainless steel s.
    Sturmdorf hemostatic s.
    Vicryl s.
suture-ligation
suture-ligature
sutures of skull
SUZI
    subzonal insemination
SVE
    sterile vaginal examination
SVT
    supraventricular
      tachyarrhythmia
    supraventricular tachycardia
swallowing
    fetal s.
swallow reflex
Swan-Ganz catheter
sweat
    s. chloride determination
    s. chloride level
    s. chloride test
Swedish porphyria
sweep
    s. gas
    s. the pelvis
    The Cell S.
Sweet syndrome
swelling
    labioscrotal s.
Swenson pull-through procedure
Swift disease
SWIM
    sperm washing insemination
      method
Swiss
    S. cheese endometrium
    S. cheese hyperplasia
switch
    genetic s.
    s. operation
swivel-arm system
swordfish test
Swyer-James-Macleod syndrome
Swyer-James syndrome
Swyer syndrome
Sydenham chorea
Sydney line
sylvian seizure

symbiotic psychosis
symbrachydactyly
symmelia
Symmetrel
symmetrical conjoined twins
symmetric communicating uterus
symmetros
    duplicitas s.
sympathectomy, sympathetectomy
    presacral s.
sympathetic nervous system
sympathomimetic
symphocephalus
symphyses (*pl. of* symphysis)
symphysiotome, symphyseotome
symphysiotomy, symphyseotomy
symphysis, pl. symphyses
    pubic s.
    s. pubis
symphysodactyly
sympodia
symptom
    premenstrual s.'s
symptomatic
    s. infection
    s. porphyria
symptomatica
    porphyria cutanea tarda s.
symptothermal method
sympus
synadelphus
Synalar
Synalgos-DC
synapsis
synaptophysin
Synarel
Synasal
syncephalus
syncheilia
synchondrotomy
synchronic
synchronized intermittent
    mandatory ventilation (SIMV)
synchronous breathing
synclitic
synclitism
syncope

syncytia (*pl. of* syncytium)
syncytial
    s. bud
    s. knot
    s. sprout
syncytiotrophoblast
    malignant s.
syncytium, pl. syncytia
syndactyly
syndrome
    Aarskog s.
    Aarskog-Scott s.
    Aase s.
    Abderhalden-Fanconi s.
    Abt-Letterer-Siwe s.
    Achard s.
    Achard-Thiers s.
    achondrogenesis s.
    achondroplasia s.
    acid aspiration s.
    acquired immune
      deficiency s. (AIDS)
    acquired
      immunodeficiency s.
      (AIDS)
    acrodysostosis s.
    acute urethral s.
    Adair-Dighton s.
    Adams-Stokes s.
    addisonian s.
    Adie s.
    adiposogenital s.
    adrenal virilizing s.
    adrenogenital s. (AGS)
    adult respiratory distress s.
      (ARDS)
    AEC s.
    aglossia-adactylia s.
    Ahumada-Del Castillo s.
    Aicardi s.
    air leak s.
    Alagille s.
    Alajouanine s.
    Albers-Schönberg s.
    Albright s.
    ALCAPA s.
    Aldrich s.

NOTES

403

syndrome *(continued)*
Allemann s.
Allen-Masters s.
Alport s.
amenorrhea-galactorrhea s.
amniotic banding s.
amniotic fluid s.
amniotic fluid embolus s.
amniotic infection s.
Andogsky s.
androgen insensitivity s.
androgen resistance s.
Angelman s.
angio-osteohypertrophy s.
anomalous left coronary
  artery from pulmonary
  artery s.
anterior chamber cleavage s.
antiphospholipid s.
Antley-Bixler s.
Apert s.
Apert-Crouzon s.
Argonz-Del Castillo s.
Arnold-Chiari s.
Asherman s.
asphyxiating thoracic
  dysplasia s.
asphyxiating
  thoracodystrophy s.
asplenia s.
ataxia-telangiectasia s.
Axenfeld s.
Babinski-Fröhlich s.
Ballantyne-Runge s.
Ballantyne-Smith s.
Baller-Gerold s.
Banti s.
Bardet-Biedl s.
Barlow s.
Bart s.
Bartter s.
basal cell nevus s.
Bassen-Kornzweig s.
battered child s.
battered fetus s.
battered wife s.
BBB s.
Beckwith s.
Beckwith-Wiedemann s.
Behçet s.
Bielschowsky s.
Biemond s.
Biglieri s.

bile-plug s.
bird-headed dwarf s.
Blackfan-Diamond s.
bladder outlet s.
blind loop s.
Bloch-Sulzberger s.
Bloom s.
blue diaper s.
blue rubber-bleb nevus s.
Bodian-Schwachman s.
Bonnevie-Ullrich s.
BOR s.
Börjeson s.
Börjeson-Forssman-
  Lehmann s.
brachio-otorenal s., brachial
  otorenal syndrome (BOR)
Brachmann-de Lange s.
brain-death s.
branchial arch s.
Brandt s.
Brentano s.
bronze baby s.
brown baby s.
Brown vertical retraction s.
Brushfield-Wyatt s.
bubbly lung s.
Budd-Chiari s.
burning vulva s.
Caffey s.
Caffey-Silverman s.
Caffey-Smyth-Roske s.
Calvé-Legg-Perthes s.
camptomelic s.
Camurati-Englemann s.
Cantrell s.
carcinoid s.
cardiac-limb s.
Carpenter s.
cat-cry s.
cat-eye s.
caudal dysplasia s.
caudal regression s. (CRS)
cerebrocostomandibular s.
cerebrohepatorenal s.
Chapple s.
Charcot-Marie-Tooth-
  Hoffmann s.
CHARGE s.
Chédiak-Higashi s.
Chiari-Arnold s.
Chiari-Frommel s.
Chilaiditi s.

CHILD s.
Chotzen s.
Christian-Opitz s.
Christ-Siemens-Touraine s.
Clarke Hadfield s.
cleidocranial dysplasia s.
Clifford s.
climacteric s.
clomiphene-resistant
  polycystic ovary s.
Clouston s.
cloverleaf skull s.
Cockayne s.
Coffin-Lowry s.
Coffin-Siris s.
congenital hypothyroidism s.
congenital rubella s.
Conn s.
Conradi s.
Conradi-Hünermann s.
contiguous gene s.
contractural
  arachnodactyly s.
Cornelia de Lange s.
corpus luteum deficiency s.
craniocarpotarsal s.
craniosynostosis-radial
  aplasia s.
CREST s.
Creutzfeldt-Jakob s.
cri-du-chat s.
Crigler-Najjar s.
Cross s.
Cross-McKusick-Breen s.
Crouzon s.
CRST s.
cryptophthalmia s.
cryptophthalmia-syndactyly s.
cryptophthalmos s.
Curtis s.
Cushing s.
cushingoid s.
Dandy-Walker s.
Danlos s.
Darrow-Gamble s.
dead fetus s.
Debré-Fibiger s.

Debré-Sémélaigne s.
De Crecchio s.
Dejerine-Klumpke s.
de Lange s.
del Castillo s.
Demons-Meigs s.
de Morsier-Gauthier s.
Dennie-Marfan s.
De Sanctis-Cacchione s.
de Toni-Fanconi s.
de Toni-Fanconi-Debré s.
De Vaal s.
Diamond-Blackfan s.
diencephalic s.
DiGeorge s.
Dighton-Adair s.
Donahue-Uchida s.
Donohue s.
DOOR s.
Down s.
Drash s.
Duane s.
Dubin-Johnson s.
duplication-deficiency s.
dwarf s.
Dyggve-Melchior-Clausen s.
Dyke-Davidoff s.
dysmaturity s.
dystocia-dystrophia s.
dysuria-sterile pyuria s.
Eagle-Barrett s.
ectrodactyly, ectodermal
  dysplasia, clefting s.
Eddowes s.
Edwards s.
EEC s.
Ehlers-Danlos s.
Eisenmenger s.
elfin facies s.
Ellis-van Creveld s.
embryonic testicular
  regression s.
EMG s.
empty scrotum s.
empty-sella s.
epidermal nevus s.
epiphyseal s.

NOTES

405

syndrome *(continued)*
   Erb-Goldflam s.
   Erlacher-Blount s.
   ethmocephaly s.
   exomphalos, macroglossia,
     and gigantism s.
   extended rubella s.
   faciodigitogenital s.
   failure-to-thrive s.
   Fallot s.
   familial aortic ectasia s.
   familial atypical multiple
     mole melanoma s.
   familial cardiac myxoma s.
   Fanconi s.
   Fanconi-Albertini
     Zellweger s.
   Fanconi-Petrassi s.
   Felty s.
   feminization s.
   feminizing testes s.
   fetal alcohol s. (FAS)
   fetal aspiration s.
   fetal distress s.
   fetal face s.
   fetal hydantoin s. (FHS)
   fetal phenytoin s.
   fetal trimethadione s.
   fetal varicella s. (FVS)
   fetal warfarin s.
   fetofetal transfusion s.
   Fèvre-Languepin s.
   FG s.
   Fibiger-Debré-Von Gierke s.
   fibrinogen-fibrin
     conversion s.
   first arch s.
   Fitz-Hugh and Curtis s.
   floppy infant s.
   focal dermal hypoplasia s.
   Forbes-Albright s.
   four-day s.
   fragile X s.
   Franceschetti s.
   Franceschetti-Jadassohn s.
   Franceschetti-Klein s.
   Francois s.
   Fraser s.
   Freeman-Sheldon s.
   Friend s.
   Fritsch s.
   Fritsch-Asherman s.
   Fröhlich s.

   Fryne s.
   functional prepubertal
     castrate s.
   Funston s.
   Gailliard s.
   galactorrhea-amenorrhea s.
   Gamble-Darrow s.
   Gardner s.
   Gasser s.
   Gee-Herter-Heubner s.
   gender dysphoria s.
   genital ulcer s.
   Gerstmann s.
   Gianotti-Crosti s.
   Gilbert-Dreyfus s.
   Gilbert-Lereboullet s.
   Gilles de la Tourette s.
   Glanzmann s.
   Glanzmann-Riniker s.
   glossopalatine ankylosis s.
   Goldenhar s.
   Goltz s.
   Goltz-Gorlin s.
   gonadal agenesis s.
   gonadotrophin-resistant
     ovary s.
   Goodman s.
   Goodpasture s.
   Gordan-Overstreet s.
   Gorlin-Psaume s.
   Gougerot-Carteaud s.
   Gradenigo s.
   gray s., gray baby s.
   Greig s.
   Griscelli s.
   Gruber s.
   Guillain-Barré-Landry s.
   HAIR-AN s.
     hyperandrogenism, insulin
     resistance, acanthosis
     nigricans syndrome
   Hajdu-Cheney s.
   Hakim s.
   Hakim-Adams s.
   Halban s.
   Halbrecht s.
   Hallermann-Streiff s.
   Hallermann-Streiff-
     François s.
   Hallervorden-Spatz s.
   Hallopeau-Siemens s.
   Hall-Pallister s.
   Hall-Riggs s.

Hamman-Rich s.
hand-foot s.
hand-foot-mouth s.
hand-foot-uterus s.
Hand-Schüller-Christian s.
Hanhart s.
happy puppet s.
HARD s.
Hart s.
Hay-Wells s.
heart-hand s.
HELLP s.
hemangioma-
  thrombocytopenia s.
hemolytic-uremic s.
hemolytic-uremic s.
hereditary benign
  intraepithelial
  dyskeratosis s.
hereditary dysplastic
  nevus s.
Hermansky-Pudlak s.
heterotaxia s.
HLHS s.
Holt-Oram s.
Hunter s.
Hurler s.
Hurler-Scheie s.
Hutchinson s.
Hutchinson-Gilford s.
hyaline membrane s.
17-hydroxylase deficiency s.
21-hydroxylase deficiency s.
hyperandrogenism, insulin
  resistance, acanthosis
  nigricans s. (HAIR-AN
  syndrome)
hyperlucent lung s.
hypertelorism-hypospadias s.
hyperviscosity s.
hypochondroplasia s.
hypoglossia-hypodactyly s.
hypoplastic congenital
  anemia s.
hypoplastic left heart s.
  (HLHS)

hypoplastic right heart s.
  (HRHS)
IADH s.
idiopathic infantile
  hypercalcemia s.
idiopathic respiratory
  distress s. (IRDS)
Imerslund s.
Imerslund-Graesback s.
immunodeficiency s.
s. of inappropriate
  antidiuretic hormone
  (SIADH)
s. of inappropriate
  antidiuretic hormone
  secretion
infantile respiratory
  distress s.
infant respiratory distress s.
infection-associated
  hemophagocytic s. (IAHS)
insensitive ovary s.
inspissated bile s.
inspissated milk s.
intrauterine parabiotic s.
Isaac s.
isolated autosomal
  dominant s.
Ivemark s.
Jacob s.
Jacobsen s.
Jacobsen-Brodwall s.
Jadassohn-Lewandowski s.
Jaffe-Gottfried-Bradley s.
Jaffe-Lichtenstein s.
Jahnke s.
Jaksch s.
Jansen s.
Jansky-Bielschowsky s.
Jarcho-Levin s.
Jensen s.
Jervell-Lange-Nielson s.
Jervis s.
Jeune s.
Job s.
Johanson-Blizzard s.
Johnson s.

NOTES

syndrome *(continued)*
Joseph s.
Josephs-Blackfan-Diamond s.
Joubert s.
Juberg-Holt s.
Junius-Kuhnt s.
Kabuki make-up s.
Kallmann s.
Kanner s.
Kartagener s.
Kasabach-Merritt s.
Kasnelson s.
Kaufman s.
Kaufman-McKusick s.
Kearns-Sayre s.
Keipert s.
Kenny-Caffey s.
Kenny-Linarelli-Caffey s.
Kesaree-Wooley s.
Kimmelstiel-Wilson s.
kinky-hair s.
Kinsbourne s.
KIO s.
kleeblattschädel s.
Klein-Waardenburg s.
Klinefelter s.
Klippel-Feil s.
Klippel-Trenaunay s.
Klippel-Trenaunay-Weber s.
Kloepfer s.
Klotz s.
Klüver-Bucy s.
Kniest s.
Koby s.
Kocher-Debré-Sémélaigne s.
Koerber-Salus-Elschnig s.
Kosenow-Sinios s.
Kostmann s.
Krause s.
Ladd s.
Landry-Guillain-Barré s.
Lange-Akeroyd s.
Langer s.
Langer-Giedion s.
Langer-Petersen-Spranger s.
Langer-Saldino s.
Laron s.
Larsen s.
late embryonic testicular
regression s.
Launois s.
Launois-Cléret s.
Laurence-Moon s.

Laurence-Moon-Bardet-
Biedl s.
Läwen-Roth s.
lazy leukocyte s.
Leigh s.
Lejeune s.
Lennox s.
Lennox-Gastaut s.
Lenz s.
LEOPARD s.
Leri s.
Leri-Weill s.
Leroy s.
Leschke s.
Lesch-Nyhan s.
lethal multiple pterygium s.
Li-Fraumeni cancer s.
Lightwood-Albright s.
limp infant s.
Lobstein s.
Löffler s.
Louis-Bar s.
Lowe oculocerebrorenal s.
Lowe-Terry-Machlachan s.
Lub s.
Lucey-Driscoll s.
lupus obstetric s.
luteinized unruptured
follicle s. (LUFS)
Lutembacher s.
Lyell s.
lymphoproliferative s.
Macleod s.
Maffucci s.
Majewski s.
malabsorption s.
Mallory-Weiss s.
Marañón s.
Marden-Walker s.
Marfan s.
Marie s.
Marinesco-Garland s.
Marinesco-Sjögren s.
Mariñon s.
Maroteaux-Lamy s.
Masters-Allen s.
maternal deprivation s.
maternal hydrops s.
Mauriac s.
Mayer-Rokitansky-Küster-
Hauser s.
McCune-Albright s.
McKusick-Kaufman s.

Meadows s.
Meckel s.
Meckel-Gruber s.
meconium aspiration s.
 (MAS)
meconium blockage s.
meconium plug s.
median facial cleft s.
megacystis-megaureter s.
megacystis, microcolon,
 intestinal hypoperistalsis s.
Meigs s.
Meigs-Kass s.
Melkersson-Rosenthal s.
Mendelson s.
Mengert shock s.
Menkes s.
menopausal s.
methionine malabsorption s.
Meyer-Schwickerath and
 Weyers s.
micrognathia-glossoptosis s.
midfetal testicular
 regression s.
Mikity-Wilson s.
Miller s.
Miller-Dieker s.
Minkowski-Chauffard s.
Minot-von Willebrand s.
MMIH s.
Möbius s.
Mohr s.
monosomy 7 s.
monosomy G s.
morning glory s.
Morquio s.
Morquio-Ulrich s.
Moynahan s.
mucocutaneous lymph
 node s. (MLNS)
mucosal neuroma s.
multiple epiphyseal dysplasia
 tarda s.
multiple lentigines s.
multiple neuroma s.
multiple synostosis s.
MURCS s.

muscular hypertrophy s.
mystery s.
Nafucci s.
Nager s.
Nager-de Reynier s.
nail-patella s.
narcotic withdrawal s.
Nelnick-Needles s.
Nelson s.
neonatal respiratory
 distress s.
neonatal small left colon s.
nephrotic s.
Netherton s.
Nettleship s.
neurocutaneous s.
newborn respiratory
 distress s.
Nezelof s.
Noack s.
Nonne-Milroy-Meige s.
nonsalt-losing
 adrenogenital s.
Noonan s.
Norman-Wood s.
Norrie s.
Obrinsky s.
oculocerebral s.
oculodentodigital s.
oculomandibulofacial s.
 (OMF)
OFD s., type I, II, III
Ohtahara s.
Oliver-McFarlane s.
Ollier s.
Omenn s.
Opitz s.
Opitz-Christian s.
Opitz-Frias s.
Oppenheim s.
orofaciodigital s., oral-facial-
 digital syndrome
orogenital s.
Osgood-Schlatter s.
osteogenesis imperfecta
 congenita s.
osteopathia striata s.

NOTES

syndrome *(continued)*
    Ostrum-Furst s.
    otopalatodigital s.
    otosclerosis s.
    otospongiosis s.
    ovarian hyperstimulation s.
    ovarian remnant s.
    ovarian vein s.
    overdistention s.
    pancreatic insufficiency s.
    Papillon-Léage-Psaume s.
    Papillon-Léfevre s.
    paraneoplastic s.
    Parenti-Fraccaro s.
    Parrot s.
    Patau s.
    Pellizzi s.
    pelvic congestion s.
    Pendred s.
    pentalogy s.
    penta-X s.
    persistent müllerian duct s.
    Peutz-Jeghers s.
    Pfaundler-Hurler s.
    Pfeiffer s.
    pickwickian s.
    Pierre Robin s.
    Pirie s.
    placental dysfunction s.
    placental hemangioma s.
    placental transfusion s.
    POEMS s.
    Poland s.
    polycystic ovary s. (PCOS)
    polyglandular s.
    polysplenia s.
    Pompe s.
    popliteal pterygium s.
    popliteal web s.
    Porak-Durante s.
    postirradiation s.
    postmaturity s.
    postmenopausal s.
    postpartum hemolytic uremic s.
    postpartum pituitary necrosis s.
    postperfusion s.
    postrubella s.
    posttubal ligation s.
    Potter s.
    Prader-Gurtner s.
    Prader-Labhart-Willi s.

    Prader-Willi s.
    premenstrual s. (PMS)
    premenstrual salivary s.
    premenstrual tension s.
    primary empty sella s.
    prolonged Q-T s.
    prune-belly s.
    pseudoachondroplasia s.
    pseudo-Turner s.
    pulmonary dysmaturity s.
    Purtilo X-linked lymphoproliferative s.
    pyknodysostosis s.
    Pyle s.
    13-q deletion s.
    radial aplasia-thrombocytopenia s.
    Ramsey-Hunt s.
    rape-trauma s.
    Refsum s.
    Reifenstein s.
    Rendu-Osler-Weber s.
    Renpenning s.
    residual ovary s.
    resistant ovary s.
    respiratory distress s. (RDS)
    respiratory distress s. of the newborn
    restless legs s.
    retinoblastoma-mental retardation s.
    retraction s.
    Rett s.
    Reye s.
    rhizomelia s.
    rhizomelic chondrodysplasia punctata s.
    Rh-null s.
    Richards-Rundle s.
    Richner-Hanhart s.
    Rieger s.
    right ovarian vein s.
    Riley-Day s.
    Riley-Schwachman s.
    Riley-Smith s.
    ring chromosome 18 s.
    ring chromosome 22 s.
    Roberts s.
    Robin s.
    Robinow s.
    Rokitansky-Küster-Hauser s.
    Rosewater s.
    Rothmann-Makai s.

Rothmund s.
Rothmund-Thomson s.
Rothmund-Werner s.
Rotor s.
round ligament s.
Roussy-Lévy s.
Rubinstein s.
Rubinstein-Taybi s.
Rud s.
rudimentary testis s.
Russell s.
Russell-Silver s.
Saethre-Chotzen s.
Sakati-Nyhan s.
Saldino-Noonan s.
salt-losing adrenogenital s.
  (SLAS)
Sanchez-Salorio s.
Sandifer s.
Sanfilippo s.
Santavuori s.
Santavuori-Haltia s.
Savage s.
scalded-skin s.
Schafer s.
Scheie s.
Scheuthauer-Marie-Sainton s.
Schmidt s.
Schwachman s.
Schwachman-Diamond s.
Schwartz-Jampel s.
Schwartz-Jampel-Aberfeld s.
scimitar s.
sea-blue histiocyte s.
Seabright bantam s.
sebaceous nevus s.
Seckel s.
Seip-Lawrence s.
Senter s.
sepsis-pneumonia s.
Sertoli-cell-only s.
shaken baby s.
shedding s.
Sheehan s.
short-bowel s.
short rib-polydactyly s.
  (SRPS)

Shprintzen s.
Shy-Drager s.
Shy-Magee s.
sicca s.
Silver s.
Silver-Russell s.
Silverskiöld s.
Simmonds s.
Sipple s.
Sjögren s.
Sjögren-Larsson s.
slick-gut s.
Slotnick-Goldfarb s.
Sly s.
small left colon s.
Smith-Lemli-Opitz s.
Sohval-Soffer s.
Sorsby s.
Sotos s.
spastic diplegia s.
splenic sequestration s.
spondylocostal dysplasia s.
spondyloepiphyseal dysplasia
  congenita s.
spondylothoracic dysplasia s.
Sprangeler-Wiedemann s.
Spurway s.
staphylococcal-scalded
  skin s.
steely-hair s.
Steinert s.
Stein-Leventhal s.
sterile pyuria s.
Stevens-Johnson s.
Stewart-Treves s.
Stickler s.
stiff-baby s.
Stilling-Türk-Duane s.
Stock-Spielmeyer-Vogt s.
straight-back s.
Sturge s.
Sturge-Kalischer-Weber s.
Sturge-Weber s.
sudden infant death s.
  (SIDS)
superior vena caval s.
supine hypotensive s.

NOTES

syndrome *(continued)*
surfactant deficiency s.
Sweet s.
Swyer s.
Swyer-James s.
Swyer-James-Macleod s.
TAR s.
Taussig-Bing s.
Taybi s.
terminal Xp deletion s.
Terry s.
testicular feminization s.
tethered cord s.
tetralogy of Fallot s.
tetrasomy 15p s.
tetra-X s.
thalidomide s.
Thiemann s.
Thomsen s.
Thomson s.
thoracic compression s.
thrombocytopenia-absent
    radius s.
thyrohypophysial s.
Tietze s.
tired housewife s.
TORCH s.
Tourette s.
Townes s.
Townes-Brocks s.
toxic shock s. (TSS)
tracheal agenesis s.
transient respiratory
    distress s. (TRDS)
translocation Down s.
Treacher Collins s.
Treacher Collins-
    Franceschetti s.
trichorhinophalangeal s.
triple-X s.
trismus-
    pseudocamptodactyly s.
trisomy 8 s.
trisomy 11q s.
trisomy 13 s.
trisomy 13-15 s.
trisomy 16-18 s.
trisomy 18 s.
trisomy 21 s.
trisomy 22 s.
trisomy C s.
trisomy D s.
trisomy E s.

trisomy G s.
Turner s.
twin transfusion s.
Ullrich s.
Ullrich-Bonnevie s.
Ullrich-Feichtiger s.
Ulrich-Turner s.
universal joint s.
Unverricht-Lundborg s.
urethral s.
uterine hernia s.
VACTERL s.
Van Buchem s.
van der Hoeve s.
Van der Woude s.
vanishing testes s.
vanishing twin s.
vascular ring s.
VATER s.
velocardiofacial s.
Verner-Morrison s.
Vogt s.
von Willebrand s.
vulvar vestibulitis s. (VVS)
Waardenburg s.
Waardenburg-Klein s.
WAGR s.
Walker-Warburg s.
Walton s.
Warburg s.
Waring blender s.
Waterhouse-Friderichsen s.
Watson-Alagille s.
Weber-Christian s.
Weill-Marchesani s.
Werdnig-Hoffmann s.
Wermer s.
Werner s.
West s.
wet lung s.
Weyers oligodactyly s.
Whipple s.
whistling face s.
whistling face-windmill vane
    hand s.
Wiedemann s.
Wildervanck s.
Wilkins s.
Willebrand-Jurgens s.
Williams s.
Williams-Beuren s.
Williams-Campbell s.
Wilms s.

Wilson-Mikity s.
Winter s.
Wiskott-Aldrich s.
Wolff-Parkinson-White s.
Wolf-Hirschborn s.
Wolfram s.
Wyburn-Mason s.
s. X
45,X s.
X-linked
  lymphoproliferative s.
XO s.
XX male s.
46,XX male s.
XXX s.
47,XXX s.
XXXX s.
XXXXX s.
XXXXY s.
49XXXXY s.
XXY s.
47,XXY s.
XYY s.
yellow vernix s.
Young s.
YY s.
Zellweger s.
Ziehen-Oppenheim s.
Zinsser-Engman-Cole s.
Zipokowski-Margolis s.
Zollinger-Ellison s.
synechia, pl. synechiae
  intrauterine s.
  s. vulvae
synencephalocele
Synevac vacuum curettage system
syngeneic tissue
syngnathia
syngraft
Synkayvite
synkinesia
  mouth-and-hand s.
Synodroy
synophthalmia
Synophylate
synorchidism

synoscheos
synostosis, pl. synostoses
  cranial s.
  multiple synostoses
  tribasilar s.
synovitis
syntenic genes
synthase
  prostaglandin s.
synthesis, pl. syntheses
  decidual prolactin s.
  estrogen s.
  ovarian estrogen s.
  progesterone s.
synthetic suture material
Synthroid
Syntocinon
syphilis
  congenital s.
  s. hereditaria tarda
  serologic test for s. (STS)
syringe
  Asepto s.
  bulb s.
  s. feeding
  FNA-21 s.
  Luer-Lok s.
  tuberculin s.
syringocele
syringoma
syringomeningocele
syringomyelocele
syrinx
syrup
  Karo s.
syssomus
system
  Abbott LifeCare PCA Plus
    II infusion s.
  ABO blood group s.
  AEGIS sonography
    management s.
  Affirm VP microbial
    identification s.
  Aggregate Neurobehavioral
    Student Health &

NOTES

system *(continued)*
    Education Review S.
        (ANSER)
    AI 5200 S Open Color
        Doppler imaging s.
    Aloka ultrasound s.
    AspenVAC smoke
        evacuation s.
    autonomic nervous s.
    Autoread centrifuge
        hematology s.
    Aviva mammography s.
    BABE OB ultrasound
        reporting s.
    Babyflex heated
        ventilation s.
    Bair Hugger patient
        warming s.
    Bethesda classification s.
    bicarbonate-carbonic acid s.
    breast leakage inhibitor s.
        (BLIS)
    bursa-dependent s.
    Capasee diagnostic
        ultrasound s.
    cardiovascular s.
    CDE blood group s.
    central nervous s. (CNS)
    Cineloop image review
        ultrasound s.
    Companion 318 Nasal
        CPAP S.
    continuous distention
        irrigation s. (CDIS)
    Cooper Surgical Monopolor
        ELSG LEEP S.
    Cryomedics electrosurgery s.
    digestive s.
    Duffy s.
    endocrine s.
    EndoMed LSS
        laparoscopy s.
    Endotek urodynamics s.
    Estraderm transdermal s.
    estradiol transdermal s.
    EUB-405 ultrasound s.
    E-Z-EM BioGun automated
        biopsy s.
    Ferriman-Gallwey hirsutism
        scoring s.
    fibrinolytic and clotting s.
    Gleeson FloVAC Hi-Flo
    laparoscopic
        suction/irrigation s.
    Glucometer Elite diabetes
        care s.
    HemoCue blood glucose s.
    HemoCue blood
        hemoglobin s.
    Histofreezer cryosurgical s.
    Hitachi EUB-405 imaging s.
    Illumina Pro Series CO2
        surgical laser s.
    image recording s.
    IMEXLAB vascular
        diagnostic s.
    immune s.
    InfraGuide delivery s.
    Innova electrotherapy s.
    Innova feminine
        incontinence treatment s.
    International Staging S.
        (INSS)
    Kagan staging s.
    Lectromed urinary
        investigation s.
    lymphatic s.
    male reproductive s.
    Mammomat C3
        mammography s.
    Mammoscan digital
        imaging s.
    Mityvac vacuum delivery s.
    Mullin s.
    musculoskeletal s.
    nervous s.
    neuroendocrine s.
    Norplant s.
    opsonization s.
    OPUS immunoassay s.
    orthogonal lead s.
    Pap-Perfect supply s.
    parasympathetic nervous s.
    Performa diagnostic
        ultrasound imaging s.
    Pregnancy Risk Assessment
        Monitoring S. (PRAMS)
    prognostic scoring s.
    prorenin-renin-angiotensin s.
    Renaissance spirometry s.
    renin-angiotensin s.
    renin-angiotensin-
        aldosterone s.
    reproductive s.
    respiratory s.

Rh blood group s.
Riechert-Mundinger
  stereotactic s.
selective no-fault s.
Shimadzu ultrasound s.
Shutt suture punch s.
Siemens Sonoline SI-400
  ultrasound s.
single-use diagnostic s.
  (SUDS)
Sirecust 404N neonatal
  monitoring s.
Sky-Boot stirrup s.
Sonicaid Vasoflow
  Doppler s.
Spect-Align laser s.
Spectra 400 extended
  surveillance and alert s.
Sperm Select sperm
  recovery s.
swivel-arm s.
sympathetic nervous s.
Synevac vacuum
  curettage s.
TroGARD electrosurgical
  blunt trocar s.
UD 2000 urodynamic
  measurement s.
ULPA/charcoal filtration s.

Ultramark ultrasound s.
UPS 2020 ambulatory
  measurement s.
urinary s.
Urocyte diagnostic
  cytometry s.
Vacutainer s.
Vakutage suction s.
Valleylab REM s.
Valley Vac smoke
  evacuation s.
VIDAS immunoanalysis
  testing s.
systemic
  s. arteriovenous fistula
  s. illness
  s. lupus erythematosus
  (SLE)
  s. vascular resistance
**systemic-active nonspecific
  immunotherapy**
systolic
  s. ejection murmur
  s. murmur
systolic/diastolic (S/D)
  s./d. ratio
Syva test
Sztehlo umbilical clamp

NOTES

T

> T band
> T cell
> T lymphocyte

T$_2$

> diiodothyronine

T$_3$

> triiodothyronine

T$_4$

> thyroxine

T2 test
T3 test
T4 test
T6 antigen
^{182}Ta

> tantalum-182

TAA

> tumor-associated antigen

TAB

> therapeutic abortion

Tabb curette
tabes

> t. infantum
> t. mesaraica
> t. mesenterica

table

> Bayley-Pinneau t.
> height t.

tablet

> hormonal pregnancy test t.'s

TACE
tachyarrhythmia

> supraventricular t. (SVT)

tachycardia

> atrial t.
> atrioventricular
>   reciprocating t.
> paroxysmal t.
> sinus t.
> supraventricular t. (SVT)
> ventricular t.

tachydysrhythmia

> supraventricular t.

tachyphylaxis
tachypnea

> transient t.

tactile

> t. fever
> t. sensory monitoring
> t. stimulation

> t. stimulus
> t. temperature

taeniasis
TAF

> tumor angiogenesis factor

tag

> hymenal t.
> skin t.

Tagamet
TAGO diagnostic kit
TAH

> total abdominal hysterectomy

tail

> axillary t.
> t. bud
> Spence axillary t.

tailgut
talc
talipes

> t. calcaneovalgus
> t. calcaneovarus
> t. calcaneus
> t. cavovalgus
> t. cavus
> t. equinovalgus
> t. equinovarus
> t. equinus
> t. hobble splint
> t. planovalgus
> t. valgus
> t. varus

talipomanus
Talwin
Tambocor
Tamm-Horsfall

> T.-H. mucoprotein
> T.-H. protein

tamoxifen citrate
tampon

> Genupak t.
> stype t.
> vaginal t.

tamponade

> cardiac t.
> pericardial t.

tandem

> afterload t.
> Fleming afterloading t.
> Fletcher-Suit afterloading t.

tandem *(continued)*
    T. Icon II hCG
    t. and ovoids (T&O)
Tangier disease
Tanner
    T. stage
    T. stages of development
    T. staging (Grade I, II, III, IV)
tantalum
    t.-182 (^{182}Ta)
tanycyte
Tanyoz sign
Tao
tap
    supraciliary t.
Tapar
Tapazole
tapir mouth
tapiroid
TAR
    thrombocytopenia-absent radius
    T. syndrome
Taractan
Tarasan
tarda
    osteopetrosis t.
    porphyria cutanea t.
Tardieu test
target
    t. cell
    molybdenum t.
    t. organ response
    tungsten t.
Tarkowski method
Tarnier axis-traction forceps
tarry cyst
tartrate
    butorphanol t.
    ergotamine t.
    metoprolol t.
    zolpidem t.
taurine
Taussig-Bing
    T.-B. disease
    T.-B. syndrome
tautomenial
Tavist
taxis
    bipolar t.
taxofere
Taxol
taxotere

Taybi syndrome
Tay-Sachs disease
Tazicef
Tazidime
tazobactam
Tazol
TB
    tuberculosis
TBG
    thyroid-binding globulin
TBLC
    term birth, living child
TBP
    thyroxine-binding protein
TC-7 adhesion barrier
T-cell subsets
TCIFTT
    transcervical intrafallopian tube transfer
tCpO$_2$
    transcutaneous partial pressure of oxygen
TDF
    testis-determining factor
TDLU
    terminal duct lobular unit
TDx-FLM
    T.-F. Assay
    T.-F. assay test
TDxFLx Assay
tdy gene
Tebamide
Tebrazid
technetium
technique
    Ayre spatula-Zelsmyr Cytobrush t.
    balloon catheter t.
    Beverly-Douglas lip-tongue adhesion t.
    Brockenbrough t.
    Brown-Wickham t.
    Bruhat t.
    clip t.
    clonogenic t.
    cobalt-60 moving strip t.
    contraceptive t.
    Counsellor-Flor modification of McIndoe t.
    Culcher-Sussman t.
    dot-blot t.
    double-freeze t.
    Dufourmentel t.

Dyban t.
Eklund t.
evoked potential t.
ferning t.
Frank t.
Gittes t.
Goebell-Frangenheim-
  Stoeckel t.
Gomco t.
gracilis flap t.
GRASS MRI t.
Hamou t.
Heaney t.
hybridoma t.
immune monitoring t.
immune separation t.
insemination swim-up t.
Jones and Jones wedge t.
Kehr t.
Kety-Schmidt t.
Kidde cannula t.
Krönig t.
Lapides t.
Lazarus-Nelson t.
Leboyer t.
Limberg t.
loss of resistance t.
Madden t.
March t.
marsupialization t.
Millen t.
minimally invasive
  surgical t. (MIST)
modified Pomeroy t.
molecular genetic t.
Pacey t.
pants-over-vest t.
Percoll t.
rollerball t.
Semm Z t.
Simonton t.
snapshot GRASS t.
soluble gas t.
Southern blot t.
Strassman t.
surveillance t.

Tompkins median
  bivalving t.
tubal ligation band t.
Wallace t.
technology
  assisted reproductive t.
    (ART)
  recombinant DNA t.
  reproductive t.
  Society for Assisted
    Reproductive T. (SART)
  Stat-Lab T.'s
tectocephaly
TED
  thromboembolic disease
    TED stockings
teeth
  Fournier t.
  milk t.
  Moon t.
  natal t.
  neonatal t.
  precocious t.
  predeciduous t.
  screwdriver t.
Teflon periurethral injection
Tegison
Tegopen
Tegretol
Teilum tumor
telangiectasia
  ataxia t.
  calcinosis cutis, Raynaud
    phenomenon,
    sclerodactyly, t. (CRST)
  calcinosis cutis, Raynaud
    phenomenon, esophageal
    motility disorders,
    sclerodactyly, t. (CREST)
  hemorrhagic t.
telangiectatic granuloma
Teldrin
telecanthus
teleologic theory
telephase
teleradiology
teletherapy

NOTES

TeLinde operation
Teline
telocentric chromosome
telogen
    t. effluvium
    t. phase
telophase
Temaril
temazepam
temperature
    absolute t.
    artificial t.
    aseptic t.
    aural t.
    axillary t.
    basal body t. (BBT)
    body t.
    core t.
    critical t.
    ephemeral t.
    eruptive t.
    maximum t. (T-max)
    normal t.
    oral t.
    rectal t.
    room t.
    skin t.
    subnormal t.
    tactile t.
    tympanic t.
temporal lobe epilepsy
temporary diverting colostomy
Tempra
tenaculum, pl. tenacula
    Braun-Schroeder single-
      tooth t.
    cervical t.
    double-tooth t.
    Emmett cervical t.
    t. hook
    t. hook loop
    Jacobs t.
    Schroeder uterine t.
    single-tooth t.
    uterine t.
Tenckhoff catheter
tendency
    familial t.
tenderness
    cervical motion t. (CMT)
    costovertebral angle t.
      (CVAT)

    lower abdominal t.
    pelvic t.
Tender-Touch
    T.-T. extractor
    T.-T. vacuum birthing cup
tendineus
    arcus t.
Tenex
teniposide
Tenney-Parker sign
Tenol
Tenoretic
Tenormin
Tensilon
tension
    carbon dioxide t.
    t. cyst
    oxygen t.
    t. pneumothorax
    premenstrual t.
    surface t.
tensor fascia lata (TFL)
tent
    CAM t.
    intracervical t.
    laminaria t.
    t. mist
    mist t.
    t. oxygen
    Silon t.
tentorial laceration
Tenuate
tenuous
Tenzel calipers
Tepanil
teras, pl. terata
teratism
teratoblastoma
teratocarcinoma
teratogen
teratogenesis
teratogenic
    t. agent
    t. effect
    t. medication
    t. outcome
    t. risk
teratogenicity
teratogen-induced malformation
Teratogen Registry
teratology
teratoma, pl. teratomata
    benign cystic ovarian t.

germ cell t.
immature ovarian t.
malignant t.
malignant ovarian t.
mature cystic ovarian t.
mature ovarian t.
ovarian t.
ovarian cystic t.
ovarian embryonal t.
pediatric ovarian t.
sacrococcygeal t.

teratophobia

teratospermia

Terazol
T. 3 vaginal cream
T. 7 vaginal cream
T. vaginal suppository

terbutaline
t. sulfate

terconazole

Terfluzine

term
t. birth, living child (TBLC)
t. delivery
t. gestation
t. infant
t. pregnancy

Term-Guard

terminal
t. cardiotocogram
t. deletion
t. duct lobular unit (TDLU)
t. hair
t. ileitis
t. neosalpingostomy
t. saccular period
t. Xp deletion syndrome

termination
selective t.

terminus
vaginal t.

Ter-Pogossian cervical applicator

Terramycin

Terry syndrome

Teslac

Tessier craniofacial operation

TEST
tubal embryo stage transfer

test, testing
Accu-Chek t.
acid elution t.
acoustic stimulation t.
(AST)
ACTH stimulation t.
Affirm VPIII t.
agglutination inhibition t.
Allen-Doisy t.
ambulatory uterine
contraction t.
Amiel-Tison t.
Amniostat-FLM t.
antiglobulin t.
antitreponemal t.
Aschheim-Zondek t.
A.-Z. t.
Ballard t.
Barlow hip dysplasia t.
Betke-Kleihauer t.
Biocept-G pregnancy t.
Biocept-5 pregnancy t.
BioStar strep A 1A t.
bitterling t.
bladder muscle stress t.
bladder neck elevation t.
blood-type t.
Bonney blue stress
incontinence t.
bovine mucus penetration t.
breast stimulation
contraction t. (BSCT)
Brouha t.
bubble stability t.
cancer antigen-125 t.
Children's Depression
Inventory t.
Chlamydiazyme t.
chlortetracycline
fluorescence t.
Clearview hCG pregnancy t.
coagulation t.
Concise Plus hCG urine t.
contraction stress t. (CST)
Coombs t.

NOTES

test *(continued)*
   Corner-Allen t.
   Cortrosyn stimulation t.
   cosyntropin stimulation t.
   DAP t.
   dehydroepiandrosterone
     sulfate loading t.
   Denver Developmental
     Screening T. (DDST)
   dexamethasone
     suppression t.
   DFA t.
     direct fluorescent antigen
      test
   Dienst t.
   diiodothyronine t.
   direct fluorescent antigen t.
     (DFA test)
   Eagle t.
   early pregnancy t. (EPT)
   Eastern blot t.
   Elispot t.
   enzyme-linked antiglobulin t.
   estrogen-progestin t.
   Farber t.
   Farris t.
   fern t.
   fetal acoustic stimulation t.
   fetal activity t.
   Fibrindex t.
   Fisher exact t.
   Fisher-Yates t.
   five-hour glucose
     tolerance t.
   Fluhmann t.
   fluorescein-conjugated
     monoclonal antibody t.
   fluorescein treponema
     antibody t.
   fluorescent treponemal
     antibody-absorption t.
   foam stability t.
   Fortel ovulation t.
   Franklin-Dukes t.
   free beta t.
   Frei t.
   Friberg microsurgical
     agglutination t.
   Friedman-Lapham t.
   Friedman rabbit t.
   FTA t.
   Galli-Mainini t.
   gelatin agglutination t.

   genetic t.
   Gen-Probe t.
   Gesell t.
   glucose challenge t.
   glucose tolerance t. (GTT)
   Gono Kwik t.
   Gonozyme t.
   Gravindex t.
   growth hormone
     stimulation t. (GHST)
   guaiac t.
   Guthrie t.
   HABA binding t.
   hanging-drop t.
   Heller t.
   hemagglutination
     treponemal t. (HATT)
   Hematest t.
   Hemoccult t.
   HemoCue glucose t.
   HemoCue hemoglobin t.
   heparin challenge t.
   Heprofile ELISA t.
   Herp-Check t.
   Hi-Gonavis t.
   Hinton t.
   Hirschberg t.
   HIV t.
   HIVAGEN t.
   Hogben t.
   home pregnancy t.
   Hooker-Farbes t.
   Huhner t.
   human immunodeficiency
     virus t.
   human ovum fertilization t.
   hypoosmotic swelling t.
   Icon serum pregnancy t.
   Icon strep B t.
   Icon urine pregnancy t.
   IgA HIV antibody t.
   immunobead t.
   immunofluorescent
     antibody t.
   immunologic pregnancy t.
   Indiclor t.
   InSight prenatal t.
   insulin tolerance t.
   Isojima t.
   Jadassohn t.
   Kahn t.
   Kapeller-Adler t.
   Kibrick t.

Kibrick-Isojima infertility t.
Kleihauer-Betke t.
Kline t.
Knobloch-Gesell t.
Kodak hCG serum t.
Kodak SureCell
  Chlamydia T.
Kodak SureCell hCG-
  Urine T.
Kodak SureCell Herpes
  (HSV) T.
Kodak SureCell LCH in-
  office pregnancy t.
Kodak SureCell Strep A t.
KOH t.
Kolmer t.
Kolmer-Kline-Kahn t.
Kruskal-Wallis t.
Kupperman t.
Kurzrok-Miller t.
Kurzrok-Ratner t.
Kveim t.
laboratory t.
Landau t.
Lange t.
latex agglutination
  inhibition t. (LAIT)
latex fixation t.
Leiter t.
leucine tolerance t.
levothyroxine t.
LH Color t.
Liddle t.
liver function t.'s
Locke-Wallace Marital
  Adjustment t.
Lumadex-FSI t.
Mann-Whitney U t.
Mantel-Cox t.
Marchetti t.
Marshall t.
Mazzini t.
McCaman-Robins t.
Meinicke t.
Metopirone t.
metyrapone t.
MicroTrak t.

Monospot t.
Monosticon Dri-Dot t.
nappy t.
Nimbus t.
nipple stimulation t.
Nitrazine t.
nitroblue tetrazolium dye t.
Noguchi t.
nonstress t. (NST)
Northern blot t.
Omniprobe t.
OncoScint t.
one-hour glucose
  tolerance t.
one-tail t.
Ortolani t.
otoacoustic emission t.
  (OAE)
OvuKIT t.
OvuQUICK Self-T.
oxytocin challenge t. (OCT)
PACE-2 t.
Pathfinder DFA t.
Paul-Bunnell-Davidsohn t.
PCR t.
phenolsulfonphthalein t.
phenylketonuria t.
Piso t.
PKU t.
plasmacrit t.
platelet function t.
Porges-Meier t.
postcoital t.
Precise pregnancy t.
predictive value of t.
pregnancy t.
Profile viral probe t.
progesterone challenge t.
PSA t.
pulmonary function t.'s
Qtest Strep t.
Q-tip t.
Quick t.
Quickpac-II OneStep hCG
  pregnancy t.
QuickVue One-Step hCG-
  Combo t.

NOTES

test *(continued)*
    QuickVue One-Step hCG-
      urine t.
    QUIDEL Group B strep t.
    radioallergosorbent t.
      (RAST)
    radioimmunosorbent t.
      (RIST)
    rapid plasma reagin card t.
    rapid slide t.
    RCA t.
    renal clearance t.
    renal function t.
    Rinne t.
    Rofsing t.
    roll-over t.
    Rotazyme t.
    routine preoperative t.
    Rubin t.
    Sabin-Feldman dye t.
    Schick t.
    Schiller t.
    Schilling t.
    Scotch-tape t.
    screening laboratory t.'s
    Sephadex binding t.
    serologic t.
    Serono t.
    Sgambati t.
    shake t.
    Sickledex t.
    Sims-Huhner t.
    SISI t.
    skin t.
    Social Support Scale for
      Children t. (SSSC)
    Sonoclot t.
    Southern blot t.
    Speck t.
    sperm agglutination t.
    sperm immobilization t.
    stimulation t.
    STORCH t.
    straight catheter t.
    stress t.
    Student t t.
    SUDS HIV-1 antibody t.
    supine pressor t.
    SureCell Herpes (HSV) T.
    surf t.
    sweat chloride t.
    swordfish t.
    Syva t.

    T2 t.
    T3 t.
    T4 t.
    Tardieu t.
    TDx-FLM assay t.
    Tes-Tape urine glucose t.
    TestPackChlamydia t.
    tetraiodothyronine t.
    Thayer-Martin gonorrhea t.
    Thomas t.
    Thorn t.
    thrombin clot t.
    Thrombo-Wellco t.
    thymol turbidity t.
    thyroid function t.'s (TFT)
    thyrotropin-releasing
      hormone stimulation t.
    thyroxine t.
    tilt t.
    tine t.
    tissue thromboplastin-
      inhibition t.
    toluidine blue t.
    TPI t.
    Treponema pallidum
      immobilization t.
    triiodothyronine t.
    triple swab t.
    Tuttle t.
    two-tail t.
    Tzanck t.
    UCG-Slide T.
    Uniscreen urine t.
    Uri-Check t.
    urinary concentration t.
    urine t.
    urine CIE t.
    urine latex t.
    Urispec GP+A t.
    Urispec 9-Way t.
    vaginal cornification t.
    vaginal mucification t.
    van den Bergh t.
    Venereal Disease Research
      Laboratory t.
    Venning-Brown t.
    Vernes t.
    ViraPap t.
    ViraPap HPV DNA t.
    ViraType t.
    Visscher-Bowman t.
    von Poehl t.
    Wampole t.

Wasserman t.
Weber t.
Wepman t.
Western blot t.
wheat sperm agglutination t.
whiff t.
Whittaker t.
Wilcoxon rank sum t.
withdrawal bleeding t.
Xenopus t.
zona-free hamster egg
penetration t.
Tes-Tape urine glucose test
tester
HemoCue Blood-Glucose t.
HemoCue Blood-
Hemoglobin t.
testes (*pl. of* testis)
t. down
testicle
testicular
t. cancer
t. differentiation
t. feminization
t. feminization syndrome
t. steroidogenesis
testing (*var. of* test)
testis, pl. testes
t. determination
gonadotropin-resistant t.
rete t.
yolk sac tumor of t.
testis-determining factor (TDF)
testolactone
Testopel Pellet
testosterone
bound t.
t. cypionate
t. enanthate
ethinyl t.
free t.
t. index
non-sex hormone-binding
globulin bound t.
plasma t.
serum t.

t. suppression
topical t.
testosterone-estrogen-binding
globulin
testosterone-secreting adrenal
adenoma
TestPackChlamydia test
Test Pack hCG
Testred
Testsimplets prestained slide
test-tube baby
TET
tubal embryo transfer
tetania
t. gravidarum
t. neonatorium
t. neonatorum
tetanism
tetanus
diphtheria, pertussis, t.
(DPT)
t. immune globulin
t. neonatorum
postpartum t.
puerperal t.
t. toxoid
t. toxoid booster
uterine t.
tetany
neonatal t.
tethered cord syndrome
tetrabenazine
tetrabrachius
Tetracap
tetrachirus
tetracycline
t. analogue
t. hydrochloride
t. pleurodesis
prophylactic t.
Tetracyn
tetrad
tetradactyly
9-tetrahydrocannabinol (THC)
tetrahydrocortisol
tetraiodothyronine test
Tetralan

NOTES

tetralogy
    t. of Fallot (TF, TOF)
    t. of Fallot syndrome
Tetram
tetramastia
tetramelus
tetranitrate
    erythrityl t.
    pentaerythritol t.
tetranophthalmos
tetraotus
tetraploid distribution
tetraploidy
tetrascelus
tetrasomy
    t. 15p syndrome
tetra-X
    t.-X. chromosomal
      aberration
    t.-X. syndrome
TF
    tetralogy of Fallot
TFL
    tensor fascia lata
TFT
    thyroid function tests
TGA
    transposition of great arteries
T-Gen
TGF
    transforming growth factor
TGFα
    transforming growth factor alpha
TGFβ
    transforming growth factor beta
TGV
    transposition of great vessels
thalassemia
    α-t.
    alpha t.
    β-t.
    t. intermedia
    Lepore t.
    t. major
    t. minor
    sickle t. (HbS-Thal)
    sickle cell t.
β-thalassemia
    -t. major
    -t. minor
α-thalassemia minor
thalassemic patient

thalidomide
    t. syndrome
thallium poisoning
THAM
    tromethamine
thanatophoric
    t. dwarfism
    t. dysplasia
Thayer-Martin gonorrhea test
THb O$_2$
    total oxyhemoglobin
THC
    9-tetrahydrocannabinol
theca
    t. cell
    t. cell tumor
    t. externa
    t. interna
    t. lutein cell
    t. lutein cyst
theca-granulosa cell cooperativity
thecal/interstitial cell
The Cell Sweep
thecoma
    luteinized t.
    ovarian t.
Theelin
thelarche
    premature t.
theleplasty
theloncus
thelorrhagia
Theo-24
Theobid
Theochron
Theoclear
    T. L.A.
Theo-Dur
Theolair
Theon
theophyllinate
    choline t.
theophylline
    t. level
theory
    clonal selection t.
    Cohnheim t.
    endorphin, dopamine, and
      prostaglandin t.
    Freud t.
    ganglion trigger t.
    gate control t.
    grandmother t.

implantation t.
Ishihara t.
Larmarck t.
skin trigger t.
teleologic t.
Trivers-Willard t.
Theospan-SR
Theostat
Theovent
Theo-X
therapeutic
  t. abortion (TAB)
  t. insemination
  t. window
therapy
  adjuvant t.
  adjuvant chemoradiation t.
  aerosol t.
  antibacterial t.
  anticoagulant t.
  antidepressant t.
  antiemetic t.
  antifungal drug t.
  antihelminthic t.
  antihypertensive t.
  antimicrobial t.
  antiparasitic drug t.
  antithyroid drug t.
  antiviral t.
  belly bath t.
  biofeedback t.
  blood component t.
  broad-spectrum antibiotic t.
  bromocriptine t.
  caffeine t.
  cancer t.
  chest physical t.
  electroshock t.
  embolization t.
  endocavitary radiation t.
  enterostomal t.
  estrogen t.
  estrogen-progestin
    replacement t.
  estrogen replacement t.
    (ERT)
  extended field irradiation t.

external radiation t.
external x-ray t.
fetal drug t.
fluid t.
fractionated radiation t.
frappage t.
gene t.
glucocorticosteroid t.
gold t.
hormonal antineoplastic t.
hormone t.
hormone replacement t.
  (HRT)
hyperbaric oxygen t.
immunosuppressive t.
internal radiation t.
interstitial t.
intraperitoneal t.
intraperitoneal radiation t.
iodide t.
laser t.
menopausal estrogen
  replacement t.
monoclonal antibody t.
neutron t.
oral hormone replacement t.
percussion t.
photodynamic t.
physical t. (PT)
polyvalent
  immunoglobulin t.
postmenopausal estrogen
  replacement t.
progestational t.
progestogen support t.
quadrantectomy, axillary
  dissection, radiation t.
  (QUART)
radiation t.
salvage t.
single-dose methotrexate t.
steroid t.
thrombolytic t.
ʟ-thyroxine t.
tocolytic t.
transdermal hormone
  replacement t.

NOTES

427

therapy *(continued)*
    vaginal estrogen t.
    vasopressin t.
    xanthochromia t.
    x-ray t.
thermal injury
Thermasonic gel warmer
thermistor thermometer
thermodilution method
thermogenesis
    brown fat nonshivering t.
thermography
thermometer
    basal body t.
    Ototemp 3000 t.
    thermistor t.
    Thermoscan tympanic
      instant t.
thermoregulation
Thermoscan tympanic instant
  thermometer
thetaiotaomicron
    Bacteroides t.
THI
    transient
    hypogammaglobulinemia of
    infancy
thiabendazole
thiamine
thiazide
    t. diuretic
thickening
    skin t.
thickness
    endometrial t.
    fetal nuchal translucency t.
    placental t.
Thiemann
    T. disease
    T. syndrome
thin-layer chromatography
ThinPrep processor
thioguanine
thiomalate
    gold sodium t.
thiopental sodium
thiopropazate
thiosulfate
    sodium t.
Thiosulfil
thiotepa
thiothixene
thiphenamil hydrochloride

third
    t. degree prolapse
    t. disease
    t. parallel pelvic plane
    t. spacing
    t. stage of labor
    t. trimester
    t. trimester bleeding
THL
    true histiocytic lymphoma
thlipsencephalus
Thomas
    T. curette
    T. test
Thomas-Gaylor biopsy forceps
Thomsen
    T. disease
    T. myotonia congenita
    T. syndrome
Thomson
    T. disease
    T. syndrome
thoracentesis
thoracic
    t. cavity
    t. clamp
    t. compression syndrome
thoracoceloschisis
thoracodelphus
thoracodidymus
thoracogastrodidymus
thoracogastroschisis
thoracolumbar sympathetic nerve
thoracomelus
thoracopagus
thoracoparacephalus
thoracoschisis
thoracotomy
thoradelphus
thorax
    amazon t.
Thorazine
Thorn
    T. maneuver
    T. test
threatened
    t. abortion
    t. miscarriage
three-day measles
three-quarter strength formula
three-vessel cord
threshold
    phenotypic t.

speech reception t. (SRT)
t. trait
thrive
failure to t. (FTT)
nonorganic failure to t.
(NOFT)
thrombasthenia
Glanzmann t.
thrombectomy
thrombi (*pl. of* thrombus)
thrombin
t. clot test
t. time
thrombocythemia
thrombocytopenia
alloimmune t.
immune t.
isoimmune t.
transfusion-induced t.
thrombocytopenia-absent radius
(TAR)
thrombocytopenia-absent radius
syndrome
thrombocytopenic purpura
thrombocytosis
thromboembolic disease (TED)
thromboembolism
pulmonary t.
venous t.
thrombolytic therapy
thrombophlebitis
deep vein t.
pelvic t.
pelvic vein t.
septic pelvic t.
superficial t.
thromboplastin
thrombosis, pl. **thromboses**
arterial t.
cavernous sinus t.
cerebral t.
coronary t.
deep vein t. (DVT)
deep venous t. (DVT)
maternal cortical vein t.
ovarian vein t.
placental t.

renal vascular t.
renal vein t.
venous t.
thrombospondin
thrombotic
t. microangiopathy
t. phlegmasia
t. purpura
t. thrombocytopenic purpura
(TTP)
Thrombo-Wellco test
thromboxane
t. A_2
t. dominance
thrombus, pl. **thrombi**
thrush
t. pneumonia
thrust
tongue t.
thumb
hitchhiker t.
t. retractor
thumbsucking
thymectomy
neonatal t.
thymic
t. aplasia
t. asthma
t. dysplasia
t. lymphocyte antigen (TL)
t. shadow
thymic-dependent deficiency
thymic-parathyroid aplasia
thymine
thymol turbidity test
thymoma
thymopoietin
thymosin
thymus gland
thyroarytenoid muscle
Thyro-Block
thyroglobulin
thyroglossal
thyrohypophysial syndrome
thyroid
t. autoantibody
t. cancer

NOTES

thyroid *(continued)*
    t. crisis
    t. deficiency
    t. disease
    t. dysfunction
    t. function
    t. function tests (TFT)
    t. gland
    t. hormone
    t. index
    t. neoplasia
    t. nodule
    t. storm
thyroid-binding globulin (TBG)
thyroidectomy
thyroiditis
    Hashimoto t.
    postpartum t.
thyroid-stimulating
    t.-s. hormone (TSH)
    t.-s. hormone assay
    t.-s. immunoglobulin
Thyrolar
thyrotoxicosis
thyrotrope
thyrotropic hormone
thyrotropin
    chorionic t.
thyrotropin-releasing
    t.-r. hormone (TRH)
    t.-r. hormone stimulation
    test
thyroxine, thyroxin (T₄) (T_4)
    t. test
ʟ-thyroxine
    -t. therapy
thyroxine-binding
    t.-b. globulin
    t.-b. protein (TBP)
Thytropar
TIA
    transient ischemic attack
TIBC
    total iron-binding capacity
tibiae
    osteochondrosis deformans t.
tibial torsion
tic
    maladie des t.'s
Ticar
ticarcillin
    t. disodium
tick fever

Ticon
tidal volume
Tietze syndrome
Tigan
Tillaux disease
tilt test
time
    activated clotting t. (ACT)
    activated partial
      thromboplastin t. (APTT)
    bleeding t.
    capillary refill t.
    cell generation t.
    circulation t.
    doubling t.
    gastric emptying t.
    inspiration t. (I-time)
    Ivy bleeding t.
    kaolin clotting t.
    Lee-White clotting t.
    partial thromboplastin t.
     (PTT)
    t. position scan
    prothrombin t. (PT)
    recovery t.
    Russell viper venom t.
    thrombin t.
Timentin
timer
    Apgar t.
Timolide
timolol
Timoptic
Tincture
    Fungoid T.
Tindal
tinea
    t. capitis
    t. corporis
    t. cruris
    t. nigra palmaris
    t. pedis
    t. versicolor
tine test
tinnitus
tioconazole
tip
    Corometrics Gold Quik
     Connect Spiral electrode t.
    Corometrics Quik Connect
     Spiral electrode t.
    nonfrosted t.
tiptoeing

tired housewife syndrome
Tischler cervical biopsy forceps
Tischler-Morgan
    T.-M. biopsy punch
    T.-M. uterine biopsy forceps
Tisit
tissue
    adipose t.
    anechoic t.
    attenuating t.
    breast biopsy t.
    connective t.
    echogenic t.
    ectopic endometrial t.
    t. factor
    fibrous connective t.
    t. forceps
    glandular t.
    granulation t.
    t. homogeneity
    t. inhibitors of
      metalloproteinase
    intralobular connective t.
    lymphoid t.
    maternal t.
    paravaginal soft t.
    perilobular connective t.
    t. pH monitoring
    placental t.
    t. regeneration
    residual ductal t.
    retroperitoneal soft t.
    scar t.
    sonolucent t.
    splenic t.
    t. study
    syngeneic t.
    t. thromboplastin-inhibition
      test
    t. tolerance to radiation
    t. transplant
    trophoblastic t.
    xenogeneic t.
tissue-specific antibody
Tis-U-Trap
titanium staple

titer
    antistreptolysin t.
    HI t.
      hemagglutination
       inhibition
Titralac
titrate
TKO
    to keep open
TL
    thymic lymphocyte antigen
    tubal ligation
TLC
    total lung capacity
      TLC antiseptic soap
T-max
    maximum temperature
TNF-α
    tumor necrosis factor-α
TNF
    tumor necrosis factor
TNM
    tumor, node, metastasis
      TNM classification
      TNM nomenclature
T&O
    tandem and ovoids
toast
    bananas, rice cereal,
      applesauce, and t. (BRAT)
Tobey ear rongeur
tobramycin
Tobrex
tococardiography
tocodynagraph
tocodynamometer
tocodynamometry
tocograph
tocography
tocology
tocolysis
tocolytic
    t. agent
    t. therapy
tocometer
tocophobia
Today vaginal contraceptive sponge

NOTES

Toddler Temperament Scale
toe
    catheter t.'s
    hammer t.
    pigeon t.
toeing
    t. in
    t. out
toe-in gait
toewalking
TOF
    tetralogy of Fallot
Tofranil
togavirus
toilet
    pulmonary t.
    respiratory t.
Toitu MT-810 cardiographic
  monitor
Tolamide
tolazamide
tolazoline
    t. hydrochloride
tolbutamide
Toldt
    line of T.
Tolectin
tolerance
    antigen t.
    carbohydrate t.
    glucose t.
    immunologic t.
    impaired glucose t. (IGT)
    radiation t.
tolfenamic acid
tolmetin
Toloxan
toluidine
    t. blue
    t. blue test
Tolzol
Tom Jones closure
tomography
    computed t. (CT)
    computed axial t. (CAT)
    hypocycloidal t.
    quantitative computed t.
     (QCT)
    Somatom Plus computed t.
Tompkins median bivalving
  technique
tongue
    black t.

    t. crib
    crocodile t.
    fern leaf t.
    geographic t.
    hairy t.
    scrotal t.
    strawberry t.
    t. thrust
tongue-tie
tonic
    t. neck reflex
    t. seizure
tonic-clonic, tonoclonic
    t.-c. movements
    t.-c. seizure
tonicocolonic seizure activity
tonsillectomy
tonsillitis
    white t.
tonsillopharyngitis
tonus
    baseline t.
Tool
    Adolescent and Pediatric
     Pain T. (APPT)
Topaz-UPS
topical
    t. iodine application
    t. testosterone
    t. treatment
Toradol
TORCH
    toxoplasmosis, other agents,
     rubella, cytomegalovirus,
     herpes simplex
    T. syndrome
Toriello-Carey sign
Torpin cul-de-sac resection
torr
torsade de pointes
torsion
    adnexal t.
    t. dystonia
    ovarian t.
    splenic t.
    tibial t.
torso presentation
torti
    pili t.
torticollis
torulosis
Totacillin
    T.-N

total
t. abdominal hysterectomy (TAH)
t. anomalous pulmonary venous return
t. ascertainment
t. body water
t. breech extraction
t. cavopulmonary connection
t. iron-binding capacity (TIBC)
t. lung capacity (TLC)
t. mastectomy
t. oxyhemoglobin (THb O$_2$, THb O$_2$)
t. parenteral nutrition (TPN)
t. pelvic exenteration
t. perineal rupture
t. peripheral parenteral nutrition (TPPN)
t. placenta previa
t. pulmonary resistance
t. testosterone index

totalis
situs inversus t.

totipotent cell
totipotential cell
Toupet fundoplication
Tourette syndrome
TOVA ADD/ADHD assessment
Towako method
towel clip
tower skull
Townes-Brocks syndrome
Townes syndrome
Townsend biopsy punch
toxemia, toxicemia
preeclamptic t.
t. of pregnancy

toxemic
t. rash of pregnancy
t. retinopathy of pregnancy

toxic
t. epidermal necrolysis
t. megacolon
t. shock

t. shock syndrome (TSS)
t. shock syndrome toxin-1

toxicemia (*var. of* toxemia)
toxicity
bone marrow t.

toxicology screen
toxicum
erythema neonatorum t.

toxin
bacterial t.
environmental t.

toxin-1
toxic shock syndrome t.-1

toxocariasis
toxoid
tetanus t.

Toxoplasma gondii
toxoplasmosis
congenital t.
fetal t.

toxoplasmosis, other agents, rubella, cytomegalovirus, herpes simplex (TORCH)
TPI
Treponema pallidum immobilization
TPI test

TPN
total parenteral nutrition

TPPN
total peripheral parenteral nutrition

trace metal
tracer
radioactive t.

trachea
tracheal
t. agenesis syndrome
t. compression
t. intubation
t. stenosis
t. web

tracheal-aspirate culture
trachelectomy
trachelitis
trachelobregmatic diameter
trachelopanus

NOTES

trachelopexia, trachelopexy
tracheloplasty
trachelorrhaphy
tracheloschisis
trachelotomy
tracheobronchial
tracheobronchitis
tracheobronchomegaly
tracheoesophageal
    t. fistula
tracheolaryngomalacia
tracheomalacia
tracheostomy
tracheotome
    Sierra-Sheldon t.
tracheotomy
trachoma
    t. inclusion conjunctivitis
    (TRIC)
trachomatis
    Chlamydia t.
tract
    gastrointestinal t.
    genital t.
    intestinal t.
    reproductive t.
    respiratory t.
traction
    t. atrophy
    axis t.
    Bryant t.
tragus, pl. tragi
    accessory t.
TRAIDS
    transfusion-related AIDS
training
    Lovas t.
trait
    autosomal dominant t.
    autosomal recessive t.
    dominant lethal t.
    familial t.
    galtonian t.
    hereditary t.
    mendelian t.
    penetrant t.
    recessive t.
    sickle cell t.
    threshold t.
    X-linked t.
Trandate
tranexamic acid
tranquilizer

transabdominal
    t. cervicoisthmic cerclage
    t. ultrasound
transaminase
    serum t.
transanimation
transcapillary
    t. fluid
    t. fluid balance
transcatheter embolization
transcephalic impedance
transcervical
    t. balloon tuboplasty
    t. division
    t. intrafallopian tube
    transfer (TCIFTT)
    t. resection
transcobalamine deficiency
transcortin
transcript
    X inactive, specific t.
    (XIST)
transcriptase
    reverse t.
transcription
    gene t.
    reverse t.
transcutaneous
    t. measurement
    t. monitor
    t. oxygen tension
    monitoring
    t. partial pressure of oxygen
    ($tCpO_2$)
Transdermal
    Estraderm T.
transdermal
    t. administration
    t. estrogen
    t. hormone replacement
    therapy
    t. medication patch
transducer
    endovaginal t.
    Oxisensor t.
    SLA t.
Transeptic cleansing solution
transesophageal electrophysiologic
  study
transfer
    direct oocyte t. (DOT)
    direct oocyte sperm t.
    (DOST)

embryo t. (ET)
embryo intrafallopian t. (EIFT)
t. factor
gamete intrafallopian t. (GIFT)
gas t.
intrafallopian t.
in vitro fertilization-embryo t. (IVF-ET)
linear energy t. (LET)
placental t.
pronucleate stage embryo t. (PROST)
t. ribonucleic acid (tRNA)
t. RNA (tRNA)
transcervical intrafallopian tube t. (TCIFTT)
tubal embryo t. (TET)
tubal embryo stage t. (TEST)
zygote intrafallopian t. (ZIFT)

transferase
gamma glutamyl t. (GGT)

transferrin

transformation
t. zone

transforming
t. growth factor (TGF)
t. growth factor alpha (TGFα)
t. growth factor beta (TGFβ)

transfusion
autologous t.
blood t.
t. controversy
double-volume exchange t.
erythrocyte t.
exchange t.
fetal t.
fetofetal t.
fetomaternal t.
fetoplacental t.
intraperitoneal blood t.
intraperitoneal fetal t.

intrauterine t.
intrauterine intraperitoneal fetal t.
intravascular t.
leukocyte t.
massive t.
percutaneous fetal t.
placental t.
platelet t.
prophylactic red-cell t.
twin-twin t.
umbilical cord t.

transfusion-induced thrombocytopenia

transfusion-related AIDS (TRAIDS)

transient
t. congenital hypothyroidism
t. erythroid hypoplasia
t. fetal distress
t. hypogammaglobulinemia
t. hypogammaglobulinemia of infancy (THI)
t. ischemic attack (TIA)
t. neonatal pustular melanosis
t. respiratory distress syndrome (TRDS)
t. tachypnea
t. tachypnea of the newborn (TTN)

transillumination
t. of head

transition
fetal-neonatal t.

translation
nick t.

translocation
autosome t.
balanced t.
t. carrier
chromosomal t.
t. chromosome
t. Down syndrome
reciprocal t.
robertsonian t.
unbalanced t.

NOTES

transmesenteric hernia
transmigration
 ovular t.
transmission
 maternal-fetal t.
 t. medium
 perinatal t.
 pressure t.
 sexual t.
 viral t.
transnasal administration
transpeptidase
 glutamyl t. (GTP)
transperineal implant
transperitoneal cesarean section
transplacental
 t. hemorrhage
 t. passage
transplant
 fetal tissue t.
 fetus-to-fetus t.
 liver t.
 organ t.
 placental tissue t.
 tissue t.
transplantation
 t. antigen
 bone marrow t.
 t. immunology
 kidney t.
 liver t.
 organ t.
 orthotopic live t.
 pituitary gland t.
 renal t.
transport
 t. disorder
 egg t.
 ovum t.
 sperm t.
transposable element
transposed adnexa
transposition
 t. of great arteries (TGA)
 t. of great vessels (TGV)
 t. of ovary
 penoscrotal t.
 Watkins t.
transposon
transpyloric enteral feeding
transrectal
 t. approach

 t. probe
 t. surgical treatment
transsexual
transsexualism
transsphenoidal
 t. microsurgical resection
 t. operation
transurethral
 t. catheter
 t. electrocautery
 t. marsupialization
transvaginal
 t. cone
 t. implant
 t. sonography (TVS)
 t. transducer probe
 t. tubal catheterization
 t. ultrasonography
 t. ultrasound
transverse
 t. arrest
 t. cervical ligament
 t. diameter
 t. fundal incision of
  Strassman
 t. incision
 t. lie
 t. lie presentation
 lower uterine segment t.
  (LUST)
 t. myelitis
 occiput t. (OT)
 t. oval pelvis
 t. presentation
 t. ridge
 t. scan
 t. vaginal septum
transversus
 situs t.
tranylcypromine
trap
 filtered specimen t.
 sterile specimen t.
trapped ovum
Trasicor
trauma, pl. **traumata, traumas**
 acoustic t.
 birth t.
 blunt t.
 childhood genital t.
 fetal t.
 genital tract t.
 maternal t.

perinatal t.
psychological t.
traumatic
    t. amenorrhea
    t. injury
    t. vaginitis
Travamine
Travamulsion IV fat emulsion
tray
    E-Z-EM PercuSet
     amniocentesis t.
    HSG t.
    Unimar HSG t.
trazodone
TRDS
    transient respiratory distress
    syndrome
Treacher
    T. Collins-Franceschetti
    syndrome
    T. Collins syndrome
treatment
    antenatal phenobarbital t.
    continuous/combined t.
    Fliess t.
    hormonal t.
    hyperbaric oxygen t.
    infertility t.
    laser t.
    military antishock
     trousers t. (MAST)
    P32 intraperitoneal t.
    prenatal t.
    Rotunda t.
    topical t.
    transrectal surgical t.
    updraft t.
    ureteral surgical t.
treatment-associated pregnancy
treatment-independent pregnancy
Trecator-SC
Treitz
    ligament of T.
Trendelenburg position
Trental
trephine, trepan

Treponema
    T. pallidum
    T. pallidum immobilization
    (TPI)
    T. pallidum immobilization
    test
treponemal
treponematosis
Tresilian sign
tretinoin
Trevor disease
Trexan
TRH
    thyrotropin-releasing hormone
triacetyloleandomycin
triad
    Currarino t.
    Hutchinson t.
trial
    Bernoulli t.
    Cetus t.
    chemotherapy phase t.
    t. forceps
    labor t.
triamcinolone acetonide
triamterene
triangle
    Burger t.
    Einthoven equilateral t.
    Hesselbach t.
    pubic t.
    Ward t.
triangular
    t. ligament
    t. uterus
Triasox
triatriatum
    cor t.
Triazole
Triban
    Pediatric T.
tribasilar synostosis
tribrachius
TRIC
    trachoma inclusion
    conjunctivitis
tricephalus

NOTES

tricheiria
trichinosis
Trichlorex
trichlormethiazide
trichloroacetic acid
trichloroethylene
2,4,5-trichlorophenoxyacetic acid
trichobezoar
trichoepithelioma
trichomonad
Trichomonas
    T. infection
    T. vaginalis
    T. vaginalis vaginitis
trichomoniasis
    t. vaginitis
trichorhinophalangeal
    t. dysplasia
    t. syndrome
trichorrhexis
    t. invaginata
    t. nodosa
trichoschisis
trichotillomania
trichuriasis
tricuspid
    t. atresia
    t. insufficiency
    t. regurgitation
Tri-Cyclen
    Ortho T.-C.
tricyclic antidepressant
tridactylism
tridermogenesis
tridihexethyl chloride
Tridione
tridymus
triencephalus
triethylenethiophosphoramide
trifluoperazine hydrochloride
triflupromazine hydrochloride
trigger point
triglyceride
trigonal
    t. plate
    t. ring
    t. urothelium
trigone
    urinary t.
trigonitis
trigonocephaly
Trihexane
Trihexy

trihexyphenidyl
trihydrate
    ampicillin t.
trihydroxycoprostanic acidemia
triiniodymus
triiodothyronine (T_3)
    reverse t.
    t. test
Trikacide
Trilafon
trilaminar blastoderm
Tri-Levlen
    T.-L. 5/
    T.-L. 6/
    T.-L. 10/
triloba
    placenta t.
trilogy of Fallot
Trimazide
trimeprazine
trimester
    first t.
    second t.
    third t.
trimethadione
trimethaphan camsylate
trimethobenzamide hydrochloride
trimethoprim
    t.-sulfamethoxazole
      (SMZ- TMP)
    t. sulfate
trimipramine
Trimox
Trimpex
Trimstat
Trimtabs
trinitrate
    glyceryl t. (GTN)
Tri-Norinyl
    T.-N. 5/
    T.-N. 7/
    T.-N. 9/
Trinsicon
trinucleotide repeat expansion
    mutation
triocephalus
triodurin
triophthalmos
triose phosphate isomerase
triotus
tripartita
    placenta t.
Tripedia

tripelennamine hydrochloride
tripe palm
triphasic oral contraceptive
Triphasil
    T. 5/
    T. 6/
    T. 10/
triphosphate
    adenosine t. (ATP)
    guanosine t. (GTP)
1,4,5-triphosphate
    inositol-1,4,5-t.
5'-triphosphate
    guanosine-5't. (GTP)
triple
    t. bromide
    t. diapers
    t. dye
    T. Sulfa vaginal cream
    t. swab test
triplet
triple-X
    t.-X. chromosomal
      aberration
    t.-X. syndrome
triploid fetus
triploidy
tripodia
tripoding
triprolidine hydrochloride
Triptil
tripus
trismus
    t. nascentium
    t. neonatorum
trismus-pseudocamptodactyly
  syndrome
trisomy
    t. 8
    t. 13
    t. 15
    t. 16
    t. 18
    t. 21
    t. 22
    autosomal t.
    t. C syndrome

t. D syndrome
t. E syndrome
t. G syndrome
t. 8 mosaicism
t. 11q syndrome
t. 8 syndrome
t. 13 syndrome
t. 13-15 syndrome
t. 16-18 syndrome
t. 18 syndrome
t. 21 syndrome
t. 22 syndrome
trisphosphate
    inositol t.
tritodrine hydrochloride
Trivers-Willard theory
Tri-Vi-Flor vitamins
Tri-Vi-Sol vitamins
tRNA
    transfer ribonucleic acid
    transfer RNA
Trobicin
trocar
    Cabot t.
    Circon-ACMI t.
    Core Dynamics
      disposable t.
    Dexide disposable t.
    Ethicon disposable t.
    Jarit disposable t.
    Marlow disposable t.
    Olympus disposable t.
    Solos disposable t.
    Stortz disposable t.
    Weck disposable t.
    Wisap disposable t.
    Wolf disposable t.
    Ximed disposable t.
trochocephaly
TroGARD electrosurgical blunt
  trocar system
troleandomycin
tromethamine (THAM)
    carboprost t.
    dinoprost t.
    ketorolac t.

NOTES

439

TrophAmine
    T. hyperalimentation
trophectoderm
    t. biopsy
trophoblast
    t. sampling
trophoblastic
    t. cell
    t. disease
    t. embolus
    t. neoplasia
    t. neoplastic disease
    t. pseudotumor
    t. tissue
    t. tumor
trophospongia
trophotropism
tropical bubo
tropicamide
tropic hormone
troponin
trousers
    antishock t.
    MAST t.
Trousseau sign
true
    t. conjugate
    t. hermaphroditism
    t. histiocytic lymphoma
      (THL)
    t. incontinence
    t. knots of umbilical cord
    t. labor
    t. precocious puberty
    t. twins
    t. uterine inertia
trumpet
    Iowa t.
truncate selection
truncus arteriosus
trunk presentation
Truphylline
Trymegen
trypanosomiasis
tryptophan
    t. malabsorption
tryptophanuria
tryptorelin
Trysul
TSH
    thyroid-stimulating hormone

T-shaped
    T.-s. constriction ring
    T.-s. uterus
TSS
    toxic shock syndrome
TSTA
    tumor-specific transplantation
      antigen
TTN
    transient tachypnea of the
      newborn
TTP
    thrombotic thrombocytopenic
      purpura
tubage
tubal
    t. abortion
    t. colic
    t. diverticulum
    t. dysmenorrhea
    t. embryo stage transfer
      (TEST)
    t. embryo transfer (TET)
    t. endometriosis
    t. endometrium
    t. factor
    t. gestation
    t. insufflation
    t. ligation (TL)
    t. ligation band technique
    t. mass
    t. metaplasia
    t. microsurgery
    t. obstruction
    t. occlusion
    t. patency
    t. pregnancy
    t. reconstruction surgery
    t. ring
    t. rupture
    t. sterilization
tubatorsion (*var. of* tubotorsion)
tube
    bilateral myringotomy t.'s
      (BMT)
    Cantor t.
    Cole endotracheal t.
    Cole orotracheal t.
    double-focus t.
    embryonic neural t.
    endotracheal t.
    eustachian t.
    fallopian t.

fimbriated end of
   fallopian t.
follicle aspiration t.
Keofeed t.
knuckle of t.
Miller-Abbott t.
molybdenum rotating anode
   x-ray t.
Moss t.
nasogastric t.
neural t.
NG t.
Pedi PEG t.
pus t.
Replogle t.
Reuter t.
Sengstaken-Blakemore t.
smoke removal t. (SRT)
tympanostomy t.
uterine t.
tubectomy
tubercle
   genital t.
   Ghon t.
   Montgomery t.'s
   Morgagni t.
   Müller t.
   Rokitansky t.
tuberculin syringe
tuberculoma
tuberculosis (TB)
   abdominal t.
   endometrial t.
   extrathoracic t.
   gastrointestinal t.
   intrathoracic t.
   miliary t.
   t. papulonecrotica
   pulmonary t.
   renal t.
tuberculous
   t. colitis
   t. dactylitis
   t. keratoconjunctivitis
   t. meningitis
   t. peritonitis
   t. salpingitis

tuberous
   t. mole
   t. sclerosis
   t. subchorial hematoma of
      the decidua
Tubex
tubing
   pressure-separator t.
tuboabdominal pregnancy
tubocornual
   t. microsurgery
   t. reanastomosis
tubocurarine
   t. chloride
tuboendometrial cell
tuboovarian
   t. abscess
   t. complex
   t. pregnancy
   t. varicocele
tuboovariectomy
tuboovaritis
tuboplasty
   balloon t.
   transcervical balloon t.
   ultrasound transcervical t.
tubotorsion, tubatorsion
tubouterine
   t. implantation
   t. pregnancy
tubular
   t. carcinoma
   t. proteinuria
   t. stenosis
tubule
   annular t.
   mesonephric t.
   seminiferous t.
tubulointerstitial disease
tuck
   tummy t.
Tucker-McLane forceps
Tucker-McLane-Luikhart forceps
tularemia vaccine
tummy tuck
tumor
   adenomatoid t.

NOTES

tumor *(continued)*
    adenomatoid oviduct t.
    adnexal t.
    adrenal t.
    adrenal cell rest t.
    androgen-producing t.
    t. angiogenesis factor (TAF)
    angiomatoid t.
    t. antigen
    t. antigenicity
    t. ascites
    autochthonous t.
    benign t.
    bladder t.
    bone t.
    borderline epithelial
      ovarian t.
    Brenner t.
    t. burden
    carcinoid t.
    central nervous system t.
    cervical stump t.
    colorectal t.
    debulking of t.
    endocervical sinus t.
    endodermal sinus t.
    endometrioid t.
    epithelial t.
    epithelial stromal t.
    Ewing t.
    feminizing adrenal t.
    genital tract t.
    germ cell t.
    germ cell testicular t.
    gestational trophoblastic t.
    Glazunov t.
    gonadal stromal ovarian t.
    t. grading
    granulosa cell t.
    granulosa-stromal cell t.
    hilar cell t.
    t. immunology
    t. immunotherapy
    intracranial t.
    islet cell t.
    Krukenberg t.
    Leydig cell t.
    lipid cell t.
    lipid cell ovarian t.
    lipoid ovarian t.
    liver t.
    malignant t.

    malignant mixed
      müllerian t. (MMMT)
    t. marker
    t. mass
    mesonephroid t.
    mixed germ cell t.
    mixed mesodermal t.
    mixed uterine t.
    monodermal t.
    mucinous t.
    t. necrosis factor-α (TNF-α)
    t. necrosis factor (TNF)
    neuroectodermal t.
    neurogenic t.
    t., node, metastasis (TNM)
    t., node, metastasis
      classification
    ovarian t.
    parovarian t.
    persistent trophoblastic t.
    pineal t.
    pituitary gland t.
    placental site
      trophoblastic t. (PSTT)
    pontine t.
    pregnancy t.
    prepubertal testicular t.
      (PPTT)
    t. progression
    pseudomucinous t.
    Recklinghausen t.
    t. regression
    Schiller t.
    Scully t.
    serous t.
    Sertoli cell t.
    Sertoli-Leydig cell t.
    sex-cord stromal t.
    sex-cord stromal germ
      cell t.
    t. size
    Steiner t.
    Teilum t.
    theca cell t.
    trophoblastic t.
    ulcerative t.
    uterine corpus t.
    virilizing t.
    virilizing adrenal t.
    vitelline t.
    Wilms t.
    yolk sac t.
tumor-associated antigen (TAA)

tumor-cloning assay
tumor-limiting factor
tumorous hyperprolactinemia
tumor-specific transplantation
  antigen (TSTA)
Tums Extra Strength
tungsten target
tunica
  t. albuginea
turcica
  sella t.
Turco posteromedial release of
  clubfoot
turgescence
turgescent
turmschädel
Turner
  T. mosaicism
  T. syndrome
turnover
  bone t.
  iron t.
turricephaly
turtle sign
Tusstat
Tuttle test
TVS
  transvaginal sonography
twenty-nail dystrophy
twilight sleep
twin
  acardiac t.
  allantoidoangiopagous t.'s
  asymmetrical conjoined t.'s
  binovular t.
  t. birth
  conjoined t.'s
  t. delivery
  dichorial t.'s
  dichorionic t.'s
  dichorionic-diamniotic t.'s
  diovular t.'s
  dissimilar t.'s
  dizygotic t.
  enzygotic t.'s
  equal conjoined t.'s
  false t.'s

false heteroovular t.'s
fraternal t.'s
t. gestation
growth-discordant t.'s
heterologous t.'s
heteroovular t.'s
identical t.'s
impacted t.'s
incomplete conjoined t.'s
locked t.'s
membranous t.'s
t. method
monoamniotic t.'s
monochorial t.'s
monochorionic t.'s
monoovular t.'s
monozygotic t.'s
omphaloangiopagous t.'s
one-egg t.'s
parabolic t.'s
t. placenta
t. pregnancy
second t.'s
Siamese t.'s
similar t.'s
symmetrical conjoined t.'s
t. transfusion syndrome
true t.'s
two-egg t.'s
unequal conjoined t.'s
uniovular t.'s
unlike t.'s
twinning
twin-twin transfusion
Two-Cal HN
two-cell
  t.-c. mechanism
  t.-c. zygote
two-dimensional echocardiogram
two-egg twins
two-tail test
Tylenol
Tylox
tympanic temperature
tympanites
  uterine t.
tympanogram

NOTES

tympanostomy tube
type
    t. 7 glycogenosis
    t. I diabetes mellitus
    t. I H/S
    mucopolysaccharidosis
    t. II diabetes mellitus
    t. III mucopolysaccharidosis
    t. II mucopolysaccharidosis
    t. II pneumonocyte
    t. IS mucopolysaccharidosis
    t. IVA, B
    mucopolysaccharidosis
    t. 16 papillomavirus
    t. VIII
    mucopolysaccharidosis
    t. VII mucopolysaccharidosis
    t. VI mucopolysaccharidosis
    t. V mucopolysaccharidosis

typhlitis
typhoid
    t. autoantibody
    t. fever
    t. vaccine
typhus fever
typing
    blood t.
Tyrode solution
tyropanoate sodium
tyrosinase-negative oculocutaneous
    albinism
tyrosinase-positive oculocutaneous
    albinism
tyrosine
    t. kinase
tyrosinemia
tyrosinosis
Tzanck test

U-500
>   Regular (Concentrated)
>   Iletin II U.

UA
>   umbilical artery

UAC
>   umbilical artery catheter

UCG
>   urinary chorionic gonadotropin

UCG-Slide Test

UDI
>   urinary diagnostic index

UD 2000 urodynamic measurement system

U-elevator
>   Gregersen U.-e.

u-hFSH
>   urinary-derived human follicle-stimulating hormone

Uhl anomaly

UICC
>   International Union Against Cancer

ulcer
>   aphthous u.
>   Curling u.
>   Cushing-Rokitansky u.
>   duodenal u.
>   genital u.
>   Lipschütz u.
>   peptic u.
>   phagedenic u.
>   rectal postradiation u.
>   vaginal u.

ulcerative
>   u. colitis
>   u. tumor

ulcus, pl. ulcera
>   u. vulvae acutum

Ullrich-Bonnevie syndrome
Ullrich-Feichtiger syndrome
Ullrich syndrome
ULPA/charcoal filtration system
Ulrich-Turner syndrome
Ultracef
Ultra Cover transducer cover
Ultralente
>   Humulin U U.
>   U. insulin
>   U. U

Ultramark
>   U. 4 Ultrasound
>   U. ultrasound system

ultrasonic
>   u. cephalometry
>   u. egg recovery
>   u. endovaginal finding
>   u. fetometry

ultrasonography
>   compression u.
>   Doppler u.
>   gray-scale u.
>   real-time u.
>   transvaginal u.

ultrasound
>   Acuson 128 Doppler u.
>   Advantage u.
>   Aloka OB/GYN u.
>   A-mode u.
>   Ansaldo AU560 u.
>   antenatal u.
>   u. assessment
>   ATL/ADR Ultramark 4/9 HDI u.
>   B-mode u.
>   Cineloop U.
>   cranial u.
>   u. diagnosis
>   Doppler u.
>   duplex u.
>   dynamic image on u.
>   Elscint ESI-3000 u.
>   fetal u.
>   u. fetometry
>   GE RT 3200 Advantage II u.
>   u. guidance
>   head u.
>   high-resolution u.
>   MAGGI disposable biopsy needle guide for u.
>   M-mode u.
>   MultiPRO 2000 disposable biopsy needle guide for u.
>   Pie Medical u.
>   prenatal u.
>   pulsed Doppler u.
>   pulsed-wave u.
>   real-time u.
>   real-time imaging on u.

ultrasound *(continued)*
   u. screening
   Shimadzu u.
   Siemens SI 400 u.
   Spectra-Diasonics u.
   u. stethoscope
   u. surveillance
   transabdominal u.
   u. transcervical tuboplasty
   transvaginal u.
   Ultramark 4 U.
   vaginal u.
   128 XP u.
ultrasound-directed egg retrieval
Ultratard
   Actrapid insulin with U.
umbilical
   u. artery (UA)
   u. artery catheter (UAC)
   u. artery catheterization
   u. artery line
   u. blood flow
   u. blood sampling
   u. circulation
   u. clamp
   u. cord
   u. cord anomaly
   u. cord transfusion
   u. cyst
   u. fistula
   u. fungus
   u. hernia
   u. ligament
   u. presentation
   u. scissors
   u. souffle
   u. vein
   u. vein catheter (UVC)
   u. vein catheterization
umbilicalis
   arteritis u.
umbilicus
Umbilicutter
umbrella
   vascular u.
Unasyn
unavoidable hemorrhage
unbalanced translocation
unborn child
underlying renal disease
undernourishment
   maternal u.
Underwood disease

undifferentiated gonad
Undritz anomaly
undulant fever
unequal conjoined twins
unexplained
   u. fever
   u. infertility
UNG
   uracil-N-glycosylase
Unicare breast pump
unicellular
unicolic uterus
unicornous, unicorn
unicornuate uterus
unilateral salpingo-oophorectomy
Unimar HSG tray
uninterrupted estrogen
uniovular twins
uniparental disomy
Unipath
Unipen
Uniphyl
unipolar electrode
Uniscreen urine test
unit
   Bovie u.
   bubble isolation u.
   calf compression u.
   Ferrold-Hisaw u.
   fetal-placental u.
   Flowtron DVT
     prophylaxis u.
   u. inheritance
   Magnetrode cervical u.
   maternal-placental u.
   maternal-placental-fetal u.
   Montevideo u.
   mouse uterine u. (MUU)
   nem (milk nutritional u.)
   neonatal intensive care u.
     (NICU)
   Nytone enuretic control u.
   pilosebaceous u.
   terminal duct lobular u.
     (TDLU)
Unitensen
universal
   u. joint syndrome
Universal vaginal probe
unlike twins
Unna
   U. mark
   U. nevus

unopposed estrogen
unpaired chromosome
unplanned pregnancy
unresponsiveness
    immunologic u.
unruptured tubal gestation
unsaturated fat
unstable lie
Unverricht disease
Unverricht-Lundborg syndrome
up
    pinked u.
u-PA
  urokinase-type plasminogen
  activator
updraft treatment
upper
    u. genital tract infection
    u. respiratory infection
    (URI)
UPS 2020 ambulatory
  measurement system
uptake
    maximum oxygen u.
    (VO$_2$max)
    minute oxygen u.
    radioactive u.
Uracel
urachal
    u. cyst
    u. fistula
urachus
Uracid
uracil-N-glycosylase (UNG)
uranoschisis
uranostaphyloschisis
urate
    u. calculus
    u. clearance
Urban operation
urea
    u. clearance
urealyticum
    Ureaplasma u.
Ureaphil

Ureaplasma
    U. culture
    U. urealyticum
Urecholine
uremia
ureter
    double u.
    ectopic u.
    u. fistula
ureteral, ureteric
    u. duplication
    u. dysmenorrhea
    u. ectopia
    u. node
    u. obstruction
    u. surgical treatment
ureterocele
ureterocervical
ureteroneocystostomy
    Glen Anderson u.
    Politano-Leadbetter u.
ureteropelvic
ureteropyelocaliectasis
ureterotubal anastomosis
ureteroureteral anastomosis
ureteroureterostomy
ureterouterine
ureterovaginal
    u. fistula
ureterovesical
    u. junction (UVJ)
    u. obstruction
    u. reflux
urethra
    imperforate u.
    lead pipe u.
    penile u.
    pipestem u.
urethral
    u. angle
    u. candle
    u. caruncle
    u. coaptation
    u. discharge
    u. diverticulum
    u. function
    u. gland

NOTES

urethral *(continued)*
  u. lumen
  u. opening
  u. pressure
  u. pressure profile
  u. prolapse
  u. sound
  u. spasm
  u. sphincter
  u. stenosis
  u. syndrome
urethritis
  anterior u.
  chlamydial u.
  follicular u.
  granular u.
  nongonococcal u.
  nonspecific u.
  u. petrificans
  posterior u.
  simple u.
  specific u.
  u. venerea
urethrocele
urethrocystometry
urethrography
urethropexy
  retropubic u.
urethroplasty
  Badenoch u.
urethroscopy
urethrotome
  Huffman-Huber infant u.
urethrovaginal fistula
urethrovesical
  u. angle
Urex
urge incontinence
urgency
  urinary u.
URI
  upper respiratory infection
uric
  u. acid
  u. acid infarct
Uri-Check test
Uridon
urinalysis
  clean-catch u.
urinary
  u. bladder
  u. bladder dysfunction
  u. calculus

  u. catheterization
  u. chorionic gonadotropin (UCG)
  u. concentrating capacity
  u. concentration test
  u. conduit
  u. diagnostic index (UDI)
  u. diversion
  u. exertional incontinence
  u. fistula
  u. free progesterone
  u. frequency
  u. glucose
  u. incontinence
  u. outlet obstruction
  u. retention
  u. sediment
  u. stasis
  u. stent
  u. steroid conjugate
  u. stress incontinence
  u. system
  u. tract abnormality
  u. tract disorder
  u. tract endometriosis
  u. tract infection (UTI)
  u. tract obstruction
  u. trigone
  u. urgency
urinary-derived human follicle-stimulating hormone (u-hFSH)
urination
  fetal u.
urine
  u. CIE test
  u. culture
  u. cytology
  u. flow
  u. latex test
  maple syrup u.
  u. output
  residual u.
  spun u.
  u. test
  u. toxicology screen
urinoma
Urispas
Urispec
  U. GP+A test
  U. 9-Way test
Urobiotic-250
Urocyte diagnostic cytometry system

urodynamic study
uroflometry
urofollitropin
urogenital
    u. anomaly
    u. atrophy
    u. diaphragm
    u. fistula
    u. fold
    u. hiatus
    u. sinus
urogram
    intravenous u. (IVU)
urokinase
urokinase-type plasminogen
  activator (u-PA)
Urolene Blue
urolithiasis
urological
    u. evaluation
    u. injury
urologic history
urology
Uro-Mag
    U.-M. capsules
uropathy
    bilateral u.
    fetal u.
    obstructive u.
urorectal
urosepsis
urothelium
    trigonal u.
Urozide
urticaria
    papular u.
    u. pigmentosa
urticarial papule
u-score method
use
    conservative drug u.
    illicit drug u.
    maternal cocaine u.
    oral contraceptive u.
    prophylactic aspirin u.
Usko pillars
US 1005 uroflow meter

uterectomy
uteri (*pl. of* uterus)
uterine
    u. abnormality
    u. absence
    u. access
    u. action
    u. activity
    u. activity alteration
    u. activity monitor
    u. angiosarcoma
    u. anomaly
    u. artery
    u. atony
    u. ballottement
    u. bleeding
    u. blood flow
    u. calculus
    u. carcinosarcoma
    u. cast
    u. cavity
    u. chondrosarcoma
    u. colic
    u. compression
    u. contraction
    u. corpus
    u. corpus tumor
    u. cough
    u. cramping
    u. cry
    u. curette
    u. decompression
    u. dysfunction
    u. dysmenorrhea
    u. elevator
    u. endolymphatic stroma
    u. endometrial stroma
    u. epithelial stroma
    u. epithelium
    u. evacuator
    u. evaluation
    u. factor
    u. fibroid
    u. fibromyoma
    u. gland
    u. hematoma
    u. hernia syndrome

NOTES

uterine *(continued)*
    u. horn
    u. incision
    u. inertia
    u. infection
    u. insufficiency
    u. leiomyomata
    u. lysosome level
    u. malposition
    u. manipulator
    u. mass
    u. massage
    u. milk
    u. müllerian sarcoma
    u. myoma
    u. myometrium
    u. necrosis
    u. papillary serous
      carcinoma
    u. pathology
    u. perforation
    u. pregnancy
    u. prolapse
    u. pyomyoma
    u. quiescence
    u. relaxation
    u. retroflexion
    u. retroversion
    u. rupture
    u. sarcoma
    u. sarcoma metastasis
    u. scar separation
    u. screening
    u. segment
    u. septa
    u. sinus
    u. size
    u. souffle
    u. sound
    u. suspension
    u. tenaculum
    u. tenaculum forceps
    u. tetanus
    u. tube
    u. tympanites
    u. vein
    u. vessel
uterinus
    vagitus u.
uterismus
uteritis
in utero
uteroabdominal pregnancy

Uterobrush endometrial sample
    collector
uterocystostomy
uterofixation
uterolith
uterometer
uteroovarian
    u. ligament
    u. varicocele
uteroperitoneal fistula
uteropexy
uteroplacental
    u. apoplexy
    u. blood flow
    u. insufficiency
    u. perfusion
    u. sinus
    u. vessel
uteroplasty
uterosacral
    u. ligament
uterosalpingography
uteroscope
uteroscopy
uterotomy
uterotonic
uterotonin
uterotropin
uterotubography
uterovaginal
    u. canal
uterus, pl. uteri
    u. acollis
    anomalous u.
    arcuate u., u. arcuatus
    AV/AF u.
    u. bicameratus vetularum
    bicornate u., u. bicornis
    bicornuate u.
    bifid u., u. bifidus
    biforate u., u. biforis
    u. bilocularis
    bipartite u., u. bipartitus
    boggy u.
    capped u.
    communicating u.
    cordiform u., u. cordiformis
    corpus u.
    Couvelaire u.
    Credé maneuver of u.
    didelphic u.
    u. didelphys
    double-mouthed u.

duplex u., u. duplex
gravid u.
heart-shaped u.
hourglass u.
incudiform u., u.
  incudiformis
large-for-dates u.
myomata u.
one-horned u.
u. parvicollis
placenta, ovary, u. (POU)
ruptured u.
septate u., u. septus
subseptate u., u. subseptus
symmetric communicating u.
triangular u., u. triangularis
T-shaped u.

unicolic u.
unicorn u., u. unicornis
unicornuate u.
UTI
  urinary tract infection
utricle
  prostatic u.
UVC
  umbilical vein catheter
uveitis
uveokeratitis
UVJ
  ureterovesical junction
uvula
  bifid u.
uvulitis

NOTES

V

V
venous
ventral
V line
VA
venoarterial
ventriculoatrial
Vabra
V. cannula
V. catheter
V. cervical aspirator
V. suction
V. suction curet
VAC
vincristine, actinomycin D,
cyclophosphamide
vaccination
v. varicella
vaccinatum
eczema v.
vaccine
ActHIB H. influenzae type
B v.
Bacille bilié de Calmette-
Guérin v.
bacillus Calmette-Guérin v.
BCG v.
cholera v.
DPT v.
Engerix-B hepatitis B v.
Escherichia coli v.
Haemophilus pertussis v.
(HPV)
hepatitis B v.
HIB polysaccharide v.
inactivated poliovirus v.
(IPV)
influenza v.
killed virus v.
live poliovirus v.
live-virus v.
measles v.
meningococcal
polysaccharide v.
Meningococcus v.
MMR v.
mumps v.
oral polio v.
Pasteur Institute bacillus
Calmette-Guérin v.

plague v.
pneumococcal v.
polyvalent pneumococcal v.
rabies v.
rubella v.
Sabin v.
Salk v.
smallpox v.
tularemia v.
typhoid v.
varicella v. (Varivax)
yellow fever v.
vacciniforme
hydroa v.
vache
coitus la v.
VACTERL
vertebral, anal, cardiac, tracheal,
esophageal, renal, limb
VACTERL anomaly
VACTERL syndrome
vacuole
vacuolization
Vacurette
Berkeley V.
vacuronium
Vacutainer system
vacuum
v. aspiration
v. aspirator
v. cannula
v. extraction
v. extractor
v. extractor delivery
vacuum-assisted delivery
vagina
apex of v.
artificial v.
dry v.
rugae of v.
vaginal
v. absence
v. adenocarcinoma
v. adenosis
v. administration
v. agenesis
v. anomaly
v. antibiotic cream
v. artery
v. atresia

vaginal *(continued)*
  v. atrophy
  v. birth after cesarean
  v. birth after cesarean
  section (VBAC)
  v. bleeding
  v. cancer
  v. candidiasis
  v. carcinoma
  v. celiotomy
  v. clear cell adenocarcinoma
  v. condom
  v. cone
  v. contraceptive
  v. cornification test
  v. cyst
  v. cystourethropexy
  v. cytology
  v. delivery
  v. dilator
  v. dimple
  v. discharge
  v. douche
  v. dysmenorrhea
  v. dysontogenetic cyst
  v. ectopic anus
  v. embryonic cyst
  v. epithelial abnormality
  v. estrogen therapy
  v. examination
  v. flora
  v. GIFT
  v. hand
  v. hematoma
  v. hood
  v. hysterectomy
  v. hysterotomy
  v. inclusion cyst
  v. infection
  v. injury
  v. intraepithelial neoplasia
  (VAIN)
  v. irrigation smear (VIS)
  v. laceration
  v. lithotomy
  v. lubricant
  v. microflora
  v. mucification test
  v. mucosa
  v. myomectomy
  v. opening
  v. outlet
  v. perineorrhaphy

  v. pH
  v. plate
  v. pool
  v. pool L/S ratio
  v. prolapse
  v. prolapse prosthesis
  v. repair
  v. retractor
  v. ring contraception
  v. secretion
  v. smear
  v. sonography
  v. speculum loop
  v. sponge
  v. squamous metaplasia
  v. stump prolapse
  v. suppository
  v. surgery
  v. tampon
  v. terminus
  v. ulcer
  v. ultrasound
  v. vault
  v. vault prolapse
  v. venous plexus
  v. wall repair
  v. wall sling procedure
  v. yeast
vaginales
  rugae v.
vaginalis
  portio v.
  vagitus v.
vaginalis
  Haemophilus v.
  Trichomonas v.
vaginapexy
vaginectomy
vaginism
vaginismus
  posterior v.
vaginitis, pl. vaginitides
  adhesive v., v. adhesiva
  amebic v.
  atrophic v.
  chlamydial v.
  Corynebacterium v.
  v. cystica
  desquamative
    inflammatory v.
  v. emphysematosa
  Gardnerella v.
  Haemophilus v.

Mobiluncus v.
monilial v.
nonspecific v.
pinworm v.
recurrent v.
senile v., v. senilis
streptococcal v.
traumatic v.
Trichomonas vaginalis v.
yeast v.
vaginocele
vaginodynia
vaginofixation
vaginohysterectomy
vaginometer
vaginomycosis
vaginopathy
vaginoperineoplasty
vaginoperineorraphy
vaginoperineotomy
vaginopexy
Norman Miller v.
vaginoplasty
Fenton v.
vaginoscope
Huffman-Huber infant v.
Huffman infant v.
vaginoscopy
pediatric v.
vaginosis
anaerobic v.
bacterial v. (BV)
mycotic v.
vaginotomy
Vagistat
Vagi-TEST
Vagitrol
vagitus
v. uterinus
v. vaginalis
VAIN
vaginal intraepithelial neoplasia
Vakutage suction system
Valadol
Valentine position

valerate
betamethasone v.
estradiol v.
Valergen
valgum
genu v.
valgus
hallux v.
talipes v.
validity
Valisone
Valium
Valle hysteroscope
Valley
V. fever
V. Vac smoke evacuation
system
Valleylab
V. ball electrode
V. Force IC electrosurgical
generator
V. loop electrode
V. pencil
V. REM system
Valorin
Valpin 50
valproate
sodium v.
valproic acid
Valrelease
Valsalva
V. maneuver
V. sinus
sinus of V.
squirming V.
value
acid-base v.
Astrup blood gas v.
baseline v.
complement v.
fetal blood v.
flail v.
maturation v.
P v.
valve
bicuspid aortic v.
mitral v.

NOTES

valve *(continued)*
    parachute mitral v.
    pulmonary v.
valvotomy
valvular
    v. heart disease
    v. prosthesis
    v. pulmonic stenosis
valvulotomy
    balloon v.
    v. procedure
van
    v. Bogaert disease
    V. Buchem syndrome
    v. den Bergh test
    v. der Hoeve syndrome
    V. der Woude syndrome
    V. Hoorn maneuver
Vancaillie uterine cannula
Vancenase
    V. AQ
Vanceril
Vancocin
Vancoled
vancomycin
    v. hydrochloride
vanillylmandelic acid (VMA)
vanishing
    v. testes syndrome
    v. twin syndrome
Vanquin
Vantin
Vantos vacuum extractor
vapocauterization
Vapo-Iso
Vaponefrin
vaporization
vara
    coxa v.
variabilis
    erythrokeratodermia v.
variability
    baseline v. of fetal heart rate
    beat-to-beat v.
    fetal heart rate v.
    interpretation v.
variable
    continuous v.
    continuous random v.
    v. decelerations
    discrete v.
    discrete random v.

    mixed discrete-continuous random v.
    random v.
variance
    analysis of v. (ANOVA)
    multivariate analysis of v. (MANOVA)
    v. ratio
variant
    albopapuloid v.
    Pasini v.
variation
    beat-to-beat v. of fetal heart rate
    coefficient of v. (CV)
    interobserver v.
    observer v.
varicella
    v. bullosa
    v. gangrenosa
    v. infection
    v. inoculata
    v. pneumonia
    pustular v.
    v. pustulosa
    vaccination v.
    v. vaccine (Varivax)
varicellae
    Herpesvirus v.
varicella-zoster
    v.-z. immune globulin (VZIG)
    v.-z. virus (VZV)
    v.-z. virus infection
varicelliform
varices (*pl. of* varix)
varicocele
    ovarian v.
    tuboovarian v.
    uteroovarian v.
varicocelectomy
varicomphalus
varicosity
variegata
    porphyria v.
variegate
    v. porphyria
variola
varioliform
Varivax
    varicella vaccine
varix, pl. varices
    esophageal v.

gelatinous v.
vulvar v.
varus
metatarsus v.
talipes v.
vas, pl. vasa
v. deferens
vasal
vascular
v. anomaly
v. calcification
v. cell adhesion molecule
v. channel
v. communication
v. complication
v. disease
v. engorgement
v. headache
v. injury
v. leiomyoma
v. malformation
v. metastasis
v. parabiosis
v. reactivity
v. resistance
v. ring syndrome
v. spider
v. umbrella
vascularization
chorionic v.
vasculitis
cutaneous v.
rheumatoid v.
vasectomy
v. reversal
vasitis
vasoactive
v. intestinal peptide (VIP)
v. intestinal polypeptide
(VIP)
vasocongestion
Vasodilan
vasopressin
arginine v.
v. infusion
v. therapy
vasopressor

Vasospan
vasospasm
Vasotec
vasotocin
arginine v.
vasovagal
v. reflex apnea
Vasoxyl
VATER
vertebral defects, imperforate
anus, tracheoesophageal fistula,
renal defects
VATER syndrome
vault
vaginal v.
VBAC
vaginal birth after cesarean
section
VBG
venous blood gas
VBP
vinblastine, bleomycin, cisplatin
VBS
venous blood sample
V-Cillin K
VCP
VCU
videocystourethrography
voiding cystourethrogram
VCUG
vesicoureterogram
voiding cystourethrogram
VDRL
Venereal Disease Research
Laboratories
VE
volume of expired gas
Vecchietti
V. method
V. operation
vectis
Veetids
vegan
vegetarian
v. diet
vegetative reproduction
Veillonella

NOTES

vein
v. compressibility
dilated collateral v.
iliac v.
maternal cortical v.
ovarian v.
umbilical v.
uterine v.
vela (*pl. of* velum)
velamen, pl. **velamina**
v. vulvae
velamentosa
placenta v.
velamentous
v. insertion
velamina (*pl. of* velamen)
Velban
vellus hair
velocardiofacial syndrome
velocimetry
Doppler v.
velocity
v. flow profile
Velosef
Velosulin Human
Veltane
velum, pl. **vela**
vena
v. cava
v. caval filter
v. caval interruption
venenata
dermatitis v.
venereal
v. bubo
v. collar
v. disease
V. Disease Research
Laboratories (VDRL)
V. Disease Research
Laboratory test
v. lymphogranuloma
v. wart
venereology
venereum
lymphogranuloma v. (LGV)
venipuncture
Venning-Brown test
venoarterial (VA)
Venodyne pneumatic compressive
device
Venoglobulin-I
Venoglobulin-S

venography
radionuclide v.
venous (V)
v. blood gas (VBG)
v. blood sample (VBS)
v. catheter
v. collateral
v. line
v. oozing
v. thromboembolism
v. thrombosis
venovenous (VV)
venter
v. propendens
vent gleet
ventilation
bag-and-mask v.
bagged mask v.
controlled mechanical v.
(CMV)
hand v.
HFJ v.
HFO v.
HFPP v.
high-frequency jet v.
(HFJV)
high-frequency oscillatory v.
(HFOV)
high-frequency positive
pressure v. (HFPPV)
intermittent mandatory v.
(IMV)
intermittent mechanical v.
(IMV)
intermittent positive
pressure v. (IPPV)
v. by mask
oscillatory v.
v. scintigraphy
synchronized intermittent
mandatory v. (SIMV)
ventilation/perfusion ($\dot{V}/\dot{Q}$)
v. mismatch
v. quotient
v. ratio
v. scan
ventilator
respirator
Amsterdam infant v.
BABYbird II v.
Babyflex v.
Bear Cub infant v.
Bennett PR-2 v.

Bourns LS104-150 infant v.
Breeze v.
CPAP v.
Healthdyne v.
HFJV v.
HFOV v.
HFPPV v.
high-frequency v.
humidification v.
HVF v.
infant Star v.
Infant Star high-
  frequency v.
nebulization v.
PEEP v.
pressure-cycled v.
pressure-preset v.
Pulmo-Aid v.
Sechrist neonatal v.
Servo 900C v.
Siemens-Elema Servo
  900C v.
Star v.
v. support
Vickers Neovent v.
Vix infant v.
volume-limited v.
Wave v.
Ventolin
ventouse
ventral (V)
  v. hernia
ventricle
  dilation of v.
  double-inlet left v.
  double-inlet right v.
  left v. (LV)
ventricular
  v. function
  v. response rate
  v. septal defect (VSD)
  v. tachycardia
ventriculoatrial (VA)
ventriculography

ventriculomegaly
ventriculoperitoneal (VP)
  v. shunt
ventroposterior (VP)
ventrosuspension
Venturi mask
Venus
  collar of V.
VEP
  visual evoked potential
VER
  visual evoked response
vera
  placenta accreta v.
  polycythemia v.
  polycythemia rubra v.
Veralba
verapamil
***Veratrum* alkaloid**
Veress needle
vergeture
Veriloid
vermiculation
Vermox
Verner-Morrison syndrome
Vernes test
vernix
  v. caseosa
  v. membrane
Vero cell
verruca
  v. acuminata
  v. plana juvenilis
verruciformis
  epidermodysplasia v.
verrucous
  v. carcinoma
versicolor
  tinea v.
version
  bimanual v.
  bipolar v.
  Braxton Hicks v.
  cephalic v.
  combined v.
  external v.
  Hicks v.

NOTES

version *(continued)*
    internal v.
    pelvic v.
    podalic v.
    postural v.
    Potter v.
    spontaneous v.
    Wigand v.
    Wright v.
vertebral
    v., anal, cardiac, tracheal, esophageal, renal, limb (VACTERL)
    v., anal, cardiac, tracheal, esophageal, renal, limb anomaly
    v. artery
    v. bone loss
    v. bone mass
    v. compression fracture
    v. defects, imperforate anus, tracheoesophageal fistula, renal defects (VATER)
vertebral,
vertebra plana
vertebrodidymus
vertex, pl. **vertices**
    v. delivery
    v. position
    v. potential
    v. presentation
vertical hymen
vertically-acquired infection
vertices (*pl. of* vertex)
vertiginous seizure
vertigo
very
    v. low birth weight (VLBW)
    v. low-density lipoprotein (VLDL)
very-low-birth-weight infant
vesical neck
vesicle
    chorionic v.
    germinal v.
    graafian v.
    nabothian v.'s
    seminal v.
vesicobullous
vesicocele
vesicocervical
    v. space

vesicofixation
vesicomyectomy
vesicomyotomy
vesicoureteral
    v. reflux
vesicoureterogram (VCUG)
vesicourethral
    v. canal
    v. primordial
vesicouterine fistula
vesicovaginal
    v. fistula
    v. repair
vesicovaginorectal
    v. fistula
vesicular
    v. mole
vessel
    chorioallantoic v.
    corkscrew v.
    great v.'s
    hairpin v.
    v. spread
    transposition of great v.'s (TGV)
    uterine v.
    uteroplacental v.
vestibular
    v. adenitis
    v. anus
    v. bulb
    v. cyst
    v. duct
    v. gland
vestibule
vestibulitis
    vulvar v.
vestigial
viability
    fetal v.
viable
    v. fetus
vial
    Nickerson Biggy v.'s
Vibramycin
Vibra-Tabs
vibroacoustic-induced fetal movement
vibroacoustic stimulation
vicarious
    v. menstruation
    v. respiration
Vickers Neovent ventilator

Vicodin
Vicryl
V. suture
Victor Gomel method
vidarabine
VIDAS immunoanalysis testing system
Vi-Daylin vitamins
videocystourethrography (VCU)
videolaparoscope
VideoZoomscope
Videx
view
axillary v.
craniocaudal v.
exaggerated craniocaudal v.
four-chamber v.
frogleg v.
lateral oblique v.
lateromedial oblique v.
long-axis v.
medial oblique v.
mediolateral v.
pulmonary artery/ductus v.
short-axis v.
spot compression v.
vigabatrin
Vignal cells
vigorous infant
villi (*pl. of* villus)
villositis
villous placenta
villus, pl. villi
chorionic villi
placental v.
vimentin
Vim-Silverman needle
VIN
vulvar intraepithelial neoplasia
vinblastine
vinblastine, bleomycin, cisplatin (VBP)
Vinca alkaloid
Vincasar PFS
vincristine
v. sulfate

vincristine, actinomycin D, cyclophosphamide (VAC)
Vineland Adaptive Behavior Scales
VIN III
vulvar carcinoma in situ
violaceous lesion
violet
crystal v.
gentian v.
VIP
vasoactive intestinal peptide
vasoactive intestinal polypeptide
voluntary interruption of pregnancy
Vipond sign
viprynium
Vira-A
viral
v. encephalitis
v. infection
v. pharyngitis
v. pneumonia
v. pneumonitis
v. shedding
v. transmission
ViraPap
V. HPV DNA test
V. test
ViraType
V. HPV DNA typing assay
V. probe
V. test
Virazole
Virchow
pneumonia alba of V.
virgin
virginal
v. breast hypertrophy
v. hymen
v. introitus
Virginia needle
virginity
viridans
Streptococcus v.
virilescence
virilism
adrenal v.

NOTES

virilization
virilizing
    v. adenoma
    v. adrenal tumor
    v. 3α-androstanediol
      glucuronide
    v. tumor
Virilon
    V. capsule
virion
    intranuclear v.
virulent bubo
virus
    acquired immunodeficiency
      syndrome-related v. (ARV)
    ECHO v.
    enteric cytopathogenic
      human orphan v.
    Epstein-Barr v. (EBV)
    hepatitis A v.
    hepatitis B v.
    herpes simplex v. (HSV)
    herpes simplex v. type II
      (HSV II)
    herpes zoster v. (HZV)
    horizontal transmission
      of v.
    human immunodeficiency v.
      (HIV)
    human papilloma v. (HPV)
    human T-cell leukemia v.
      (HTLV)
    human T-cell leukemia v.
      type I (HTLV-I)
    human T-cell leukemia v.
      type II (HTLV-II)
    human T-cell leukemia v.
      type III (HTLV-III)
    influenza v.
    lymphadenopathy-
      associated v. (LAV)
    molluscum contagiosum v.
      (MCV)
    mouse mammary tumor v.
      (MMTV)
    mumps v.
    respiratory syncytial v.
      (RSV)
    RS v.
    rubella v.
    varicella-zoster v. (VZV)
VIS
    vaginal irrigation smear

visceral
    v. cleft
    v. peritoneum
viscerale
    cranium v.
visceromegaly
viscerum
    situs inversus v.
viscoelastic
viscous semen
Visicath
Visken
Visscher-Bowman test
Vista disposable skin stapler
Vistaril
visual
    v. analog scale for stress
    v. change
    v. disturbance
    v. evoked potential (VEP)
    v. evoked response (VER)
    v. field
    v. stimulation
visualization
Vitabee 6
vital
    v. capacity
    v. sign
vitamin
    v. B_6
    B complex v.'s
    v. B complex
    Bronson chewable
      prenatal v.'s
    v. C
    v. D
    v. D-binding protein
    v. D-resistant rickets
    v. E
    Fer-In-Sol v.'s
    v. K
    v. K prophylaxis
    Materna prenatal v.
    v. metabolism
    Poly-Vi-Flor v.'s
    Poly-Vi-Sol v.'s
    v. requirement
    Stuart Prenatal v.'s
    v. supplement
    Tri-Vi-Flor v.'s
    Tri-Vi-Sol v.'s
    Vi-Daylin v.'s
Vita Plus E

vitelliform degeneration
vitelline
> v. cord
> v. duct
> v. duct cyst
> v. fistula
> v. membrane
> v. sac
> v. tumor

vitellinum
> mesoblastoma v.

vitellointestinal cyst
vitello-intestinal duct
vitiligo
vitreoretinopathy
> familial exudative v.

vitreous
vitro
> in v.

vitronectin
Vivactil
Vivigen diagnostics
viviparity
viviparous
vivo
> ex v.
> in v.

Vivol
Vix infant ventilator
VLBW
> very low birth weight

VLDL
> very low-density lipoprotein

V-line
VM-26
VMA
> vanillylmandelic acid

Vogt
> V. cephalodactyly
> V. syndrome

Vogt-Spielmeyer disease
voiding
> v. cystourethrogram (VCU, VCUG)
> v. dysfunction

voiding dysfunction

volatile
> v. acid
> v. anesthetic

Volkmann
> V. deformity
> V. disease

volt
> electron-v. (eV, ev)
> megaelectron v. (MeV)

Voltaren
Voltolini disease
volume
> amniotic fluid v.
> blood v.
> closing v.
> v. of dead space
> v. expansion
> v. of expired gas (VE)
> fetal blood v.
> v. flow
> forced expiratory v. (FEV)
> intrauterine v.
> lung v.
> mean corpuscular v. (MCV)
> minute ventilatory v.
> v. overload
> plasma v.
> red cell v.
> residual v.
> semen v.
> tidal v.

volume-limited ventilator
voluntary
> v. interruption of pregnancy (VIP)
> v. sterilization

volvulus
> gastric v.
> midgut v.
> v. neonatorum

VO$_2$max
> maximum oxygen uptake

vomiting
> nausea and v.
> v. of pregnancy
> projectile v.

vomitus

NOTES

von

V. Fernwald sign
v. Gierke disease
v. Gierke glycogenolysis
v. Graefe sign
v. Hippel-Lindau disease
V. Jaksch anemia
v. Poehl test
v. Recklinghausen disease
v. Recklinghausen neurofibromatosis
v. Willebrand disease
v. Willebrand factor (vWF)
v. Willebrand syndrome

Voorhees bag
VP

ventriculoperitoneal
ventroposterior
VP shunt

VP-16
V̇/Q̇

ventilation/perfusion
V̇/Q̇ mismatch
V̇/Q̇ ratio
V̇/Q̇ scan

Vrolik disease
VSD

ventricular septal defect

vu

jamais v.

vulgaris

acne v.
ichthyosis v.
lupus v.
pemphigus v.

Vulpe Assessment Battery
vulsellum clamp
vulva, pl. **vulvae**

noma vulvae
synechia vulvae

vulvar

v. adenoid cystic adenocarcinoma
v. angiokeratoma
v. atrophy
v. atypia
v. biopsy
v. carcinoma
v. carcinoma in situ (VIN III)
v. contact dermatitis
v. cyst
v. dystrophy

v. edema
v. endometriosis
v. fibroma
v. hemangioma
v. hematoma
v. hydatidiform mole
v. inclusion cyst
v. infection
v. intraepithelial neoplasia (VIN)
v. lipoma
v. lymph node
v. malignancy
v. melanoma
v. nevus
v. pigmented lesion
v. pruritus
v. psoriasis
v. sarcoma
v. seborrheic dermatitis
v. skin
v. squamous hyperplasia
v. varix
v. vestibulitis
v. vestibulitis syndrome (VVS)

vulvectomy

Basset radical v.
Parry-Jones v.
radical v.
simple v.
skinning v.

vulvismus
vulvitis

adhesive v.
chronic atrophic v.
chronic hypertrophic v.
creamy v.
erosive v.
follicular v.
leukoplakic v.
plasma cell v.

vulvodynia
vulvoperianal
vulvoplasty
vulvovaginal

v. anus
v. candidiasis
v. carcinoma
v. cystectomy
v. lesion
v. outlet
v. premenarchal infection

vulvovaginitis
    candidal v.
    premenarchal v.
vulvovaginoplasty
    Williams v.
Vumon
VV
    venovenous
VVS
    vulvar vestibulitis syndrome

V.V.S.
vWF
    von Willebrand factor
Vytone
VZIG
    varicella-zoster immune globulin
VZV
    varicella-zoster virus

NOTES

Waardenburg-Klein syndrome
Waardenburg syndrome
Wachendorf membrane
Wade
    Roe v. W.
Wadia elevator
WAGR
    Wilms tumor, aniridia,
        gonadoblastoma, mental
        retardation
    WAGR syndrome
waist:hip ratio
Walcher position
Waldenstrom macroglobinemia
Waldeyer
    W. fossae
    germinal epithelium of W.
    W. preurethral ligament
Walker chart
Walker-Warburg syndrome
walking
    automatic w.
    chromosome w.
    w. epidural anesthetic
wall
    opposing w.
wallaby pouch
Wallace technique
Wallach
    W. Endocell collection
        device
    W. Endocell endometrial
        cell sampler
    W. LL100 cryosurgical
        cryogun
Wallach-Papette disposable cervical
    cell collector
Walt Disney dwarfism
Walthard cell rest
Walther dilator
Walton
    W. report
    W. syndrome
Wampole
    W. Laboratories
    W. test
wandering ovary
Wangensteen needle holder
Warburg syndrome
Wardill four-flap method

Wardill-Kilner advancement flap
    method
Ward-Mayo vaginal hysterectomy
Ward triangle
warfarin
    w. embryopathy
Warfilone
Waring
    W. blender sound
    W. blender syndrome
warmer
    Kreiselman infant w.
    Ohio w.
    overhead w.
    radiant w.
    Thermasonic gel w.
Warren flap
wart
    anogenital w.
    flat w.
    genital w.
    plantar w.
    venereal w.
    water w.
washed
    w. intrauterine insemination
    w. sperm
    w. spermatozoa
washer
    Gravlee jet w.
washings
    peritoneal w.
washout
    nitrogen w.
    w. pyelogram
Wassel classification
Wasserman test
wastage
    early pregnancy w.
    fetal w.
    pregnancy w.
    reproductive w.
wasting
    salt w.
water
    bag of w.'s (BOW)
    dextrose in w.
    w. excretion
    false w.'s
    w. intoxication

water *(continued)*
    w. loss
    w. metabolism
    total body w.
    w. wart
Waterhouse-Friderichsen syndrome
waterseal drainage
Waters operation
Waterston shunt
Watkins transposition
Watson-Alagille syndrome
Watson-Crick
    W.-C. helix
    W.-C. method
Watson method
wave
    fluid w.
    rolandic sharp w.'s
waveform
    arterial w.
    discordant artery flow
     velocity w.
    Doppler w.
    flow velocity w.
Wave ventilator
Way operation
W chromosome
wean
wean-and-feed protocol
weaning
    w. brash
web
    laryngeal w.
    tracheal w.
webbed
    w. finger
    w. neck
Weber-Christian syndrome
Weber test
webspace
Webster operation
Wechsler
    W. Intelligence Scale for
     Children-Revised (WISC-R)
    W. Preschool and Primary
     Scale of Intelligence-
     Revised (WPPSI-R)
Weck
    W. disposable cannula
    W. disposable trocar
Weck-sel sponge

wedge
    pulmonary artery w. (PAW)
    w. resection
Weerda laparoscope
Wegener granulomatosis
Wegner disease
Wehamine
Wehdryl
Wehless
weight
    birth w. (BW)
    body w.
    estimated fetal w. (EFW)
    fetal w.
    w. gain
    w. loss
    low birth w. (LBW)
    maternal w.
    placental w.
    w. reduction
    very low birth w. (VLBW)
weightbearing bone
weighted speculum
Weightrol
Weil disease
Weill-Marchesani syndrome
Weill sign
Weinberg rule
Weitlaner retractor
well-being
    fetal w.-b.
well-born
    right to be w.-b.
well-circumscribed carcinoma
Wellcovorin
well-defined mass
well-hydrated baby
well-oxygenated infant
well-perfused baby
Wenckebach
    W. heart block
    W. phenomenon
Wepman test
Werdnig-Hoffmann
    W.-H. disease
    W.-H. muscular atrophy
    W.-H. paralysis
    W.-H. syndrome
Werlhof disease
Wermer syndrome
Werner syndrome
Wernicke aphasia
Wertheim operation

Wertheim-Schauta operation
West
    W. Haven-Yale
    Multidimensional Pain
    Inventory
    W. Nile fever
    W. syndrome
West-Engstler skull
Western
    W. blot
    W. blot test
wet
    w. burp
    w. lung syndrome
    w. mount
    w. nurse
    w. prep
    w. rales
    w. smear
Weyers oligodactyly syndrome
Wharton jelly
wheal
wheal-and-flare reaction
Wheaton Pavlik harness
wheat sperm agglutination test
whiff test
Whipple
    W. disease
    W. syndrome
whipworm
whistle-tip catheter
whistling
    w. face syndrome
    w. face-windmill vane hand
    syndrome
white
    w. blood cell
    W. class, B through RF
    W. classification
    w. epithelium
    w. infarct
    w. leg
    w. matter necrosis
    w. pupillary reflex
    w. sponge nevus
    w. tonsillitis
Whittaker test

WHO
    World Health Organization
whole
    w. abdominal radiation
    w. blood
whole-abdomen irradiation
whole-body irradiation
whole-pelvis irradiation
Whoo Noz
whooping cough
whorl
WI-38 cells
wick
    gauze w.
wide plane
Wiedemann syndrome
Wiegernick culdocentesis
Wigand
    W. maneuver
    W. version
Wilcoxon rank sum test
Wildermuth ear
Wildervanck syndrome
wild-type gene
Wilkins
    W. disease
    W. syndrome
Willebrand-Jurgens syndrome
Willett
    W. clamp
    W. forceps
Williams
    W. disease
    W. syndrome
    W. vulvovaginoplasty
Williams-Beuren syndrome
Williams-Campbell syndrome
Willy Meyer mastectomy
Wilms
    W. syndrome
    W. tumor
    W. tumor, aniridia,
    gonadoblastoma, mental
    retardation (WAGR)
Wilson disease
Wilson-Mikity syndrome
Winckel disease

NOTES

window
    aortopulmonary w.
    square w.
    therapeutic w.
wink
    anal w.
Winkler body
Winkler-Waldeyer
    closing ring of W.-W.
Winston cervical clamp
Winter
    W. placental forceps
    W. syndrome
Wintrobe index
wipe
    povidone-iodine w.
wire
    iridium w.
Wisap
    W. disposable cannula
    W. disposable trocar
WISC-R
    Wechsler Intelligence Scale for
    Children-Revised
Wiskott-Aldrich syndrome
witch's milk
withdrawal
    w. bleeding
    w. bleeding test
    estrogen w.
withdrawal-like activity
Wittner biopsy punch
Wolf
    W. Castroviejo needle
    holder
    W. disposable cannula
    W. disposable trocar
    W. laparoscope
Wolfe
    W. classification of breast
    cancer
    W. classification of breast
    carcinoma
wolffian
    w. duct
    w. duct carcinoma
    w. rest
    w. ridge
Wolff-Parkinson-White syndrome
Wolf-Hirschborn syndrome
Wolfram syndrome
Wolf-Veress needle
Wolman disease

woman
    androgenized w.
    battered w.
    euprolactinemic w.
    hirsute w.
    hypoestrogenic w.
    hypogonadal w.
    infertile w.
    lactating w.
    perimenopausal w.
    postmenopausal w.
womb
    falling of the w.
    scarred w.
    w. stone
Wood
    W. lamp
    W. light
Wood-Downes asthma score
Woods
    W. maneuver
    W. screw maneuver
wooly-hair
    w.-h. disease
    w.-h. nevus
Word-Bartholin gland catheter
Word bladder catheter
**World Health Organization
(WHO)**
wormian bones
wound
    w. breakdown
    w. dehiscence
    w. infection
    stab w.
WPPSI-R
    Wechsler Preschool and Primary
    Scale of Intelligence-Revised
Wramsby hypothesis
Wreden sign
Wright
    W. peak flow meter
    W. stain
    W. version
wrist
    gymnast's w.
wrongful
    w. birth and life
    w. conception
wryneck
Wullstein retractor
Wyamycin-S
Wyanoids

Wyburn-Mason syndrome
Wycillin
Wydase

Wygesic
Wymox
Wytensin

NOTES

X

X chromatin
X chromosome
X inactivation center
(XIC)
X inactive, specific
transcript
(XIST)

45,X

45,X karyotype
45,X syndrome

Xanax
xanthelasmas
xanthine
xanthinuria, xanthiuria
xanthochromia
x. therapy
xanthochromic
x. specimen
xanthogranuloma
juvenile x. (JXG)
xanthoma striata palmaris
xanthomatosis
xanthosis cutis
xanthous
xanthurenic aciduria
X-chromosome abnormality
Xe
xenon
xenogeneic
x. antibody
x. tissue
xenograft
xenon (Xe)
Xenopus test
xeroderma pigmentosum
xerodermic idiocy
xerography
xeromammography
xeromenia
xerophthalmia
xerosis
x. conjunctiva
x. cornea
xerostomia
xerotocia
XIC
X inactivation center

Ximed
X. disposable cannula
X. disposable trocar
xinafoate
salmeterol x.
xiphoid
xiphopagus
XIST
X inactive, specific transcript
X-linked
X.-l. agammaglobulinemia
X.-l. disease
X.-l. disorder
X.-l. dominant condition
X.-l. dominant disease
X.-l. dominant inheritance
X.-l. gene
X.-l. heredity
X.-l.
hypogammaglobulinemia
X.-l. ichthyosis
X.-l. lymphoproliferative
syndrome
X.-l. phenomenon
X.-l. recessive condition
X.-l. recessive disease
X.-l. recessive dysgenesis
X.-l. recessive inheritance
X.-l. trait
XO
X. chromosome
X. syndrome
45,XO
XomaZyme-H65
XP
128X. ultrasound
X. Xcelerator ultrasound
enhancer
X-Prep
Senna X.-P.
Xq13.1
x-ray
x-r. absorptiometry
chest x-r. (CXR)
x-r. mammogram
x-r. mammography
x-r. pelvimetry
x-r. therapy
X-tra
AFP X.-t.

XX
- X. chromosome
- X. hermaphroditism
- X. karyotype
- X. male syndrome
- X. and XY Turner
  phenotype

46,XX
- 46,XX karyotype
- 46,XX male
- 46,XX male syndrome

XXX
- X. karyotype
- X. syndrome

47,XXX
- 47,XXX syndrome

XXXX syndrome
XXXXX syndrome
XXXXY
- X. aneuploidy
- X. syndrome

49XXXXY syndrome
XXY
- X. male
- X. syndrome

47,XXY
- 47,XXY karyotype
- 47,XXY syndrome

69,XXY
XY
- X. gonadal dysgenesis
- X. karyotype

46,XY
- 46,XY karyotype

Xylocaine
xylulose dehydrogenase deficiency
XYY
- X. male
- X. syndrome

X-zone

Y
- Y chromatin
- Y chromosome
- Y chromosome-specific DNA sequence

YAG
- yttrium-aluminum-garnet
- YAG laser
- YAG pellet

Yale Optimal Observation Score

yaws

year
- y. of birth (YOB)
- postnatal y.

yeast
- y. infection
- vaginal y.
- y. vaginitis

Yellen clamp

yellow
- y. fever
- y. fever vaccine
- y. vernix syndrome

Yeoman forceps

Yersinia
- *Y. enterocolitica*
- *Y. pestis*
- *Y. pseudotuberculosis*

yew
- English y.
- Pacific y.

Y-incision
Y-linkage
Y-linked
- Y.-l. character
- Y.-l. gene

YOB
- year of birth

Yocon
Yodoxin
yogurt douche
yohimbine
Yohimex
yolk
- accessory y.
- y. cells
- formative y.
- y. membrane
- y. sac
- y. sac carcinoma
- y. sac tumor
- y. sac tumor of testis
- y. space
- y. stalk

York-Mason repair
Yotopar
Young syndrome
Yp53.3
Y-plasty
YSI neonatal temperature probe
Y-specific
- Y.-s. DNA
- Y.-s. DNA amplification

yttrium-aluminum-garnet (YAG)
- y.-a.-g. laser

Yutopar
Yuzpe regimen
YY
- Y. syndrome

Zancolli clawhand deformity repair
Zantac
Zarontin
Zaroxolyn
Zaufal sign
Zavanelli maneuver
Z chromosome
ZDV
    zidovudine
Zeiss colposcope
Zellweger syndrome
Zenate
Zephrex LA
zero end-expiratory pressure
Zetran
zidovudine (ZDV)
Ziehen-Oppenheim syndrome
ZIFT
    zygote intrafallopian transfer
ZIG
    zoster immune globulin
zigzagplasty
Zimmerman arch
zinc
    z. oxide
    z. oxide ointment
    z. peroxide
    z. poisoning
Z-incision
Zinsser-Engman-Cole syndrome
Zipokowski-Margolis syndrome
zipper ring
Zithromax
Zixoryn
Z-line
Z-linked gene
zobactam sodium
Zoladex
Zolicef
Zollinger-Ellison syndrome
Zoloft
zolpidem tartrate
zomepirac sodium
zona, pl. zonae
    z. basalis
    z. compacta
    z. drilling
    z. functionalis
    z. pellucida

    z. protein
    z. reaction
    z. spongiosa
zonae pellucidae
zona-free hamster egg penetration
    test
zonary placenta
zone
    Barnes z.
    basement membrane z.
      (BMZ)
    cervical z.
    cervical transformation z.
    large loop excision of
      transformation z. (LLETZ)
    normal transformation z.
    transformation z.
zonoskeleton
zonula, pl. zonulae
    z. adherens
    z. occludens
zoogonous
zoogony
Zoomscope colposcope
Zoon erythroplasia
zoosperm
zoster
    herpes z.
    z. immune globulin (ZIG)
zosteriform
Zosyn
Zovirax
Z-plasty
    four-flap Z.-p.
Z-Sampler endometrial suction
    curette
zuclopenthixol
Zuspan regimen
Zwanck pessary
Zweifel-DeLee cranioclast
zygodactyly
zygomycosis
zygopodium
zygosity
zygote
    frozen z.
    z. intrafallopian transfer
      (ZIFT)
    two-cell z.

zygotene
    z. phase of meiosis
    z. stage

ZZ male
Z,Z,'Z″ degree of contractions

Anatomical Illustrations

The Female

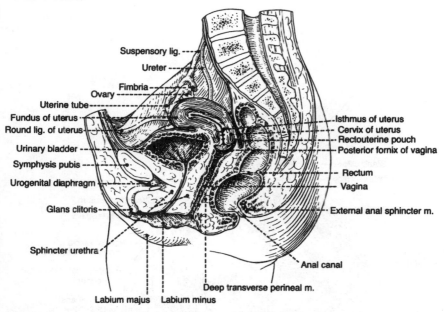

Figure 1. Sagittal section of the female pelvis. From Chung KW. Gross anatomy, 2nd ed. Baltimore: Williams & Wilkins, 1991.

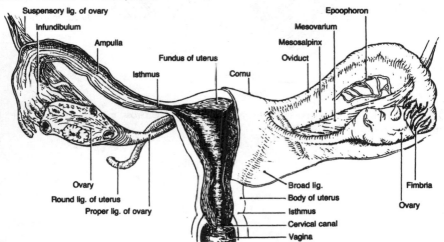

Figure 2. *Female reproductive tract.* The posterior aspect of the female reproductive tract is shown. The ligamentous supports of the uterus, right oviduct, and the right ovary are depicted intact. The left side of the uterus, left oviduct, and left ovary are shown dissected. From April EW. Anatomy, 2nd ed. Baltimore, Williams & Wilkins, 1990.

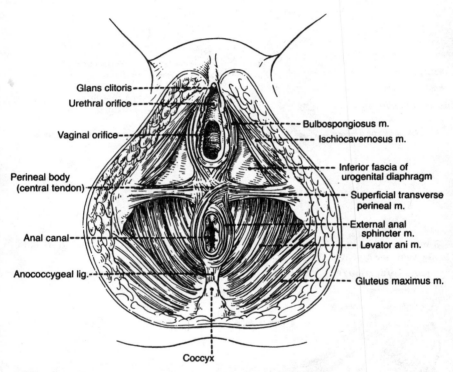

Figure 3. Muscles of the female perineum. From Chung KW. Gross anatomy, 2nd ed. Baltimore: Williams & Wilkins, 1991.

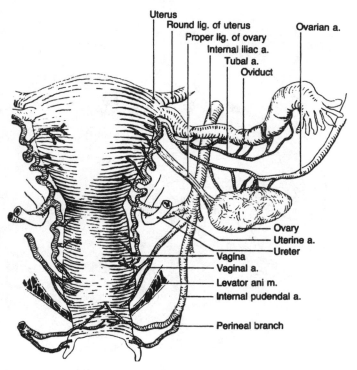

Figure 4. *Vasculature of the female reproductive tract.* The ovarian, uterine, and pudendal arteries supply the female tract and genitalia with anastomoses occurring between the ovarian and uterine arteries as well as between the uterine arteries and deep perineal branches of the pudendal arteries. From April EW. Anatomy, 2nd ed. Baltimore, Williams & Wilkins, 1990.

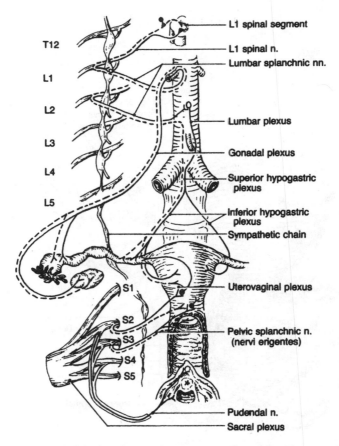

T12
L1
L2
L3
L4
L5

L1 spinal segment
L1 spinal n.
Lumbar splanchnic nn.
Lumbar plexus
Gonadal plexus
Superior hypogastric plexus
Inferior hypogastric plexus
Sympathetic chain
Uterovaginal plexus
Pelvic splanchnic n. (nervi erigentes)
Pudendal n.
Sacral plexus

S1
S2
S3
S4
S5

Figure 5. *Innervation of the female reproductive tract and genitalia.* The sympathetic pathways arise from the lower thoracic and upper lumbar spinal levels. (*black triangle*). There are no white rami below L2. These reach the aortic plexus via thoracic and lumbar splanchnic nerves. Synapse occurs in the aortic plexus (*white circles*). The postsynaptic neurons reach the pelvic viscera via hypogastric plexuses. The parasympathetic pathways arise from the midsacral spinal levels and reach the pelvic viscera via the pelvic splanchnic nerves. Synapse occurs in the walls of the viscera (*white circles*). Visceral afferent fibers (*dashed*) from the pelvic viscera travel specifically along either one or the other autonomic pathways, have their cell bodies in the dorsal root ganglia, and produce specific patterns of referred pain. The pudendal nerve provides somatic innervation to and from the perineum. From April EW. Anatomy, 2nd ed. Baltimore, Williams & Wilkins, 1990.

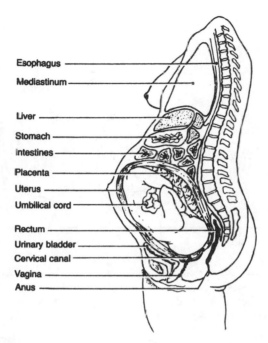

Esophagus
Mediastinum
Liver
Stomach
Intestines
Placenta
Uterus
Umbilical cord
Rectum
Urinary bladder
Cervical canal
Vagina
Anus

Figure 6. *Pregnant uterus.* Fetal development at approximately 35 weeks illustrates the relationships within the abdominal cavity. From April EW. Anatomy, 2nd ed. Baltimore, Williams & Wilkins, 1990.

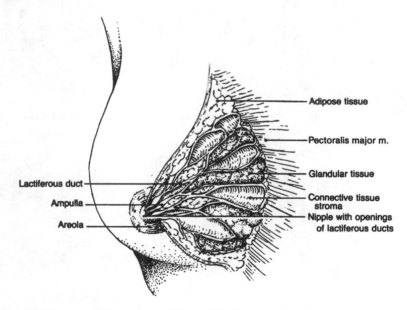

Adipose tissue
Pectoralis major m.
Glandular tissue
Connective tissue stroma
Nipple with openings of lactiferous ducts

Lactiferous duct
Ampulla
Areola

Figure 7. *The breast.* The right breast is partially dissected, showing the secretory portion. From April EW. Anatomy, 2nd ed. Baltimore, Williams & Wilkins, 1990.

The Fetus

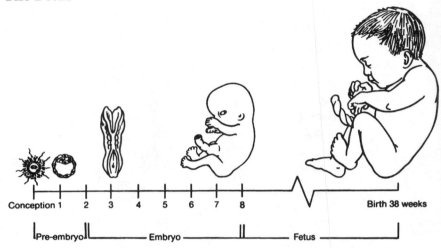

Figure 8. The periods of human development. From Johnson KE. Human developmental anatomy. Baltimore: Williams & Wilkins, 1988.

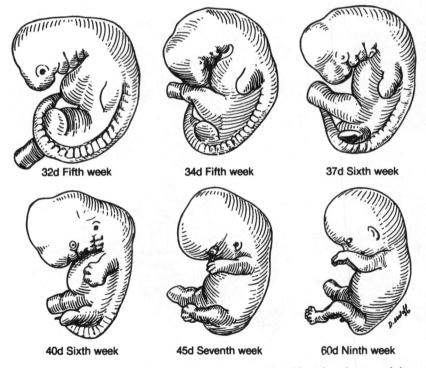

Figure 9. Human embryos and a 9-week fetus showing some of the salient features of changes in the external morphology. These are not drawn to proportional scale. From Johnson KE. Human developmental anatomy. Baltimore: Williams & Wilkins, 1988.

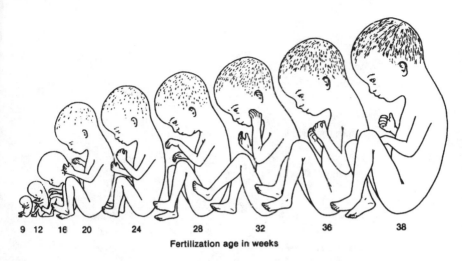

Figure 10. Changes in the relative size of the fetus throughout the fetal period. (Reprinted with permission from Moore K: *The Developing Human,* 5th ed. Philadelphia, Saunders, 1993, p. 94.)

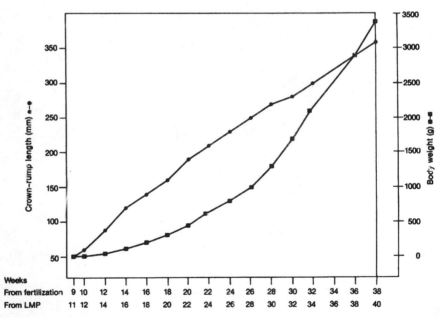

Figure 11. Graph showing the increase in crown-rump length (*circles*) and weight (*squares*) during the fetal period. Note that there is a linear increase in length but an exponential increase in weight. *LMP,* last menstrual period. From Johnson KE. Human developmental anatomy. Baltimore: Williams & Wilkins, 1988.

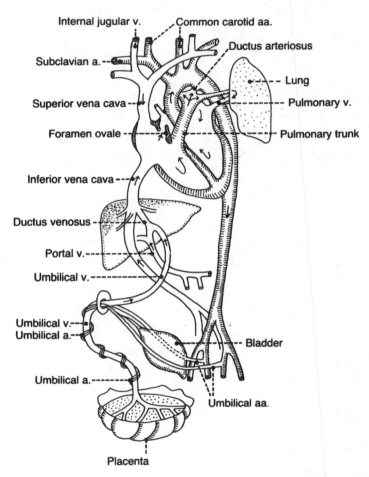

Figure 12. Fetal circulation. From Chung KW. Gross anatomy, 2nd ed. Baltimore: Williams & Wilkins, 1991.

Appendix 2
Fetal Presentations

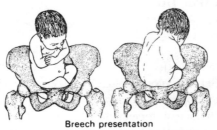

Breech presentation
Right sacroposterior   Right sacroanterior

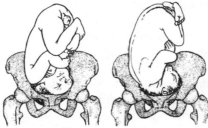

Vertex presentation
Right occipitoposterior   Right occipitoanterior

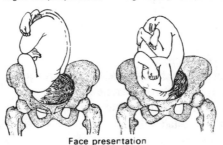

Face presentation
Right mentoposterior   Right mentoanterior

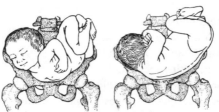

Transverse presentation
Right scapuloposterior   Right scapuloanterior

Presentations

Appendix 3

OB/GYN Drug Names by
Therapeutic Class

ABORTION (THERAPEUTIC)
dinoprostone
dinoprost tromethamine
oxytocin
Pitocin Injection (oxytocin)
Prepidil Vaginal Gel (dinoprostone)
Prostin E_2 Vaginal Suppository (dinoprostone)
Prostin F_2 Alpha (dinoprost tromethamine)
Syntocinon Injection (oxytocin)
Syntocinon Nasal Spray (oxytocin)

AMENORRHEA
Amen Oral (medroxyprogesterone acetate)
Aygestin (norethindrone)
bromocriptine mesylate
Curretab Oral (medroxyprogesterone acetate)
Cycrin Oral (medroxyprogesterone acetate)
cyproheptadine hydrochloride
Depo-Provera Injection (medroxyprogesterone acetate)
Duralutin Injection (hydroxyprogesterone caproate)
Factrel Injection (gonadorelin)
Gesterol (progesterone)
gonadorelin
hydroxyprogesterone caproate
Hy-Gestrone Injection (hydroxyprogesterone caproate)
Hylutin Injection (hydroxyprogesterone caproate)
Hyprogest Injection (hydroxyprogesterone caproate)
Lutrepulse Injection (gonadorelin)
medroxyprogesterone acetate
Micronor (norethindrone)
norethindrone
Norlutate (norethindrone)
Norlutin (norethindrone)
NOR-Q.D. (norethindrone)
Parlodel (bromocriptine mesylate)
Periactin (cyproheptadine hydrochloride)
Pro-Depo Injection (hydroxyprogesterone caproate)
Prodrox Injection (hydroxyprogesterone caproate)
progesterone
Provera Oral (medroxyprogesterone acetate)

CANDIDIASIS (VULVOVAGINAL)
Breezee Mist Antifungal (miconazole)
butoconazole nitrate
clotrimazole
Femstat (butoconazole nitrate)
Fungoid Creme (miconazole)
Fungoid HC Creme (miconazole)
Fungoid Tincture (miconazole)
Genapax Vaginal (gentian violet)
gentian violet
Gyne-Lotrimin (clotrimazole)
Lotrimin AF Cream (clotrimazole)
Lotrimin AF Lotion (clotrimazole)
Lotrimin AF Powder (miconazole)
Lotrimin AF Solution (clotrimazole)
Lotrimin AF Spray Liquid (miconazole)
Lotrimin AF Spray Powder (miconazole)
Lotrimin (clotrimazole)
Maximum Strength Desenex Antifungal Cream (miconazole)
Micatin Topical (miconazole)
miconazole
Monistat-Derm Topical (miconazole)
Monistat i.v. Injection (miconazole)
Monistat Vaginal (miconazole)
Mycelex (clotrimazole)
Mycelex-G (clotrimazole)
Mycostatin Oral (nystatin)
Mycostatin Topical (nystatin)
Mycostatin Vaginal (nystatin)
Nilstat Oral (nystatin)
Nilstat Topical (nystatin)
Nilstat Vaginal (nystatin)
nystatin
Nystat-Rx (nystatin)
Nystex Oral (nystatin)
Nystex Topical (nystatin)
O-V Staticin Oral/Vaginal (nystatin)
Terazol Vaginal (terconazole)
terconazole
tioconazole
Vagistat Vaginal (tioconazole)
Zeasorb-AF Powder (miconazole)
CARCINOMA (BREAST)
Anabolin Injection (nandrolone)

Andro-Cyp Injection (testosterone)
Android (methyltestosterone)
Andro Injection (testosterone)
Andro-L.A. Injection (testosterone)
Androlone-D Injection (nandrolone)
Androlone Injection (nandrolone)
Andronate Injection (testosterone)
Andropository Injection (testosterone)
Deca-Durabolin Injection (nandrolone)
Delatest Injection (testosterone)
Delatestryl Injection (testosterone)
Depotest Injection (testosterone)
Depo-Testosterone Injection (testosterone)
Durabolin Injection (nandrolone)
Duratest Injection (testosterone)
Durathate Injection (testosterone)
Everone Injection (testosterone)
fluoxymesterone
Halotestin (fluoxymesterone)
Histerone Injection (testosterone)
Hybolin Decanoate Injection (nandrolone)
Hybolin Improved Injection (nandrolone)
Metandren (methyltestosterone)
methyltestosterone
nandrolone
Neo-Durabolic Injection (nandrolone)
Oreton Methyl (methyltestosterone)
Teslac (testolactone)
Testoderm Transdermal System (testosterone)
testolactone
Testopel Pellet (testosterone)
testosterone
Testred (methyltestosterone)
Virilon (methyltestosterone)
CARCINOMA (CERVIX)
Blenoxane (bleomycin sulfate)
bleomycin sulfate
carboplatin
cisplatin
mitomycin
Mutamycin (mitomycin)
Oncovin Injection (vincristine sulfate)
Paraplatin (carboplatin)
Platinol-AQ (cisplatin)

Platinol (cisplatin)
Vincasar PFS Injection (vincristine sulfate)
vincristine sulfate
CARCINOMA (ENDOMETRIUM)
Adriamycin PFS (doxorubicin hydrochloride)
Adriamycin RDF (doxorubicin hydrochloride)
Adrucil Injection (fluorouracil)
Alkeran (melphalan)
altretamine
Amen Oral (medroxyprogesterone acetate)
carboplatin
chlorambucil
cisplatin
Cosmegen (dactinomycin)
Curretab Oral (medroxyprogesterone acetate)
cyclophosphamide
Cycrin Oral (medroxyprogesterone acetate)
Cytoxan Injection (cyclophosphamide)
Cytoxan Oral (cyclophosphamide)
dactinomycin
Depo-Provera Injection (medroxyprogesterone acetate)
doxorubicin hydrochloride
Duralutin Injection (hydroxyprogesterone caproate)
Efudex Topical (fluorouracil)
Emcyt (estramustine phosphate sodium)
estramustine phosphate sodium
Fluoroplex Topical (fluorouracil)
fluorouracil
Gesterol (progesterone)
Hexalen (altretamine)
Hydrea (hydroxyurea)
hydroxyprogesterone caproate
hydroxyurea
Hy-Gestrone Injection (hydroxyprogesterone caproate)
Hylutin Injection (hydroxyprogesterone caproate)
Hyprogest Injection (hydroxyprogesterone caproate)
Leukeran (chlorambucil)
mechlorethamine hydrochloride
medroxyprogesterone acetate
Megace (megestrol acetate)
megestrol acetate
melphalan
mitoxantrone hydrochloride
Mustargen Hydrochloride (mechlorethamine hydrochloride)

Neosar Injection (cyclophosphamide)
Novantrone (mitoxantrone hydrochloride)
paclitaxel
Paraplatin (carboplatin)
Platinol-AQ (cisplatin)
Platinol (cisplatin)
Pro-Depo Injection (hydroxyprogesterone caproate)
Prodrox Injection (hydroxyprogesterone caproate)
progesterone
Provera Oral (medroxyprogesterone acetate)
Rubex (doxorubicin hydrochloride)
Taxol (paclitaxel)
teniposide
thiotepa
Vumon Injection (teniposide)
CERVICITIS
Achromycin Ophthalmic (tetracycline)
Achromycin Topical (tetracycline)
Achromycin V Oral (tetracycline)
azithromycin dihydrate
Bio-Tab Oral (doxycycline)
ceftriaxone sodium
Doryx Oral (doxycycline)
Doxychel Injection (doxycycline)
Doxychel Oral (doxycycline)
doxycycline
Doxy Oral (doxycycline)
E.E.S. Oral (erythromycin)
E-Mycin Oral (erythromycin)
Eryc Oral (erythromycin)
EryPed Oral (erythromycin)
Ery-Tab Oral (erythromycin)
Erythrocin Oral (erythromycin)
erythromycin
Ilosone Oral (erythromycin)
Monodox Oral (doxycycline)
Nor-tet Oral (tetracycline)
Panmycin Oral (tetracycline)
PCE Oral (erythromycin)
Robitet Oral (tetracycline)
Rocephin (ceftriaxone sodium)
Sumycin Oral (tetracycline)
Teline Oral (tetracycline)
Tetracap Oral (tetracycline)

tetracycline
Tetralan Oral (tetracycline)
Tetram Oral (tetracycline)
Topicycline Topical (tetracycline)
Vibramycin Injection (doxycycline)
Vibramycin Oral (doxycycline)
Vibra-Tabs (doxycycline)
Zithromax (azithromycin dihydrate)

ECLAMPSIA
Barbita (phenobarbital)
diazepam
Luminal (phenobarbital)
magnesium sulfate
phenobarbital
Solfoton (phenobarbital)
Valium (diazepam)
Valrelease (diazepam)
Zetran Injection (diazepam)

HYPOGONADISM, FEMALE (TREATMENT)
Brevicon (ethinyl estradiol and norethindrone)
Demulen (ethinyl estradiol and ethynodiol diacetate)
ethinyl estradiol and ethynodiol diacetate
ethinyl estradiol and levonorgestrel
ethinyl estradiol and norethindrone
Genora (ethinyl estradiol and norethindrone)
Levlen (ethinyl estradiol and levonorgestrel)
Loestrin (ethinyl estradiol and norethindrone)
Modicon (ethinyl estradiol and norethindrone)
N.E.E. 1/35 (ethinyl estradiol and norethindrone)
Nelova (ethinyl estradiol and norethindrone)
Norcept-E 1/35 (ethinyl estradiol and norethindrone)
Nordette (ethinyl estradiol and levonorgestrel)
Norethin 1/35E (ethinyl estradiol and norethindrone)
Norinyl 1+35 (ethinyl estradiol and norethindrone)
Norlestrin (ethinyl estradiol and norethindrone)
Ortho-Novum 1/35 (ethinyl estradiol and norethindrone)
Ortho-Novum 7/7/7 (ethinyl estradiol and norethindrone)
Ortho-Novum 10/11 (ethinyl estradiol and norethindrone)
Ovcon (ethinyl estradiol and norethindrone)
Tri-Levlen (ethinyl estradiol and levonorgestrel)
Tri-Norinyl (ethinyl estradiol and norethindrone)
Triphasil (ethinyl estradiol and levonorgestrel)

INFERTILITY (FEMALE)
A.P.L. (chorionic gonadotropin)

bromocriptine mesylate
Chorex (chorionic gonadotropin)
chorionic gonadotropin
Choron (chorionic gonadotropin)
Clomid (clomiphene citrate)
clomiphene citrate
Follutein (chorionic gonadotropin)
Glukor (chorionic gonadotropin)
Gonic (chorionic gonadotropin)
menotropins
Milophene (clomiphene citrate)
Parlodel (bromocriptine mesylate)
Pergonal (menotropins)
Pregnyl (chorionic gonadotropin)
Profasi HP (chorionic gonadotropin)
Serophene (clomiphene citrate)
LABOR INDUCTION
carboprost tromethamine
dinoprostone
dinoprost tromethamine
Hemabate (carboprost tromethamine)
oxytocin
Pitocin Injection (oxytocin)
Prepidil Vaginal Gel (dinoprostone)
Prostin E_2 Vaginal Suppository (dinoprostone)
Prostin F_2 Alpha (dinoprost tromethamine)
Syntocinon Injection (oxytocin)
Syntocinon Nasal Spray (oxytocin)
LABOR (PREMATURE)
Brethaire Inhalation Aerosol (terbutaline sulfate)
Brethine Injection (terbutaline sulfate)
Brethine Oral (terbutaline sulfate)
Bricanyl Injection (terbutaline sulfate)
Bricanyl Oral (terbutaline sulfate)
Pre-Par (ritodrine hydrochloride)
ritodrine hydrochloride
terbutaline sulfate
Yutopar (ritodrine hydrochloride)
LACTATION (SUPPRESSION)
bromocriptine mesylate
oxytocin
Parlodel (bromocriptine mesylate)
Pitocin Injection (oxytocin)

Syntocinon Injection (oxytocin)
Syntocinon Nasal Spray (oxytocin)
NIPPLE CARE
glycerin, lanolin and peanut oil
Massé Breast Cream (glycerin, lanolin and peanut oil)
OVARIAN FAILURE
Aquest (estrone)
Delestrogen Injection (estradiol)
depGynogen Injection (estradiol)
Depo-Estradiol Injection (estradiol)
Depogen Injection (estradiol)
Dioval Injection (estradiol)
Dura-Estrin Injection (estradiol)
Duragen Injection (estradiol)
Estrace Oral (estradiol)
Estraderm Transdermal (estradiol)
Estra-D Injection (estradiol)
estradiol
Estra-L Injection (estradiol)
Estratab (estrogens, esterified)
Estratest H.S. Oral (estrogens with methyltestosterone)
Estratest Oral (estrogens with methyltestosterone)
Estro-Cyp Injection (estradiol)
estrogens, conjugated
estrogens, esterified
estrogens with methyltestosterone
Estroject-L.A. Injection (estradiol)
estrone
estropipate
Estrovis (quinestrol)
Gynogen L.A. Injection (estradiol)
Kestrone (estrone)
Menest (estrogens, esterified)
Ogen (estropipate)
Ortho-Est (estropipate)
Premarin (estrogens, conjugated)
Premarin With Methyltestosterone Oral (estrogens with methyltestosterone)
quinestrol
Theelin (estrone)
Valergen Injection (estradiol)
OVULATION
A.P.L. (chorionic gonadotropin)
Chorex (chorionic gonadotropin)

chorionic gonadotropin
Choron (chorionic gonadotropin)
Clomid (clomiphene citrate)
clomiphene citrate
Follutein (chorionic gonadotropin)
Glukor (chorionic gonadotropin)
Gonic (chorionic gonadotropin)
menotropins
Milophene (clomiphene citrate)
Pergonal (menotropins)
Pregnyl (chorionic gonadotropin)
Profasi HP (chorionic gonadotropin)
Serophene (clomiphene citrate)

PELVIC INFLAMMATORY DISEASE (PID)

Achromycin Ophthalmic (tetracycline)
Achromycin Topical (tetracycline)
Achromycin V Oral (tetracycline)
AKTob Ophthalmic (tobramycin)
amikacin sulfate
Amikin Injection (amikacin sulfate)
ampicillin sodium and sulbactam sodium
Bio-Tab Oral (doxycycline)
Cefobid (cefoperazone sodium)
cefoperazone sodium
cefotaxime sodium
cefoxitin sodium
ceftriaxone sodium
Claforan (cefotaxime sodium)
Cleocin HCl (clindamycin)
Cleocin Pediatric (clindamycin)
Cleocin Phosphate (clindamycin)
Cleocin T (clindamycin)
Clinda-Derm Topical Solution (clindamycin)
clindamycin
Doryx Oral (doxycycline)
Doxychel Injection (doxycycline)
Doxychel Oral (doxycycline)
doxycycline
Doxy Oral (doxycycline)
E.E.S. Oral (erythromycin)
E-Mycin Oral (erythromycin)
Eryc Oral (erythromycin)
EryPed Oral (erythromycin)
Ery-Tab Oral (erythromycin)

Erythrocin Oral (erythromycin)
erythromycin
Garamycin Injection (gentamicin sulfate)
Garamycin Ophthalmic (gentamicin sulfate)
Garamycin Topical (gentamicin sulfate)
Genoptic Ophthalmic (gentamicin sulfate)
Genoptic S.O.P. Ophthalmic (gentamicin sulfate)
Gentacidin Ophthalmic (gentamicin sulfate)
Gent-AK Ophthalmic (gentamicin sulfate)
gentamicin sulfate
Gentrasul Ophthalmic (gentamicin sulfate)
G-myticin Topical (gentamicin sulfate)
Ilosone Oral (erythromycin)
Jenamicin Injection (gentamicin sulfate)
Mefoxin (cefoxitin sodium)
Mezlin (mezlocillin sodium)
mezlocillin sodium
Monodox Oral (doxycycline)
moxalactam disodium
Moxam (moxalactam disodium)
Nebcin Injection (tobramycin)
netilmicin sulfate
Netromycin Injection (netilmicin sulfate)
Nor-tet Oral (tetracycline)
Panmycin Oral (tetracycline)
PCE Oral (erythromycin)
penicillin g, parenteral
Pfizerpen Injection (penicillin g, parenteral)
piperacillin sodium
piperacillin sodium and tazobactam sodium
Pipracil (piperacillin sodium)
Robitet Oral (tetracycline)
Rocephin (ceftriaxone sodium)
Sumycin Oral (tetracycline)
Teline Oral (tetracycline)
Tetracap Oral (tetracycline)
tetracycline
Tetralan Oral (tetracycline)
Tetram Oral (tetracycline)
ticarcillin and clavulanate potassium
ticarcillin disodium
Ticar (ticarcillin disodium)
Timentin (ticarcillin and clavulanate potassium)
tobramycin

Tobrex Ophthalmic (tobramycin)
Topicycline Topical (tetracycline)
Unasyn (ampicillin sodium and sulbactam sodium)
Vibramycin Injection (doxycycline)
Vibramycin Oral (doxycycline)
Vibra-Tabs (doxycycline)
Zosyn (piperacillin sodium and tazobactam sodium)

PRE-ECLAMPSIA
magnesium sulfate

PREGNANCY (PROPHYLAXIS)
Amen Oral (medroxyprogesterone acetate)
Aygestin (norethindrone)
Because (nonoxynol 9)
Brevicon (ethinyl estradiol and norethindrone)
Curretab Oral (medroxyprogesterone acetate)
Cycrin Oral (medroxyprogesterone acetate)
Delfen (nonoxynol 9)
Demulen (ethinyl estradiol and ethynodiol diacetate)
Depo-Provera Injection (medroxyprogesterone acetate)
Desogen (ethinyl estradiol and desogestrel)
Emko (nonoxynol 9)
Encare (nonoxynol 9)
Enovid (mestranol and norethynodrel)
ethinyl estradiol and desogestrel
ethinyl estradiol and ethynodiol diacetate
ethinyl estradiol and levonorgestrel
ethinyl estradiol and norethindrone
ethinyl estradiol and norgestimate
ethinyl estradiol and norgestrel
Genora (ethinyl estradiol and norethindrone)
Gynol II (nonoxynol 9)
Intercept (nonoxynol 9)
Koromex (nonoxynol 9)
Levlen (ethinyl estradiol and levonorgestrel)
levonorgestrel
Loestrin (ethinyl estradiol and norethindrone)
Lo/Ovral (ethinyl estradiol and norgestrel)
medroxyprogesterone acetate
mestranol and norethindrone
mestranol and norethynodrel
Micronor (norethindrone)
Modicon (ethinyl estradiol and norethindrone)
N.E.E. 1/35 (ethinyl estradiol and norethindrone)
Nelova (ethinyl estradiol and norethindrone)

nonoxynol 9
Norcept-E 1/35 (ethinyl estradiol and norethindrone)
Nordette (ethinyl estradiol and levonorgestrel)
Norethin 1/35E (ethinyl estradiol and norethindrone)
norethindrone
norgestrel
Norinyl 1+35 (ethinyl estradiol and norethindrone)
Norinyl 1+50 (mestranol and norethindrone)
Norlestrin (ethinyl estradiol and norethindrone)
Norlutate (norethindrone)
Norlutin (norethindrone)
Norplant Implant (levonorgestrel)
NOR-Q.D. (norethindrone)
Ortho-Cept (ethinyl estradiol and desogestrel)
Ortho-Cyclen (ethinyl estradiol and norgestimate)
Ortho-Novum 1/35 (ethinyl estradiol and norethindrone)
Ortho-Novum 1/50 (mestranol and norethindrone)
Ortho-Novum 7/7/7 (ethinyl estradiol and norethindrone)
Ortho-Novum 10/11 (ethinyl estradiol and norethindrone)
Ortho Tri-Cyclen (ethinyl estradiol and norgestimate)
Ovcon (ethinyl estradiol and norethindrone)
Ovral (ethinyl estradiol and norgestrel)
Ovrette (norgestrel)
Provera Oral (medroxyprogesterone acetate)
Ramses (nonoxynol 9)
Semicid (nonoxynol 9)
Shur-Seal (nonoxynol 9)
Tri-Levlen (ethinyl estradiol and levonorgestrel)
Tri-Norinyl (ethinyl estradiol and norethindrone)
Triphasil (ethinyl estradiol and levonorgestrel)
VAGINITIS
Aquest (estrone)
AVC Vaginal Cream (sulfanilamide)
AVC Vaginal Suppository (sulfanilamide)
chlorotrianisene
Delestrogen Injection (estradiol)
depGynogen Injection (estradiol)
Depo-Estradiol Injection (estradiol)
Depogen Injection (estradiol)
dienestrol
diethylstilbestrol
Dioval Injection (estradiol)
Dura-Estrin Injection (estradiol)
Duragen Injection (estradiol)

DV Vaginal Cream (dienestrol)
Estinyl (ethinyl estradiol)
Estrace Oral (estradiol)
Estraderm Transdermal (estradiol)
Estra-D Injection (estradiol)
estradiol
Estra-L Injection (estradiol)
Estratest H.S. Oral (estrogens with methyltestosterone)
Estratest Oral (estrogens with methyltestosterone)
Estro-Cyp Injection (estradiol)
estrogens, conjugated
estrogens with methyltestosterone
Estroject-L.A. Injection (estradiol)
estrone
Estrovis (quinestrol)
ethinyl estradiol
Gyne-Sulf (sulfabenzamide, sulfacetamide, and sulfathiazole)
Gynogen L.A. Injection (estradiol)
Kestrone (estrone)
Ortho Dienestrol Vaginal (dienestrol)
Premarin (estrogens, conjugated)
Premarin With Methyltestosterone Oral (estrogens with methyltestosterone)
quinestrol
Stilphostrol (diethylstilbestrol)
sulfabenzamide, sulfacetamide, and sulfathiazole
sulfanilamide
Sultrin (sulfabenzamide, sulfacetamide, and sulfathiazole)
TACE (chlorotrianisene)
Theelin (estrone)
Trysul (sulfabenzamide, sulfacetamide, and sulfathiazole)
Vagitrol Vaginal (sulfanilamide)
Valergen Injection (estradiol)
V.V.S. (sulfabenzamide, sulfacetamide, and sulfathiazole)
VAGINOSIS, BACTERIAL
  Cleocin HCl (clindamycin)
  Cleocin Pediatric (clindamycin)
  Cleocin Phosphate (clindamycin)
  Cleocin T (clindamycin)
  Clinda-Derm Topical Solution (clindamycin)
  clindamycin
  Flagyl Oral (metronidazole)
  MetroGel Topical (metronidazole)
  MetroGel-Vaginal (metronidazole)
  Metro I.V. Injection (metronidazole)

metronidazole
Protostat Oral (metronidazole)
VULVOVAGINITIS
AVC Vaginal Cream (sulfanilamide)
AVC Vaginal Suppository (sulfanilamide)
sulfanilamide
Vagitrol Vaginal (sulfanilamide)

From Quick look drug book 1995. Baltimore: Williams & Wilkins, 1995.

Common Instruments by OB/GYN Procedure

Cesarean Section Delivery Terms

Adson forceps
Adson pickups
Allis clamp
Army-Navy retractor
Babcock clamp
Balfour retractor
bandage scissors
Billroth tumor forceps
bipolar electrocautery
bladder blade
bladder retractor
Bookwalter retractor
clamp
Crile-Wood needle holder
curved hemostat
DeLee Universal retractor
Foley catheter
forceps
Heaney-Ballentine forceps
Heaney needle holder
hemostat
Kelly clamp

Kocher clamp
Lister scissors
malleable retractor
Mayo curved scissors
Mayo-Hegar needle holder
Mayo straight scissors
Metzenbaum scissors
Murless head retractor
Ochsner forceps
O'Sullivan-O'Connor retractor
Pennington clamp
Phaneuf uterine artery forceps
pickups
rat tooth pickups
retractor
Richardson retractor
Rochester-Péan forceps
Schroeder tenaculum forceps
Schroeder vulsella forceps
Singley forceps
skin staples
sponge forceps
sponge stick
thumb retractors
tissue forceps

Vaginal Delivery Terms

Allen stirrups
Allis clamp
Amniohook
Auvard speculum
Backhaus clamp
Barton forceps
Baumberger forceps
Billroth tumor forceps
Bill traction handle forceps
Bird vacuum extractor
Braun episiotomy scissors
clamp
clip
Crile forceps
DeLee forceps
DeWeese forceps
Dewey forceps
dressing forceps
Elliot forceps
English lock
extractor
forceps
French lock
Gelpi perineal retractor
German lock
Haig-Fergusson forceps
Halsted mosquito forceps
Hawk-Dennen forceps
Heaney-Ballentine forceps
Heaney needle holder
hemostat

Hodge forceps
Kelly clamp
Kelly retractor
Kjelland-Barton forceps
Kjelland forceps
Kjelland-Luikart forceps
Kobayashi vacuum extractor
Luikart forceps
Malmström vacuum extractor
Mayo-Hegar needle holder
Mayo scissors
McLane forceps
Mityvac vacuum extractor
Murless head extractor
Naegele forceps
Ochsner forceps
Piper forceps
pivot lock
Russian tissue forceps
Schroeder tenaculum
Shute forceps
Silastic cup extractor
Simpson forceps
speculum
sponge stick
stick
straight scissors
Tarnier axis-traction forceps
tenaculum
tissue forceps
towel clip
Tucker-McLane-Luikart forceps

Hysteroscopy/Pelviscopy Terms

Baggish hysteroscope
Baloser hysteroscope
bipolar cautery
cannula
Ciroon ACMI hysteroscope
electrocautery
endocoagulator
double-tooth tenaculum
grasper
Hamou hysteroscope
Hanks dilator
Hasson cannula
Hegar dilator
hysteroscope
Jacobs hysteroscope
Olympus hysteroscope
pelviscope
probe
Rubin cannula
single-tooth tenaculum
sleeve
straight Foley catheter
tenaculum
trocar
Valle hysteroscope
Veress needle
weighted vaginal speculum

Dilatation and Curettage (D & C) Terms

Auvard speculum
Backhaus clamp
Bozeman uterine dressing forceps
Braun-Schroeder single-tooth tenaculum
clamp
clip
Crile forceps
Crile hemostat
curette
Deaver retractor
dilator
double-tooth tenaculum
dressing forceps
Duncan curette
forceps
Goodell uterine dilator
Graves bivalve speculum
Green uterine curette
Hanks dilator
Heaney curette
Hegar dilator
hemostat
Jackson right-angle retractor
Jacobs tenaculum
Kelly clamp
Kelly-Gray curette

Kevorkian curette
Kevorkian-Younge biopsy forceps
Kevorkian-Younge curette
Laufe polyp forceps
Mayo-Hegar needle holder
Mayo scissors
Pratt dilator
Randall stone forceps
retractor
Rochester-Péan forceps
Schroeder uterine tenaculum
Schubert uterine biopsy forceps
serrated curette
sharp curette
Sims curette
single-tooth tenaculum
sound
speculum
sponge forceps
sponge stick
tenaculum
Thomas curette
Thomas-Gaylor biopsy forceps
tissue forceps
towel clip
uterine sound
weighted vaginal speculum
Wittner uterine forceps

Laparoscopic Tubal Ligation Terms

Band-Aids
blunt trocar
cannula
Ciroon camera
Cohen uterine cannula
cutting needle
double-tooth tenaculum
electrocautery
Falope ring
Falope-ring applicator
fiberoptic laparoscope
Foley catheter
Jacobs tenaculum
Kahn cannula
light source
pencil electrocautery
sharp trocar
Silastic ring
single-tooth tenaculum
sleeve
Storz laparoscope
uterine manipulator
Veress needle
Weerda laparoscope

Vaginal Hysterectomy Terms

Allis clamp
Allis forceps
Babcock clamp
bipolar electrocautery
Deaver retractor
duckbill retractor
duckbill speculum
electrocautery
Foley catheter
Heaney clamp
Heaney needle holder
Heaney retractor
hemostat
Jacobs tenaculum
Jorgenson scissors
Kelly clamp
Kocher clamp
Lahey clamp
long dissecting scissors
long tissue forceps
Mayo scissors
Metzenbaum scissors
needle holder
Ochsner clamp
O'Hanlon clamp
pedicle clamp
right-angle scissors
single-tooth tenaculum
Sims retractor
speculum
sponge stick
tapered needle
tissue forceps
uterine tenaculum
weighted vaginal speculum

Total Abdominal Hysterectomy and Bilateral Salpingo-oophorectomy Terms

Adson ganglion scissors
Allis clamp
Allis forceps
Army-Navy retractor
Babcock clamp
Balfour bladder blade
Balfour retractor
Ballentine clamp
Billroth tumor forceps
blade
Bookwalter retractor
clamp
Deaver retractor
DeBakey clamp
DeBakey tissue forceps
double-tooth tenaculum
dressing forceps
Foley catheter
forceps
Goulet retractor
Harrington retractor
Heaney-Ballentine forceps
Heaney clamp
Heaney-Hyst forceps
Heaney needle holder
Jacobs tenaculum
Jorgenson scissors
Kelly clamp
Kocher clamp
lap pack
Mayo scissors
metallic skin staples
Metzenbaum scissors
Ochsner forceps
O'Sullivan-O'Connor retractor
Péan forceps
pedicle clamp
retractor
right-angle scissors
Roberts thumb retractor
Rochester-Ochsner forceps
Russian tissue forceps
Schroeder tenaculum
Schroeder tenaculum forceps
Schroeder vulsella forceps
single-tooth tenaculum
sponge forceps
sponge-holding forceps
tenaculum
thoracic clamp
tissue forceps
Wagenstein needle holder

Appendix 5
Sample Reports of Common OB/GYN Procedures

Sample Low Transverse Cesarean Section

TITLE OF OPERATION: 1. Repeat low transverse cesarean section with upper midline vertical uterine extension.

PROCEDURE IN DETAIL: The patient was taken to the operating room after a successful epidural anesthesia had been placed in Labor and Delivery. She was placed in the supine position on the operating room table with her right side elevated and supported with a bag. The patient's abdomen was then prepared and draped in a sterile manner. An Allis clamp was used to check for an appropriate level of anesthesia, and the patient's breathing was noted to unlabored. A scalpel was used to make a Pfannenstiel incision through the old scar which was excised and removed in toto. The incision was extended through the subcutaneous tissue with the scalpel, and bleeding was controlled with a electrocautery device. The fascia of the abdomins muscle was identified and was nicked transversely with the scalpel. The incision in the fascia was extended transversely with the Mayo scissors. Kocher clamps were placed on the proximal fascial flap which was bluntly and sharply dissected from the rectus abdominis muscle. Kocher clamps were then placed on the lower fascial flap which was bluntly and sharp dissected free from the rectus abdominis muscle. The median raphe was then bluntly and sharply dissected in a careful manner. The parietal peritoneum was visualized and grasped with hemostats using a three-point technique, nicked with a scalpel, and the incision extended both cephalad and caudad. There were omental adhesions present to the anterior abdominal wall presumed due to the previous cesarean section. These were carefully lysed with electrocautery. A bladder blade was positioned, and the peritoneal serosa was grasped with pickups, nicked with the Metzenbaum scissors, and the incision extended transversely with the Metzenbaum scissors. A scalpel was used to score a low transverse uterine incision which was then extended utilizing blunt dissection. The surgeon's hand was placed into the uterus to remove the fetal head, but it was necessary to extend the incision through the rectus muscles, the fascia, and the skin in order to remove the fetal head safely. There was a nuchal cord times two which was reduced, and the nares and oropharynx were bulb suctioned prior to removing the remainder of the fetus. The infant cried spontaneously, the cord was clamped and cut, and the neonate was handed off the field to the waiting neonatologist in attendance. The infant weighted 8 lb.-3 oz. and had Apgars of 9 at 1 minute and 10 at 5 minutes. Cord gases were obtained as was cord blood. At this time the uterus was exteriorized and wrapped in a moist towel. The vertical upper midline extension in the uterus was reapproximated using #1 chromic in a running locked fashion. The second layer was reapproximated using #1 chromic sutures in a simple fashion. Hemostasis was excellent. The peritoneal serosa was reapproximated with 3-0 Vicryl in a running fashion. The low transverse uterine incision was closed in two layers with the first being a #1 chromic running locked stitch and the second being a #1 chromic running imbricating stitch. Cautery was used to assure complete hemostasis. After copious irrigation with normal saline, the bladder flap was reapproximated with 3-0 Vicryl in a running fashion. The cul-de-sacs were wiped free of all blood and clots, and the uterus was returned to the abdominal cavity. An Interceed barrier was placed over the upper vertical uterine incision, and the pelvic gutters were freed of all blood and clots. Once again the uterine incision was inspected and found to have excellent hemostasis. The parietal peritoneum was reapproximated with 3-0 Vicryl in a running fashion. The rectus muscles were reapproximated with 2-0 chromic in a running fashion. After irrigating the area once again with normal saline and noting that hemostasis was excellent, the rectus muscles were reapproximated using 3-0 Vicryl in a running fashion. The Scarpa fascia was reapproximated using 3-0 Vicryl in a running fashion, and the skin was reapproximated utilizing metallic skin staples. A sterile mildly compressive dressing was applied. The Foley catheter was noted at this time to be draining clear urine. The sponge, needle, instrument and lap counts were reported as being correct times two prior to the final closure. The patient was taken to the recovery room in stable condition with an estimated blood loss of 700 cc. She tolerated the procedure well. The neonate was sent to the newborn nursery in excellent condition.

Sample Controlled Vaginal Delivery

TITLE OF OPERATION: 1. Controlled vaginal delivery.
                         2. Repair of episiotomy

PROCEDURE IN DETAIL: The patient is primigravida 27-year-old white female who received prenatal care during her first trimester of pregnancy. She has remained normotensive throughout her pregnancy, and dipsticks remained negative. Maternal blood type is O negative, so RhoGAM was administered post delivery.

The patient arrived in Labor and Delivery in active labor with a good mechanism at 0430 hours. She was 80% effaced with cervix dilated to 4 cm. The fetus was noted to be in a vertex presentation at a -2 station. She progressed rapidly in labor, and by 1045 hours she was 100% effaced and dilated to 2 cm. An epidural was started by Anesthesia at the patient's request. The fetus remained in the vertex presentation and had normal fetal monitoring strips throughout labor with a heart rate ranging from 120–152.

At 1205 hours, the patient was moved to Delivery. The epidural was continued. The patient's vagina and perineum were prepped, and drapes were applied after the patient was placed in Allen stirrups in the lithotomy position. It was felt necessary to do a midline episiotomy to prevent tearing. The infant's head was delivered, and the nose and oropharynx were suctioned with a bulb. The shoulders were gently rotated, and the infant was delivered and placed on the mother's abdomen. The infant cried spontaneously and vigorously. The mouth and nose were once again suctioned. The cord was clamped and cut. Cord blood was obtained from a 3-vessel cord. The infant was handed off the field to the neonatologist in attendance. The infant's blood type will be determined, and the infant will be closely monitored for any signs of Rh incompatibility, but none were apparent at birth.

The patient delivered a viable male infant weighing 7 lb.-9 oz. with Apgars of 8 at 1 minute and 10 at 5 minutes. RhoGAM will be administered. The midline episiotomy was repaired without complications. The infant was sent to the Newborn Nursery, and the mother will be closely observed prior to returning to her room for postpartum recovery.

Sample Hysteroscopy and Dilatation and Curettage

TITLE OF OPERATION: 1. Examination under anesthesia.

                                       2. Hysteroscopy.

                                       3. Dilatation and curettage.

PROCEDURE IN DETAIL: Following routine preoperative preparation, the patient was brought to the operating room and general endotracheal anesthesia was administered. The patient was then sterilely prepped and draped in the dorsal lithotomy position. The bladder was emptied via straight catheterization. Bimanual examination under anesthesia was performed revealing the uterus to be anterior in position and normal in size and smooth in contour. Adnexal structures were unremarkable. A weighted speculum was introduced into the posterior portion of the vagina. The anterior lip of the cervix was visualized and grasped with a Jacobs double-tooth tenaculum. Using carbon dioxide insufflation, a 30-degree hysteroscope was inserted into the endocervical canal and was advanced into the endometrial cavity without difficulty. Inspection of the endometrial cavity revealed a slightly septated appearance of the upper portion of the fundus. There was a polypoid-type excrescence off the left fundal region. There was bloody mucoid material noted in the endometrial cavity. The scope was then withdrawn down the endocervical canal which was seen to be unremarkable.

Following hysteroscopic evaluation, the uterus was sounded to 7 cm, and the cervix was dilated to a #7 Hegar dilator. A sharp medium curette was introduced, the uterus was curetted, and then explored with Randall stone forceps. A moderate amount of normal-appearing endometrial tissue was removed and sent for pathologic evaluation. At this point, the procedure was terminated. The Jacobs tenaculum was removed from the cervix with only minimal oozing noted from the tenaculum sites. The weighted speculum was removed from the vagina, and the patient was taken down from the dorsal lithotomy position and returned to the recovery room in satisfactory condition with stable vital signs. The patient tolerated the procedure well without complications.

Sample Dilatation and Curettage, Pelviscopy, Biopsy, and Coagulation

TITLE OF OPERATION:
1. Fractional dilatation and curettage.
2. Pelviscopy.
3. Biopsy of right uterosacral ligament.
4. Coagulation of endometriosis of the left adnexal area.

PROCEDURE IN DETAIL: Following preoperative informed consent and preoperative sedation with Versed, the patient was taken to the operating room and general endotracheal anesthesia was induced without difficulty. The patient was examined under anesthesia and was found to have a normal-sized, anteverted uterus with normal adnexa. She was then placed in the dorsal lithotomy position and prepped and draped in a normal sterile fashion. The urinary bladder was drained of clear urine which was sent for urinalysis and culture and sensitivity because of the patient's history of recurrent urinary tract infections. A weighted speculum was inserted in the vagina, and the anterior lip of the cervix was grasped with a single-tooth tenaculum. After this a small sharp curette was inserted into the cervical canal and curettage was done yielding a small amount of tissue that was sent to Pathology. This was followed by progressive cervical dilatation using Hegar dilators to a #8. A small curette was inserted in the endometrial cavity and curettage was performed yielding a moderate amount of hyperplastic endometrial tissue which was sent as a separate specimen to Pathology for evaluation. The endometrial cavity sounded to a depth of 8 cm. There was no deformation of the uterine cavity discovered during this procedure. At this point a Rubin cannula was inserted into the cervical canal for better manipulation of the uterus during the pelviscopic procedure. The weighted speculum was removed.

Attention was directed to the patient's abdomen which had been prepped with Betadine and draped sterilely. A 12 mm skin incision was made in the umbilical fold. A Veress needle was inserted, and a pneumoperitoneum was obtained by insufflating the peritoneal cavity with carbon dioxide. The Veress needle was removed, and a trocar and sleeve were carefully advanced with intraabdominal placement being confirmed by the hanging-drop technique. The second and third 5 mm trocars were placed, and inspection of the patient's pelvis and abdomen revealed a uterus of normal size with normal tubes and ovaries bilaterally. Both ovaries had luteal cysts. The right ovarian surface and a small area of the right tube contained small implants of endometriosis which were coagulated using the endocoagulator. The examination of the posterior uterus showed that there was extensive areas of varicosities on both sides, but especially on the left side consistent with Allen-Masters syndrome. Examination of the uterosacral ligaments revealed a small area of scar tissue consistent with endometriosis. A biopsy of this area was done, and bipolar cautery was used to coagulate all bleeders until the field was dry. Examination of the abdominal contents revealed normal-appearing liver and gallbladder. The area was then irrigated and all irrigant was suctioned out of the pelvis with hemostasis being confirmed. Hyskon was then instilled before removing the final trocar to minimize adhesions in the pelvis. All instruments were removed, and the incisions were repaired with 3-0 Vicryl simple sutures followed by application of Band-Aids. The Rubin cannula and tenaculum were removed from the vagina with no bleeding noted from the cervix. The sponge, needle and instrument counts were reported as correct times three. The patient had tolerated the procedure well and was returned to the recovery room in stable condition.

Sample Laparoscopic Tubal Ligation

TITLE OF OPERATION: 1. Laparoscopic tubal ligation

PROCEDURE IN DETAIL: The patient was brought into the operating room and placed on the operating table in the dorsal lithotomy position. General endotracheal anesthesia was successfully induced. The patient's vagina and abdomen were prepped and draped in a routine sterile fashion. The anterior lip of the cervix was grasped with a single-tooth tenaculum, a uterine manipulator was inserted, and the tenaculum was removed. The abdomen was then entered through a small paraumbilical incision with a #15 scalpel blade. Two towel clips were used to grasp the abdominal wall which was tented up to avoid underlying structures. The Veress needle was inserted through the abdominal wall. A small amount of sterile saline solution was used to verify entry into the abdominal cavity via the hanging-drop technique. Approximately 3.5 L of CO_2 gas were insufflated into the abdominal cavity to create an adequate pneumoperitoneum. The Veress needle was withdrawn, and a large trocar and sleeve were inserted through the incision. The trocar was removed, and the sleeve was left in place. The Wolf laparoscope was inserted and attached to the light source. The contents of the abdominal cavity were inspected and found to be normal. Both tubes and ovaries appeared normal. A second small incision was made at the symphysis pubis for insertion of the Falope-ring applicator. First the right tube was grasped and followed to its fimbriated end. The Falope-ring applicator was inserted through the lower incision, and a single Falope ring was applied. The left fallopian tube was then grasped and followed to its fimbriated end. The Falope-ring applicator was inserted, and a Falope ring was applied. Since this ring did not appear to completely occlude the tube, a second Falope ring was applied and did occlude the tube successfully. The area was irrigated with warm saline solution and suctioned dry. Hemostasis was secure. Photographs were taken to confirm the presence of the Falope rings on each tube. The CO_2 gas was allowed to escape from the abdomen. The uterine manipulator was removed from the vagina. Both sleeves were removed, and the incisions were closed with subcuticular sutures of 3-0 Dexon. The wounds were dressed with Band-Aids. The anesthesia was reversed, and the patient was extubated and taken to the recovery room in stable condition.

Sample Vaginal Hysterectomy and Anterior and Posterior Colporrhaphy

TITLE OF OPERATION: 1. Vaginal hysterectomy.
                                    2. Anterior and posterior colporrhaphy.

PROCEDURE IN DETAIL: The patient was taken to the operating room and placed on the operating table in the supine position. General anesthesia was induced, and endotracheal intubation was accomplished without difficulty. She was placed in the dorsal lithotomy position. The perineum was prepped and draped in a standard fashion for vaginal surgery. A Foley catheter was inserted into the bladder for continuous drainage. The cervix was grasped with two Lahey clamps, and a weighted speculum was placed into the posterior fornix. The cervix was circumscribed with an electrocautery device set at 30 watts of coagulation current. Then by sharp dissection, the cervix was dissected back into the posterior cul-de-sac. A long duckbill retractor was then placed into the peritoneal cavity in the posterior cul-de-sac. Attention was then turned to the anterior cul-de-sac, where sharp dissection was utilized to identify the peritoneum and its reflection between the bladder and the anterior lower uterine segment. This was entered after transilluminating the area to ensure that it was the peritoneum. A Deaver retractor was placed into the anterior cul-de-sac and into the peritoneal cavity. Heaney clamps were placed on each uterosacral ligament, and each ligament was cut and ligated with #0 Vicryl. The cut ends were tagged with hemostats. Progressive placement of Heaney clamps on the broad ligament sequentially on each side was accomplished followed by cutting and ligating with #0 Vicryl. The uterus was then able to be removed from the field. The most superior pedicle was double ligated with #0 Vicryl and tagged with a hemostat. Bilaterally, all pedicles were inspected for hemostasis, and hemostasis was found to be excellent. The uterosacral pedicles were then attached to the right and left vaginal cuffs, respectively, for support of the vaginal cuff. The peritoneum was closed with a running pursestring suture of 2-0 Vicryl.

Next, the anterior colporrhaphy was performed by progressive placement of Allis clamps along the vertical incision from the vaginal cuff to approximately 2 cm from the urethral meatus. The vaginal mucosa was dissected laterally with sharp dissection. Three sequential Kelly plication sutures were then made with #0 Vicryl at the uterovesical junction progressing upward along the urethra. The excessive vaginal mucosa was trimmed and removed. The anterior vaginal mucosa was closed with a running stitch of 2-0 Vicryl. Adequate hemostasis was maintained throughout this portion of the procedure.

Attention was then turned to the posterior cul-de-sac, where a vertical incision was made in the posterior vaginal mucosa down to the top of the perineal body.

The vaginal mucosa was dissected off of the perirectal space and trimmed with Metzenbaum scissors. A plication suture was placed at the level of the sphincter, and several supporting sutures were placed with 2-0 Vicryl superior to this. The vaginal cuff was then closed with a running locked stitch of #0 Vicryl. The posterior colporrhaphy mucosal incision was closed with 2-0 chromic suture. Excellent hemostasis was noted at this time. She was placed in the supine position prior to being awakened from general anesthesia. She was extubated in the operating room and was taken to the recovery room in excellent condition.

Sample Total Abdominal Hysterectomy and Bilateral Salpingo-oophorectomy

TITLE OF OPERATION: 1. Total abdominal hysterectomy.
2. Bilateral salpingo-oophorectomy.

PROCEDURE IN DETAIL: The patient was taken to the operating room and placed on the operating table in the supine position. A Foley catheter was inserted, and the abdomen, vagina, and perineum were prepped and draped with Betadine in the usual manner. Under adequate general anesthesia, a Pfannenstiel incision was made using a #15 blade. The abdominal wall was opened in layers, and the parietal peritoneum was cut in a vertical fashion under direct visualization to avoid the bladder, bowel, and other underlying abdominal structures. Upon entering the abdominal cavity, a visual inspection revealed a normal liver, spleen, and kidneys, but a surgically absent gallbladder. The pelvis was explored and found to contain a slightly enlarged and irregularly shaped uterus with normal-appearing tubes and ovaries bilaterally. However, there was no evidence of pelvic inflammatory disease, endometriosis implants or other obvious pelvic pathology. An O'Connor-O'Sullivan retractor was placed in the wound, and the bowel was packed into the upper abdomen using wet lap packs to prevent injury and provide good visualization. Large Kelly clamps were placed along the uterine fundus bilaterally for added mobilization and for hemostasis purposes. The round ligaments were first suture-ligated on both sides using stick ties of #1 chromic catgut, and then the round ligaments were cut medial to the ties to enter the broad ligament on both sides. The anterior cul-de-sac was then sharply incised transversely, and the bladder sharply and bluntly dissected free from the lower uterine cervix using the surgeon's fingers and Metzenbaum scissors. The right ovary was picked up, and the infundibulopelvic ligament was doubly clamped, cut, and tied using free ties and stick ties of #1 chromic catgut. The right ovary and tube were removed. The left ovary and tube were then removed by doubly clamping the infundibulopelvic ligament on that side, cutting it, and tying it with free ties and stick ties. The uterosacral ligaments were then clamped, cut, and tied with #0 chromic sutures. The uterine artery pedicles were skeletonized, clamped, cut, and ligated with stick ties of #1 chromic catgut on both sides down to the level of the vaginal angle bilaterally. Heaney clamps were used to cross-clamp the apex of the vaginal wall, and then the uterus and cervix were sharply excised from the pelvis using Jorgenson scissors. The uterus and cervix were removed en bloc and sent to Pathology for examination and diagnosis. The vaginal angles were secured using modified Richardson stitches for added hemostasis. The vaginal cuff was then closed by using multiple interrupted figure-of-eight sutures of #0 chromic catgut. The pelvic floor was then irrigated with copious amounts of sterile saline solution. Hemostasis was noted to be adequate at this time. The area was then reperitonealized using a running locked suture of 2-0 chromic catgut. The pelvis was once again irrigated copiously with hemostasis noted to be excellent. All laps and retractors were removed from the operative field, and the abdominal wall was closed in layers. The perietal peritoneum was closed with a running locked stitch of #0 chromic catgut. After the second lap, needle, and instrument count was correct, the deep fascia was closed using multiple interrupted figure-of-eight sutures of #0 Vicryl. The subcutaneous tissue was closed using multiple interrupted sutures of 3-0 Vicryl. The original skin incision was closed using large sterile staples with a pressure dressing applied over the wound. The patient tolerated the procedure well with an estimated blood loss of 200 cc. She was taken to the recovery room in excellent condition awaking and with stable vital signs.